ADVANCED PERFORMANCE IMPROVEMENT IN HEALTH CARE

Principles and Methods

DONALD E. LIGHTER, MD, MBA, FAAP, FACHE
Director
The Institute of Healthcare Quality
Research and Education
Knoxville, Tennessee

Professor
The University of Tennessee
Knoxville, Tennessee

Vice President for Quality
WellCare, Inc.
Tampa, Florida

JONES AND BARTLETT PUBLISHERS
Sudbury, Massachusetts
BOSTON   TORONTO   LONDON   SINGAPORE

World Headquarters
Jones and Bartlett Publishers
40 Tall Pine Drive
Sudbury, MA 01776
978-443-5000
info@jbpub.com
www.jbpub.com

Jones and Bartlett Publishers
  Canada
6339 Ormindale Way
Mississauga, Ontario L5V 1J2
Canada

Jones and Bartlett Publishers
  International
Barb House, Barb Mews
London W6 7PA
United Kingdom

Jones and Bartlett's books and products are available through most bookstores and online booksellers. To contact Jones and Bartlett Publishers directly, call 800-832-0034, fax 978-443-8000, or visit our website, www.jbpub.com.

Substantial discounts on bulk quantities of Jones and Bartlett's publications are available to corporations, professional associations, and other qualified organizations. For details and specific discount information, contact the special sales department at Jones and Bartlett via the above contact information or send an email to specialsales@jbpub.com.

This publication is designed to provide accurate and authoritative information in regard to the Subject Matter covered. It is sold with the understanding that the publisher is not engaged in rendering legal, accounting, or other professional service. If legal advice or other expert assistance is required, the service of a competent professional person should be sought.

Production Credits
Publisher: Michael Brown
Editorial Assistant: Catie Heverling
Editorial Assistant: Teresa Reilly
Senior Production Editor: Tracey Chapman
Associate Production Editor: Kate Stein
Senior Marketing Manager: Sophie Fleck
Manufacturing and Inventory Control
  Supervisor: Amy Bacus

Composition: diacriTech
Art: diacriTech
Cover Design: Scott Moden
Cover Image: © Artida/Dreamstime.com
Printing and Binding: Malloy, Inc.
Cover Printing: Malloy, Inc.

Library of Congress Cataloging-in-Publication Data
Lighter, Donald E.
  Advanced performance improvement in health care: principles and methods/Donald E. Lighter.
    p. ; cm.
  Includes bibliographical references and index.
  ISBN-13: 978-0-7637-6449-4 (pbk.)
  ISBN-10: 0-7637-6449-3 (pbk.)
  1. Medical care—United States—Quality control. I. Title.
  [DNLM: 1. Quality Assurance, Health Care—organization & administration—United States.
  2. Health Services Administration—United States. 3. Outcome and Process Assessment (Health Care)—methods—United States. 4. Quality Control—United States. 5. Quality Indicators, Health Care—organization & administration—United States. W 84.4 AA1 L723a 2010]
  RA399.A3L485 2010
  362.1068—dc22
                                                    2009029061
6048

Printed in the United States of America
13 12   10 9 8 7 6 5 4

Dedication

Dedicated to my family, to my wife, to all those working daily to ensure that we provide the highest quality care to every patient, and to those who teach coming generations the principles and methods needed to make that happen.

Contents

CHAPTER 5 ■ Essentials of Statistical Thinking and Analysis   173

Preface

Quality health care has become a worldwide goal. Societies around the world have become increasingly intent on actualizing the value proposition in health care, and the science of healthcare quality is advancing rapidly. But we still face stiff headwinds. The percent of the U.S. economy allocated to health care is large and continues to grow, ergo:

- Healthcare spending in the United States in 2008 rose to $2.4 trillion (16% of Gross Domestic Product), with projections of $3.1 trillion in 2012 and $4.3 trillion by 2016.[1] By 2017, healthcare expenditures are projected to reach 20% of GDP. In comparison, the Organisation for Economic Cooperation and Development (OECD) reports that healthcare spending accounted for 10.9% of the GDP in Switzerland, 10.7% in Germany, 9.7% in Canada, and 9.5% in France.[2]
- Spending on health care was 4.3 times the amount spent on national defense in 2004. Nearly 46 million Americans are uninsured, but the United States spends more on health care than other industrialized nations that provide universal health coverage to all their citizens.[3]

These facts, combined with the current economic challenges caused by a worldwide recession, have created perfect conditions for change. The bridge is burning with flames nipping at our heels, and the healthcare delivery system now faces the crucial decision of effecting substantive change or watch as the system is wrested from our hands to be managed by those who may have a much narrower perspective (i.e., cost savings) rather than ensuring adequate resources to improve the quality, as well as the cost, of care. W. Edwards Deming, one of the pantheons of quality in the United States and many other countries, stated: "It is not necessary to change. Survival is not mandatory." The U.S. automobile industry has learned this lesson convincingly, having shrunk from world domination to be surpassed by the Japanese powerhouse Toyota and to see two of the three major automakers fall financially to bankruptcy. The healthcare delivery system faces a similar fate as consumers become savvier about healthcare costs and quality measurement.

The need to reduce costs and improve quality over the next few years has become the mantra for the healthcare industry, and the magnitude of the task will require an "all hands on deck" approach. My goal in writing this book is to provide healthcare leaders, clinicians, and executives with the knowledge and tools to guide meaningful change and to provide a "deep dive" into the culture and technology of quality that is needed to achieve the goals that society is setting for us in the next decade and beyond. Not only must we face the reality that the growth in expenditures is unsustainable, but societal expectations of quality and safety are peaking at the same time. My question to my colleagues in the industry is simple: If other industries can do it, why can't we? Air safety is at an all-time high, reaching six sigma levels, even if baggage handling isn't quite there yet. If someone can get on an airplane—a complex machine requiring hundreds or thousands of people to manufacture and maintain—and reasonably expect to travel from one location to another and arrive unharmed, why can't we in health care provide the same assurance? The answer, of course, is that we can. If for some reason a healthcare organization or provider can't reach those levels of safety, society, through Medicare, Medicaid, and other payers, is saying "We won't pay you anymore." Additionally, these "never events" will ultimately be the source of weeding out the poor quality and inefficient players in the marketplace and replacing them with those who can deliver on the value proposition.

An old maxim states that health care, like politics, is local. However, health care is gradually seeing the same pressure that brought the U.S. automobile industry to its knees through what Tom Friedman artfully describes as a "flattening" of the world.[4] His perceptive recognition of the effects of technology and travel on a number of industries is resonating in health care as medical tourism, which describes the increasingly common practice of individuals in the United States who travel to other countries for medical care that matches the safety and quality in the United States but usually costs from 75% to 90% less than in the United States. Technologies like "teleradiology," in which a digitized radiograph is sent to radiologists at a different site—even a different country—for interpretation, have intervened in traditional healthcare delivery models to insert competition in a traditionally noncompetitive marketplace. The response to these innovations has been mixed, but they are being adopted at an increasing pace, requiring physicians and healthcare organizations to adapt rapidly. Companies like Nighthawk Radiology Services (NHWK–NASDAQ) have leveraged these new techniques to develop innovative business models that compete with traditional models of care and create financial returns that make them attractive to investors. In short, globalization of health care is becoming a major force that necessitates not only innovation but also agility.

Another important trend in health care is the increasingly blurry lines between the services rendered by providers. The trend toward broadening the scope of practice of nonphysician providers has created alarm in some medical and surgical specialties, but the era of the advance practice nurse and other competent practitioners has arrived. These care providers will assume responsibility for many medical and surgical modalities that once were the province of physicians, requiring adaptation of the system to this new reality. Although some professional societies have tried to resist this evolution to a more efficient and openly competitive system, such opposition has been ineffectual. The U.S. public is voting with its pocketbook and demanding a more systematic approach to care that leverages all talent in the medical community.

The forces impinging on health care are undeniable, and change is in the offing. Leading change is the challenge of true leaders, and this book is designed to support those efforts by providing readers with an intensive information resource to support innovation and transformative systems for developing truly competitive and sustainable healthcare entities that deliver the value proposition that satisfies society's demands. Developing the leaders of today and tomorrow must be our greatest undertaking, and the book you hold in your hands is a contribution to making that happen.

■ References

1. Keehan S, Sisko A, Truffer C, et al. Health spending projections through 2017: the baby-boom generation is coming to Medicare. *Health Affairs.* 2008; 27(2): x146. http://www.healthaffairs.org/WebExclusives.php. Accessed July 2009.
2. Pear R. U.S. Health care spending reaches all-time high: 15% of GDP. *The New York Times* January 9, 2004: p. 3.
3. California Health Care Foundation. Health care costs 101, 2005. http://www.chcf.org/topics/healthinsurance/index.cfm?itemID=133630. Accessed July 2009.
4. Friedman T. *The world is flat: A brief history of the 21st century.* New York: Farrar, Straus, & Giroux; 2007.

Contributor

Sally A. Lighter, JD
Executive Director
The Institute for Healthcare Quality Research and Education
Knoxville, Tennessee

About the Author

Dr. Donald E. Lighter completed his board certification in pediatrics in 1978 and practiced in private and university settings for nearly 30 years. Presently, he serves as the Vice President for Quality at WellCare Health Plans in Tampa, where he is responsible for performance improvement activities for the Medicare and Medicaid health plans in multiple states. Before this position, Dr. Lighter was the Chief Quality Officer for the Shriners Hospitals for Children, a 22-hospital system, and he worked in the areas of medical staff performance and compensation, leadership training, and medical affairs strategic planning.

In addition to those positions, Dr. Lighter has also served in the following capacities:

- Medical Director, Quality Management, Blue Cross Blue Shield of Tennessee (commercial, Medicare lines)
- Physician Advisor, MidSouth Foundation for Medical Care (Medicare managed care and quality improvement)
- Medical Director, External Quality Review Organization, TennCare (Tennessee Medicaid managed care)
- Medical Director, University of Tennessee Health Plan (Medicaid managed care)
- Medical Director, Heritage National Health Plan (commercial managed care)
- Senior Examiner, Malcolm Baldrige National Quality Award

In addition to these medical leadership positions, Dr. Lighter has served as professor and a member of the core faculty for the Physicians' Executive MBA program at the University of Tennessee and has coauthored a widely used textbook on healthcare quality improvement, *Principles and Methods of Quality Management in Health Care*, now in its second edition. Over the course of his career Dr. Lighter has led the formation of two IPAs and three HMOs as well as the development of a physician–hospital organization of university physicians. He has also served as a consultant to the Board of the American Academy of Pediatrics on medical informatics and has received the Academy's highest award for his work in medical information systems.

Dr. Lighter and his wife, Sally, an attorney, reside in Knoxville, Tennessee, and have four children and five grandchildren.

The Business Case for Quality

The healthcare industry is finally awakening to the fact that we are far from perfection. Take for example these events in the early part of the new century:

- Twins Thomas Boone and Zoe Grace Quaid nearly died in November 2007 at Cedars-Sinai Hospital in Los Angeles when they were mistakenly given a massive overdose of heparin. Instead of using Hep-Lock, the highly diluted solution of the drug to maintain patency of an indwelling line, the twins instead received therapeutic heparin, which is 10 times more concentrated. Hemorrhaging from every possible site, the babies nearly exsanguinated before the error was discovered and action taken to correct the mistake. The infants are the children of actor Dennis Quaid and his wife Kimberly, who have set up a foundation to discover ways to prevent medical errors.[1]

- Three-year-old Sebastian Ferrero succumbed to a 10-fold overdose of arginine during a test to evaluate human growth hormone deficiency at the University of Florida Pediatric Outpatient Clinic. Not only did Sebastian receive the overdose, but when his parents took him to the Shands Hospital emergency department with vomiting and seizures, they waited 4 hours for treatment. By the time a computed tomography (CT) was performed, Sebastian was near death, and after a misread CT the child was transferred to the intensive care unit brain dead. Sebastian's parents, Horst and Luisa, received an $850,000 settlement, but they have begun a fund-raising campaign to build a new children's hospital in Gainesville within the next 5 years.[2]

- Alyssa Shinn, a baby born prematurely to a mother who had undergone in vitro fertilization, received a fatal overdose of zinc in her hyperalimentation solution, prepared by a part-time pharmacist at Summerlin Hospital in Las Vegas.[3] The error occurred because of multiple failures in the hospital pharmaceutical ordering system, including a failure of a pharmacy team to check the dose of zinc, which turned out to be 1,000 times the dose prescribed and reasonable for the baby. Multiple checks in the system failed, causing the lethal dose of zinc to be administered, resulting in the baby's death. The error resulted in an undisclosed financial settlement between the hospital and the family.

In addition to the estimated 98,000 deaths due to medical errors each year reported in the Institute of Medicine's (IOM) landmark 1999 study, *To Err Is Human: Building a Safer Health Care System*,[4] the World Health Organization published statistics on estimated error rates in other countries as well. For example, the probability of patients suffering from an error in Australian hospitals is a distressing 16.6%, whereas in Denmark the rate is around 10%. Thus the risk of injury from medical error is not limited to the United States but is recognized as a worldwide problem. The World Health Organization (WHO) statistics indicate that stories of errors like those described above are repeated many times each year around the world. Many doctors, nurses, and other professionals are alarmed at these figures but are also concerned that the reports represent only the tip of the iceberg: Counted errors are almost always in hospital settings, leaving the outpatient setting, where the bulk of care in the United States is provided, largely unmonitored.

To counter this distressing reality, healthcare professionals have begun to adopt methods developed by the manufacturing and other service industries to reduce the frequency of mistakes that harm people who seek health care. The quality improvement approaches pioneered by Shewhart, Deming, Juran, Ohne, and many others are being applied to healthcare services, with increasing recognition that the provision of health services consists of linked, interdependent processes amenable to the same approaches for achieving safety and higher value that have been applied in other industries for decades.

Another issue gnawing at the healthcare industry for the past four decades is the unsustainable growth in the cost of providing care to the U.S. population. U.S. health care has become the most costly in the world. As shown in FIGURE 1.1, U.S. healthcare costs have grown from 5.1% of the gross domestic product in 1960 to 15.3% in 2003 (adjusted for inflation).[5] The United States spends more per capita on health care than any other country in the world (see FIGURE 1.2), and in spite of that fact, the number of people who do not have health insurance has trended higher in recent years, as shown in FIGURE 1.3. These statistics would not be especially bothersome if the outcomes of care, such as overall mortality rates or infant survival rates, had improved commensurately or if the United States was exporting a substantial volume of these services to other countries (e.g., those that supply the United States with oil). However, these costs add substantially to the price of U.S. goods and services, making them less competitive in the world market. Large companies like General Motors and Caterpillar have lost market share to their competitors in other countries, in part because the cost of their products has risen to excessive levels. Economists warn that if the United States hopes to remain a dominant player on the world economic stage, healthcare costs must be stabilized and the value of health services must grow. For that reason health insurers have morphed from intermediaries that process health claims and simply transfer payments from payers to providers into active participants in cost-containment activities in an effort to stem skyrocketing price increases. U.S. companies have

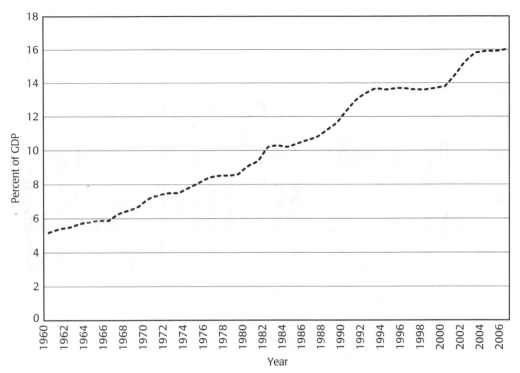

FIGURE 1.1 Growth in U.S. Healthcare Costs as a Percent of Gross Domestic Product

Source: Centers for Medicare and Medicaid Services, Office of the Actuary.

http://www.cms.hhs.gov/NationalHealthExpendData/02_NationalHealthAccountsHistorical.asp#TopOfPage. Accessed April 2008.

increasingly come to the point of reducing their healthcare costs through consumer-directed health plans that have high deductibles and copayment schedules and that start to shift the cost of care back onto employees.

What are these expenditures buying, or, in other words, what value does the U.S. population derive from health care compared with international benchmarks? Data from the National Center for Healthcare Statistics show that for several important outcome measures, the United States still lags the world. For example, the United States ranks 37th among developed nations for infant mortality rates (see FIGURE 1.4). Data for life expectancy at birth compared across several developed nations in 2004 (see FIGURE 1.5) show that U.S. life expectancy is in the bottom third of the comparison. Additionally, respiratory death rates rank in the top three in a comparison performed by the Organisation for Economic Cooperation and Development (see FIGURE 1.6). Deaths from diabetes are of great concern to public health officials, and the data in FIGURE 1.7 indicate that the United States has one of the highest rates among developed countries. One factor that relates to this increase in diabetes prevalence is the higher rate of obesity in the U.S. population, as shown in FIGURE 1.8.

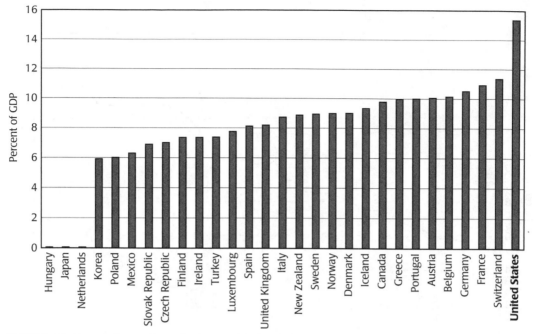

FIGURE 1.2 Comparison of per Capita Health Care Costs by Nation

Source: Stat Extracts. Organization for Economic Cooperation and Development Web Site. http://stats.oecd.org/wbos/default.aspx?DatasetCode=HEALTH. Accessed April, 2008.

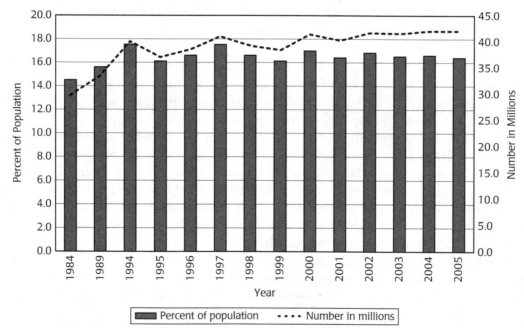

FIGURE 1.3 Uninsured U.S. Citizens as a Percent of the Population

Source: Health United States 2007. Centers for Disease Control and Prevention Web Site. http://www.cdc.gov/nchs/products/pubs/pubd/hus/uninsured.htm. Accessed April, 2008.

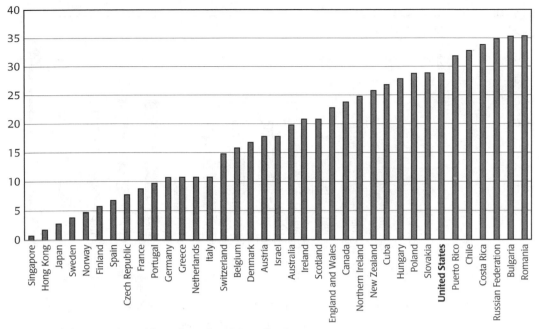

FIGURE 1.4 **National Rankings for Infant Mortality Rates**

Source: Centers for Disease Control, National Center for Health Statistics.
http://www.cdc.gov/nchs/fastats/infant_health.htm. Accessed April, 2008.

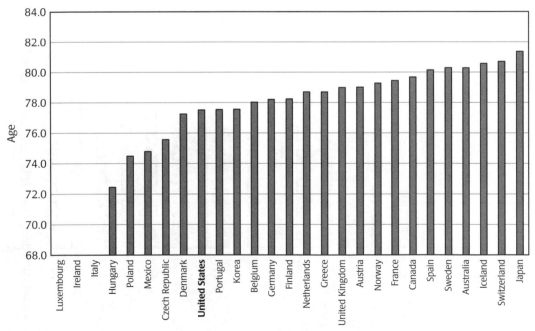

FIGURE 1.5 **Life Expectancy at Birth by Nation, 2004**

Source: Health Data. Organisation for Economic Cooperation and Development Web Site.
http://www.oecd.org/document/16/0,3343,en_2825_495642_2085200_1_1_1_1,00.html. Accessed April, 2008.

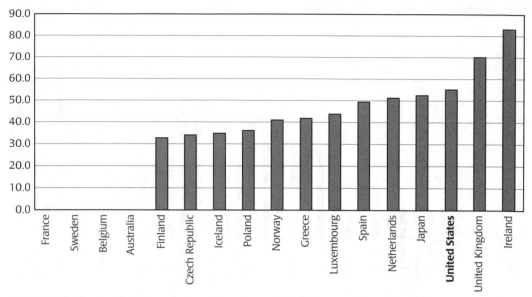

FIGURE 1.6 Deaths from Respiratory Disease per 100,000 Population, 2004

Source: Health Data. Organisation for Economic Cooperation and Development Web Site.
http://www.oecd.org/document/16/0,3343,en_2825_495642_2085200_1_1_1_1,00.html. Accessed April, 2008.

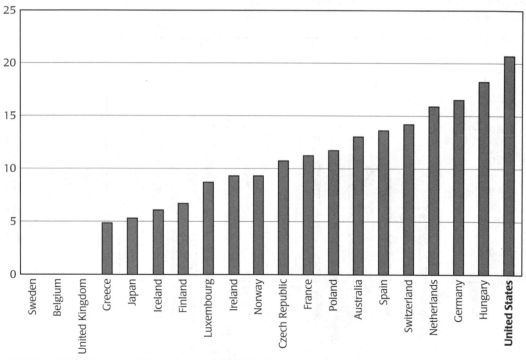

FIGURE 1.7 Deaths from Diabetes per 100,000 Population, 2003

Source: Health Data. Organisation for Economic Cooperation and Development Web Site.
http://www.oecd.org/document/16/0,3343,en_2825_495642_2085200_1_1_1_1,00.html. Accessed April, 2008.

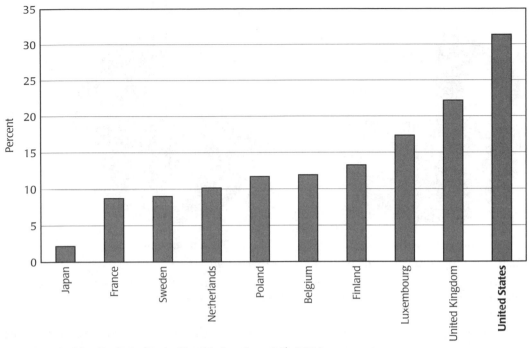

FIGURE 1.8 Obesity Rate (Body Mass Index Over 30), 2004

Source: Health Data. Organisation for Economic Cooperation and Development Web Site.
http://www.oecd.org/document/16/0,3343,en_2825_495642_2085200_1_1_1_1,00.html. Accessed April, 2008.

■ Mandate for Improvement

All these factors have led to a new mandate in U.S. society for improving the way health care is financed and delivered. For many years employers paid the bulk of health insurance premiums and thus financed the healthcare services provided to employees. Not only did those premiums cover healthcare costs for their employees, but in many cases employers paid more than the cost of services and plan administration to offset the costs that providers incurred to treat the uninsured population. Over the past 40 years, however, employers have increasingly resisted higher premiums and pushed to limit their costs through analyzing the cost of care for their employees and using data to reduce employer-paid premiums to the lowest possible amounts. That approach has had a ripple effect through the healthcare industry, forcing insurers to use cost-containment measures like restricted fees for services or even prepayment or flat rates for certain services (e.g., capitation).

Enter the federal and state governments, through Medicare and Medicaid programs, to serve as a safety net for the elderly and the poor, many of whom do not have access to health insurance. These programs have grown over the past 45 years to immense proportions, and, since 2005, state and federal government programs now represent the majority of funding for the U.S. healthcare industry (see FIGURE 1.9).

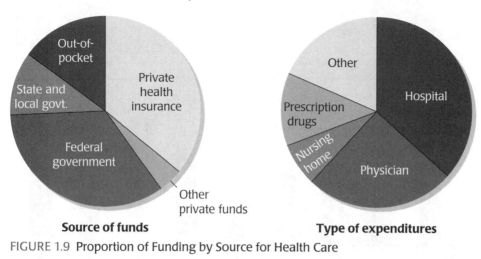

Expenditures: $1.7 trillion

Source of funds **Type of expenditures**

FIGURE 1.9 Proportion of Funding by Source for Health Care

Sources: Centers for Disease Control and Prevention, National Center for Health Statistics, United States, 2007, data from Centers for Medicare and Medicaid Services. *http://www.cdc.gov/nchs/fastats/hinsure.htm.* Accessed April, 2008.

Hospital and physician services consumed the majority of the healthcare dollar, but prescription drug costs have become increasingly important in recent years. As these socially popular governmental programs have grown, the effect on federal and state budgets has been crippling in some cases, leading to governmental efforts to contain costs. Reductions in payments to providers have been gradual but relentless, leading to a refusal by some providers to participate in state Medicaid programs, making access to some health services difficult for Medicaid beneficiaries. Additionally, in spite of these extensive governmental programs, a sizable number of U.S. citizens (approximately 46 million) remain uninsured.[6] Ethically, legally, and sometimes by necessity, hospitals must care for these uninsured people, even though there is a very small likelihood of being paid for those services.

Therefore the high number of uninsured people in the United States adds to the cost of care for private and governmental payers, leading to even greater pressure on providers to contain costs and become more efficient. This efficiency mandate has become even more acute as the federal government aggressively tries to limit health expenditures and employers shift more costs to employees.

■ Value Proposition: How Does Quality Relate to Performance?

To understand the relationship between quality and efficiency, the first step is to understand the value proposition. Think of the way most people buy something important in their lives. They start by determining how much they can spend, either by figuring how much cash they can put together for the purchase or by how much debt they can support. Then, using that number, they optimize the purchase to get the best product or service available—that is, they shop. That process of optimizing quality within cost constraints produces the value proposition, which can be thought of mathematically as follows:

$$Value = \frac{Quality}{Cost}$$

This relationship fundamentally links a consumer's perception of value directly to the quality of the good or service and inversely to the cost. In other words, purchasers look for the highest quality at the lowest cost to optimize value. The value proposition drives performance improvement across the business world, including health care, but until the past 10 to 15 years the numerator (quality) has been difficult to measure. In fact, many providers still argue that health services involve so much "art" that quality is difficult to quantify. In some cases that argument may be justified, but surrogates for precise metrics, such as patient satisfaction, are now frequently used to at least attempt to approximate the quality of health services. This approach has become acceptable to all but a minority of providers, and these types of measures are widely used in health care.

A key question, however, tries to characterize the relationship between quality improvement efforts and their associated costs and the benefits realized in organizational performance. In short, does quality pay? Comprehensive studies in health care have not yet been done, but research performed in other industries indicates that quality improvement efforts do, indeed, generate a return on investment. Consider these examples:

- The Profit Impact of Market Strategy study performed by Bradley Gale and Robert Buzzell[7] collected business strategy and financial results from over 450 companies and 3,000 business units starting in 1972 and found that the most significant factor in defining organizational success is quality. Companies that produce high-quality goods and services have a short-term advantage in premium pricing, which then leads to a long-term benefit through market share growth. These factors lead to greater profitability, providing greater customer loyalty and less vulnerability to penetration pricing by competitors that would erode margins.
- The federal General Accounting Office studied applicants for the Malcolm Baldrige National Quality Award (MBNQA) in 1991.[8] The Baldrige Award honors organizations that demonstrate superior performance in seven categories of performance: (1) leadership; (2) strategic planning; (3) customer and market focus; (4) measurement, analysis, and knowledge management; (5) workforce focus; (6) process management; and (7) results. This prestigious award requires a rigorous application and review process, culminating in a site visit for a select few organizations before their being chosen as award recipients. (The Baldrige Award is

examined in more depth in Chapter 8.) At the request of Congress, the 1991 General Accounting Office study evaluated 20 Baldrige applicants that had moved to a site visit to determine the impact of formal total quality management practices on performance. The study reported that companies that had implemented total quality management practices had better employee relations, greater productivity, higher market share, and improved profitability due to greater customer satisfaction and loyalty.

- The Baldrige Index, a hypothetical index of stock prices of publicly traded Baldrige Award recipients that has been tracked by the MBNQA program since 1995,[9] has been compared with the Standard & Poor's 500 Index (S&P 500) since its inception. In 8 of 10 years, the Baldrige Index's annual percentage increase outperformed the S&P 500 by a substantial margin, often by a factor of three to four times the S&P 500.

- A study by Easton and Jarrell[10] reported in the text by Stahl, sampled 108 firms for the impact of total quality management on corporate financial performance and stock return over a 5-year period after deployment of total quality management programs. The authors reported that improved performance was consistent among these organizations for both accounting-based indicators and return on equity. The study used an interview approach that helped characterize the companies' quality improvement systems into those that were more advanced and contrasted the results with those that were not as sophisticated, and this analysis demonstrated that level of performance was directly related to the individual firm's commitment to the quality approach and the degree of implementation of the quality system.

- Hendricks and Singhal used a surrogate measure for quality program implementation: the winning of quality awards.[11] These researchers reasoned that those companies that actually received awards for quality management should demonstrate higher market value. They published the results of a study in 2001 that validated a 38% to 46% better average performance of stock prices compared with control groups. Another study by this research team showed that operating income among award-winning firms was 79% higher than for control groups and they showed a 43% higher improvement in sales revenues.[12]

Comprehensive studies have not yet been published for the healthcare industry, but Baldrige Award recipients in the healthcare category have reported exceptional performance that they attribute to their efforts in continually improving performance. For example, SSM Health Care has increased market share in St. Louis to 18% in the 3-year period after receiving the Baldrige Award. Additionally, SSM's financial performance has earned an AA investment rating, placing them in the upper 1% of all hospitals in the United States. Kansas City's Saint Luke's Hospital system, a 2003 Baldrige recipient, was ranked 35th out of 4,500 U.S. hospitals in the 2002 Consumer's Checkbook. A review of the applications of these and other Baldrige recipients reveals a number of performance zeniths in areas such as the Centers for Medicare and Medicaid Services (CMS) performance metrics and the Joint Commission's ORYX and core measures. Senior leaders at these organizations attribute superior results to establishment and maintenance of improvement processes and systems.

■ How Do Organizations Measure the Value Proposition?

Both the numerator and denominator must be measured to demonstrate value. Both quality and cost present major challenges for healthcare organizations. The IOM defines quality as "the degree to which health services for individuals and populations increase the likelihood of desired health outcomes and are consistent with current professional knowledge."[13] Additionally, the IOM set six standards to be achieved by the healthcare industry for ensuring that the definition was met by the industry's services:

1. *Safe:* The IOM states that patient safety is not solely about ensuring that systems are designed and monitored to prevent failure of a procedure or process or the use of the wrong intervention (e.g., wrong medication or test) to achieve a diagnostic or therapeutic goal. Safe care ensures correct diagnoses, avoidance of unnecessary risks, and ensuring that patients are completely informed (informed consent) about the nature of diagnostic and therapeutic interventions and their attendant risks. One important element of the informed consent process is to understand the patient's cultural milieu, ensuring that communications are conducted in a way that a patient and caretakers can understand. More effective communication through the use of cultural training and use of interpreters can improve safety by enhancing diagnostic accuracy, reducing exposure to unnecessary risks due to a provider misunderstanding a patient's history or physical findings, and allowing patients to participate in clinical decisions regarding their care by being truly well-informed partners in the care process.

2. *Effective:* The IOM's landmark work, *Crossing the Quality Chasm*, emphasizes the importance of using evidence-based guidelines to provide high-quality care. This approach to care, often called "evidence-based practice," incorporates the most current valid research evidence into decision making and combines these clinical guides with clinical experience and, importantly, patient values. This approach also reinforces the need for the provider to be culturally competent, as described under the safety principle, but it also calls on the system of care to better understand the disparities in health needs and programs of care based on ethnic and racial differences. This cultural competence, which encompasses both clinical and system capabilities, is one key factor in ensuring that care is effective. In addition to cultural competence, though, the systems of care

(e.g., availability of supplies, lack of wasted resources in processes, adequate staffing, and high-performing capital equipment) also must be optimized to gain the efficiency in care that will ensure effectiveness of health services.

3. *Patient-centered: Crossing the Quality Chasm* states that compassion, empathy, and responsiveness to the needs, values, and expressed preferences of the individual patient are the hallmarks of patient-centeredness. Many would agree that these attitudes and skills are also central to clinical cultural competence.

4. *Timely:* A timely system prevents customers from experiencing harmful delays in receiving needed diagnostic or therapeutic interventions. One of the major complaints of health system clients is the wait time for procedures or for interaction with a medical professional. Language barriers may contribute to increased length of stay in the hospital or longer wait times in an emergency department. Systemic cultural competence could thus improve the timeliness and efficiency of a system by getting patients the services that are appropriate in an expeditious fashion.

5. *Efficient:* Business efficiency is always balanced with effectiveness as an organization is examining performance. Nearly any manager can achieve 100% effectiveness at unlimited cost, but optimizing the interaction between the two parameters requires maximizing quality and eliminating waste. A great deal of later chapters is devoted to reduction in waste, particularly in the lean sense of eliminating the "seven deadly wastes" (discussed in Chapter 6). However, one of the most difficult tasks for contemporary healthcare managers is reducing or eradicating waste while maintaining quality and operational effectiveness.

6. *Equitable: Crossing the Quality Chasm* states that a system exhibits high quality if it provides care that does not vary because of personal characteristics such as gender, ethnicity, geographic location, and socioeconomic status. Systemic cultural competence, which entails processes to monitor the quality of care and detect disparities by stratifying measures by race/ethnicity, must be at the foundation of targeted quality improvement activities. Ignoring the differences in any population based on these characteristics inevitably leads to inequity, inefficiency, and reduced effectiveness. Many healthcare systems now have special programs to deal with cultural diversity as a way of addressing this important factor.

Thus the stage has been set for organizations to measure the elements of the value proposition, and many accrediting and certification bodies have worked to gain preeminence in the field through efforts to establish standard, system-wide metrics. For example, the CMS has put forward a number of measures that are used in its continuing effort to ensure quality care for Medicare and Medicaid beneficiaries. The current measures are listed in Appendix 1.1, and updates are published on the CMS website (www.cms.gov).

Measurement Is the Key to Performance Incentives

Healthcare reimbursement programs have undergone tremendous changes in the past 50 years. Shortly after Medicare became a reality, hospitals were paid fees according to "cost-based reimbursement," which led to tremendous increases in the cost of care, because providers had little incentive to reduce or avoid unnecessary expenditures. In the 1970s the diagnosis-related group (DRG) concept was devised as a new method for paying hospitals, which at least promoted some efficiency in hospitals. Under the DRG payment system, hospitals were paid a fixed amount for each DRG, which was a statistically created grouping of diagnoses that were related based on an analysis performed by a research group at Yale University in the 1970s. This method of payment was used initially by Medicare starting in the 1980s but has since been adopted in some manner by many other payers. Capitation, another major payment scheme initiated about the same time, has not survived as well as has the DRG system. Capitation payment involves paying a fixed amount per individual being treated for a fixed basket of services. So, for example, a primary care provider might receive a capitation payment of $10 per member per month to provide all of an individual's primary care, including office visits, tests, and inpatient services that the provider renders if the person is admitted to the hospital. Thus the payer's risk is reduced, but if a beneficiary requires more than just the routine level of care, the provider may lose money on that individual. In theory, capitation arrangements are much like "mini-insurance plans" in which provider costs are spread across a population of people so that providers must consider the entire population that is capitated, rather than just an individual, and determine if the total payments offset the total costs.

Many providers had problems with capitation, because use of medical services can be unpredictable in any group of people, more so with small populations. Therefore the experiment with prospective payment did not fare well in general, and other approaches to motivating providers to become more efficient became necessary. As before, the Medicare program led the industry and in 2005 initiated a pay for performance (P4P) program for physician practices that uses the results of quality metrics to set amounts of incentive payments for Medicare providers who achieve certain levels on these metrics. Private insurers quickly followed suit, and providers are now being deluged with these programs. The concept of P4P has now become an industry standard and likely will persist into the future. The approach has only a short history at the present time, and so results are yet to be determined.[14,15]

Medicare's P4P approach bases incentives on quality measures, but many commercial insurers include cost and volume measures in the incentive program as well. By combining the cost and quality measures, insurers seem to be addressing the value proposition more completely, but in many cases these payers often emphasize the cost metrics over those designed to measure quality.[16] When the factors of the value proposition are not balanced, customer value is not optimized, leading to dissatisfaction and loss of the customer's patronage. Healthcare customers can have interesting views from the standpoint of their understanding of quality. Studies have shown that healthcare customers value time with the physician, indications of a physician's interest in them as individuals, and shorter wait times,[17,18] whereas payers are interested in performance on measures such as prescription of a beta-blocker after a heart attack or use of an angiotensin-converting enzyme inhibitor in congestive heart failure. This disconnection between the actual customer of services and those who pay for services has added increased complexity to the value proposition, and providers often have difficulty serving these occasionally conflicting requirements. Although some states and payers have made provider clinical performance information available via the Internet,[19–21] most consumers still use word-of-mouth referrals from friends or from their own physician to select a provider for healthcare services.[22] However, a combination of improved public knowledge of provider measures and use of metrics that are more easily understood and applicable to individual consumers should begin to make these publicly available data useful for customers making decisions about their health care.

The increasing use of these types of metrics has provided the momentum of change for implementing advanced performance improvement approaches like the Toyota Production System (lean processing), six sigma, and the relatively new combined approach, lean six sigma. These newer methods have enhanced efforts by healthcare institutions to make quantum leaps in efficiency and effectiveness and to improve value for customers, payers, and accreditation agencies. Because lean six sigma has just started to create value in the healthcare marketplace, quality improvement staff members are learning a new vocabulary of performance enhancement but are also demonstrating increased value to the organization as well.

■ The Marketplace Wins in the End

Although many forces are at work in the healthcare industry presently, in the end consumers determine the structure of the system in the future. The growth of consumer-determined health plans places far more economic leverage in the hands of individuals, and the use of P4P programs to improve efficiency and effectiveness will exert the greatest influence over the industry. Alternative and complementary approaches to health have become reimbursable by some payers, changing the demand profile for traditional medical services, and a competitive marketplace has changed the philosophical underpinnings of health professions. The business case for quality has never been stronger, as consumers will apply the value proposition to health purchases just as they do for other professional services, leading to higher quality at lower costs. At no time in the history of U.S. health care has the need for improving the quality of care been more compelling. The subject of this book includes approaches such as lean six sigma and other methods, but in the end quality practitioners must remember the underlying force behind these efforts—the consumer, the client, the customer—what we call patients.

■ Discussion Questions

1. The risk of medical errors has been estimated to cause 98,000 unnecessary deaths in the hospital each year. Do you believe the risk of medical care in ambulatory settings is the same, greater, or less? Why?
2. Discuss the reasons for healthcare costs being higher per capita in the United States than in any other country. Will the upward trend continue or decline? Why?
3. Medicare and Medicaid have traditionally been leaders in designing and implementing cost containment and quality initiatives in the healthcare industry. What are the reasons for this leadership? Name one approach pioneered by Medicare for reducing the cost of care.
4. Describe the value proposition. How does it apply to your life?
5. What are the six standards of quality health care defined by the Institute of Medicine? Explain one of the standards and give examples.
6. What is pay for performance? How should the approach influence the quality and cost of healthcare services?

■ References

1. Hernandez G. Quaid fights common medical errors. *Los Angeles Daily News*. Retrieved March 2008 from http://www.dailynews.com/news/ci_8579598
2. Word R. Parents of Florida boy killed by hospital error hope to prevent similar accidents. *Associated Press*. Retrieved March 2008 from http://www.nctimes.com/articles/2008/03/16/health/9_56_273_15_08
3. "Deadly Dose," ABC News. Retrieved March 2008 from http://abcnews.go.com/Video/playerIndex?id=4308939
4. Institute of Medicine. *To Err Is Human: Building a Safer Health Care System*. Retrieved March 2008 from http://www.iom.edu/CMS/8089/5575.aspx
5. Assistant Secretary for Planning and Evaluation, U.S. Department of Health and Human Services. ASPE Issue Briefings: Long-term growth of medical expenditures—Public and private, May 2005. Retrieved April 2008 from http://aspe.hhs.gov/health/MedicalExpenditures/index.shtml
6. Center on Policy and Budget Priorities. Poverty and share of americans without health insurance were higher in 2007—and median income for working-age households was lower—than at the bottom of last recession. Retrieved June 2009 from http://www.cbpp.org/cms/?fa=view&id=621
7. Buzzell RD, Gale BT. *The PIMS Principles: Linking Strategy to Performance*. New York: The Free Press; 1987.
8. U.S. General Accounting Office (GAO/NSIAD-91-190). *Management Practices: U.S. Companies Improve Performance Through Quality*. Washington, DC: U.S. General Accounting Office; 1994.
9. Malcolm Baldrige Index. Retrieved March 2008 from http://www.baldrige.gov

10. Easton GS, Jarrell SL. The emerging academic research on the link between total quality management and corporate financial performance: A critical review. In Stahl MJ, ed. *Perspectives in Total Quality*. Malden, MA: Blackwell, in association with ASQ Quality Press; 1999.

11. Hendricks KB, Singhal VR. The long run stock performance of firms with effective TQM programs. *Management Science*. 2001;47:359–368.

12. Hendricks KB, Singhal VR. Does implementing an effective TQM program actually improve operating performance? Empirical evidence from firms that have won quality awards. *Management Science*. 1997;43:1258–1274.

13. Institute of Medicine. *Crossing the Quality Chasm*. Retrieved March 2008 from http://www.iom.edu/CMS/8089.aspx

14. Stulberg J. The physician quality reporting initiative—A gateway to pay for performance: What every health care professional should know. *Quality Management in Health Care*. 2008;17:2–8.

15. Hagland M. The long run. As the P4P race continues, providers integrate EBM with data-gathering systems to cross the finish line. *Healthcare Informatics*. 2007;24:36–39.

16. Green J. Pay for performance: Quality and cost control go arm in arm. *Trustee*. 2006;59:6–11.

17. Pines JM, Garson C, Baxt WG, Rhodes KV, Shofer FS, Hollander JE. ED crowding is associated with variable perceptions of care compromise. *Academy of Emergency Medicine*. 2007;14:1176–1181.

18. Kong MC, Camacho FT, Feldman SR, Anderson RT, Balkrishnan R. Correlates of patient satisfaction with physician visit: Differences between elderly and non-elderly survey respondents. *Health Quality and Life Outcomes*. 2007;24:62.

19. Gearon CJ. State-by-state guide to health care provider performance. Retrieved April 2008 from http://www.aarp.org/health/doctors/articles/statebystate_guide_healthcare_provider_performance.html

20. HealthGrades physician evaluation website. Retrieved April 2008 from http://www.healthgrades.com

21. Integrated Health Care Association. Physician group clinical care report card. Retrieved April 2008 from http://iha.ncqa.org/reportcard

22. Wynne S, Wells R. Hospital quality report cards: Ready for prime time? Retrieved April 2008 from http://jdc.jefferson.edu/cgi/viewcontent.cgi?article=1451&context=hpn

■ Additional Resources

Bodenheimer T, Grumbach K. *Understanding Health Policy*. New York: McGraw-Hill; 2005.

Institute of Medicine. *Crossing the Quality Chasm: A New Health System for the 21st Century*. Washington, DC: National Academy Press; 2001.

Kohn L, Donaldson M, Corrigan J, eds. *To Err Is Human: Building a Safer Health System*. Washington, DC: National Academy Press; 2000.

■ Appendix 1.1

CMS Physicians Quality Reporting Initiative (PQRI) Measures

Please note: Gaps in measure numbering reflect retired 2007 and 2008 PQRI measures that were not included in the 2009 PQRI.

1. **Hemoglobin A1c Poor Control in Type 1 or 2 Diabetes Mellitus**

   Description: Percentage of patients aged 18 through 75 years with diabetes mellitus who had most recent hemoglobin A1c greater than 9.0%

2. **Low Density Lipoprotein Control in Type 1 or 2 Diabetes Mellitus**

   Description: Percentage of patients aged 18 through 75 years with diabetes mellitus who had most recent LDL-C level in control (less than 100 mg/dl)

3. **High Blood Pressure Control in Type 1 or 2 Diabetes Mellitus**

   Description: Percentage of patients aged 18 through 75 years with diabetes mellitus who had most recent blood pressure in control (less than 140/80 mmHg)

4. **Screening for Future Fall Risk**

   Description: Percentage of patients aged 65 years and older who were screened for future fall risk (patients are considered at risk for future falls if they have had 2 or more falls in the past year or any fall with injury in the past year) at least once within 12 months

5. **Heart Failure: Angiotensin-Converting Enzyme (ACE) Inhibitor or Angiotensin Receptor Blocker (ARB) Therapy for Left Ventricular Systolic Dysfunction (LVSD)**

   Description: Percentage of patients aged 18 years and older with a diagnosis of heart failure and left ventricular systolic dysfunction (LVSD) who were prescribed ACE inhibitor or ARB therapy

6. **Oral Antiplatelet Therapy Prescribed for Patients with Coronary Artery Disease**

   Description: Percentage of patients aged 18 years and older with a diagnosis of coronary artery disease who were prescribed oral antiplatelet therapy

7. **Beta-blocker Therapy for Coronary Artery Disease Patients with Prior Myocardial Infarction (MI)**

   Description: Percentage of patients aged 18 years and older with a diagnosis of coronary artery disease and prior myocardial infarction (MI) who were prescribed beta-blocker therapy

8. **Heart Failure: Beta-blocker Therapy for Left Ventricular Systolic Dysfunction**

   Description: Percentage of patients aged 18 years and older with a diagnosis of heart failure who also have left ventricular systolic dysfunction (LVSD) and who were prescribed beta blocker therapy

9. **Antidepressant Medication During Acute Phase for Patients with New Episode of Major Depression**

   Description: Percentage of patients aged 18 years and older diagnosed with new episode of major depressive disorder (MDD) and documented as treated with anti-depressant medication during the entire 84-day (12 week) acute treatment phase

10. **Stroke and Stroke Rehabilitation: Computed Tomography (CT) or Magnetic Resonance Imaging (MRI) Reports**

    Description: Percentage of final reports for CT or MRI studies of the brain performed within 24 hours of arrival to the hospital for patients aged 18 years and older with either a diagnosis of ischemic stroke or transient ischemic attack (TIA) or intracranial hemorrhage or at least one documented symptom consistent with ischemic stroke or TIA or intracranial hemorrhage that includes documentation of the presence or absence of each of the following: hemorrhage and mass lesion and acute infarction

11. **Stroke and Stroke Rehabilitation: Carotid Imaging Reports**

    Description: Percentage of final reports for carotid imaging studies (neck MR angiography [MRA], neck CT angiography [CTA], neck duplex ultrasound, carotid angiogram) performed for patients aged 18 years and older with the diagnosis of ischemic stroke or transient ischemic attack (TIA) that include direct or indirect reference to measurements of distal internal carotid diameter as the denominator for stenosis measurement

12. **Primary Open Angle Glaucoma: Optic Nerve Evaluation**

    Description: Percentage of patients aged 18 years and older with a diagnosis of primary open-angle glaucoma (POAG) who have an optic nerve head evaluation during one or more office visits within 12 months

13. **Age-Related Macular Degeneration: Dilated Macular Examination**

    Description: Percentage of patients aged 50 years and older with a diagnosis of age-related macular degeneration who had a dilated macular examination performed which included documentation of the presence or absence of macular thickening or hemorrhage AND the level of macular degeneration severity during one or more office visits within 12 months

14. **Diabetic Retinopathy: Documentation of Presence or Absence of Macular Edema and Level of Severity of Retinopathy**

    Description: Percentage of patients aged 18 years and older with a diagnosis of diabetic retinopathy who had a dilated macular or fundus exam performed which included documentation of the level of severity of retinopathy and the presence or absence of macular edema during one or more office visits within 12 months

15. **Diabetic Retinopathy: Communication with the Physician Managing Ongoing Diabetes Care**

    Description: Percentage of patients aged 18 years and older with a diagnosis of diabetic retinopathy who had a dilated macular or fundus exam performed with documented communication to the physician who manages the ongoing care of the patient with diabetes mellitus regarding the findings of the macular or fundus exam at least once within 12 months

16. **Perioperative Care: Timing of Antibiotic Prophylaxis—Ordering Physician**

    Description: Percentage of surgical patients aged 18 years and older undergoing procedures with the indications for prophylactic parenteral antibiotics, who have an order for prophylactic antibiotic to be given within one hour (if fluoroquinolone or vancomycin, two hours), prior to the surgical incision (or start of procedure when no incision is required)

17. **Perioperative Care: Selection of Prophylactic Antibiotic—First OR Second Generation Cephalosporin**

    Description: Percentage of surgical patients aged 18 years and older undergoing procedures with the indications for a first OR second generation cephalosporin prophylactic antibiotic, who had an order for cefazolin OR cefuroxime for antimicrobial prophylaxis

18. **Perioperative Care: Discontinuation of Prophylactic Antibiotics (Non-Cardiac Procedures)**

    Description: Percentage of non-cardiac surgical patients aged 18 years and older undergoing procedures with the indications for prophylactic antibiotics AND who received a prophylactic antibiotic, who have an order for discontinuation of prophylactic antibiotics within 24 hours of surgical end time

19. **Perioperative Care: Venous Thromboembolism (VTE) Prophylaxis (When Indicated in ALL Patients)**

    Description: Percentage of patients aged 18 years and older undergoing procedures for which VTE prophylaxis is indicated in all patients, who had an order for Low Molecular Weight Heparin (LMWH), Low-Dose Unfractionated Heparin (LDUH), adjusted-dose warfarin, fondaparinux or mechanical prophylaxis to be given within 24 hours prior to incision time or within 24 hours after surgery end time

20. **Osteoporosis: Communication with the Physician Managing Ongoing Care Post-Fracture**

    Description: Percentage of patients aged 50 years and older treated for a hip, spine, or distal radial fracture with documentation of communication with the physician managing the patient's on-going care that a fracture occurred and that the patient was or should be tested or treated for osteoporosis

21. **Aspirin at Arrival for Acute Myocardial Infarction (AMI)**

    Description: Percentage of patients, regardless of age, with an emergency department discharge diagnosis of AMI who had documentation of receiving aspirin within 24 hours before emergency department arrival or during emergency department stay

22. **Perioperative Care: Timing of Prophylactic Antibiotics—Administering Physician**

    Description: Percentage of surgical patients aged 18 and older who have an order for a parenteral antibiotic to be given within one hour (if fluoroquinolone or vancomycin, two hours) prior to the surgical incision (or start of procedure when no incision is required) for whom administration of prophylactic antibiotic has been initiated within one hour (if fluoroquinolone or vancomycin, two hours) prior to the surgical incision (or start of procedure when no incision is required)

23. **Stroke and Stroke Rehabilitation: Deep Vein Thrombosis Prophylaxis (DVT) for Ischemic Stroke or Intracranial Hemorrhage**

    Description: Percentage of patients aged 18 years and older with a diagnosis of ischemic stroke or intracranial hemorrhage who received DVT prophylaxis by end of hospital day two

24. **Stroke and Stroke Rehabilitation: Discharged on Antiplatelet Therapy**

    Description: Percentage of patients aged 18 years and older with a diagnosis of ischemic stroke or transient ischemic attack (TIA) who were prescribed antiplatelet therapy at discharge

25. **Stroke and Stroke Rehabilitation: Anticoagulant Therapy Prescribed for Atrial Fibrillation at Discharge**

    Description: Percentage of patients aged 18 years and older with a diagnosis of ischemic stroke or transient ischemic attack (TIA) with documented permanent, persistent, or paroxysmal atrial fibrillation who were prescribed an anticoagulant at discharge

26. **Stroke and Stroke Rehabilitation: Tissue Plasminogen Activator (t-PA) Considered**

    Description: Percentage of patients aged 18 years and older with a diagnosis of ischemic stroke whose time from symptom onset to arrival is less than 3 hours who were considered for t-PA administration

27. **Stroke and Stroke Rehabilitation: Screening for Dysphagia**

    Description: Percentage of patients aged 18 years and older with a diagnosis of ischemic stroke or intracranial hemorrhage who underwent a dysphagia screening process before taking any foods, fluids, or medication by mouth

28. **Stroke and Stroke Rehabilitation: Consideration of Rehabilitation Services**

    Description: Percentage of patients aged 18 years and older with a diagnosis of ischemic stroke or intracranial hemorrhage for whom consideration of rehabilitation services is documented

29. **Screening or Therapy for Osteoporosis for Women Aged 65 Years and Older**

    Description: Percentage of female patients aged 65 years and older who have a central dual-energy X-ray absorptiometry (DXA) measurement ordered or performed at least once since age 60 or pharmacologic therapy prescribed within 12 months

30. **Osteoporosis: Management Following Fracture**

    Description: Percentage of patients aged 50 years and older with fracture of the hip, spine or distal radius who had a central dual-energy X-ray absorptiometry (DXA) measurement ordered or performed or pharmacologic therapy prescribed

31. **Osteoporosis: Pharmacologic Therapy**

    Description: Percentage of patients aged 50 years and older with a diagnosis of osteoporosis who were prescribed pharmacologic therapy within 12 months

32. **Use of Internal Mammary Artery (IMA) in Coronary Artery Bypass Graft (CABG) Surgery**

    Description: Percentage of patients aged 18 years and older undergoing isolated coronary artery bypass graft (CABG) surgery using an internal mammary artery (IMA)

33. **Preoperative Beta-blocker in Patients with Isolated Coronary Artery Bypass Graft (CABG) Surgery**

    Description: Percentage of patients aged 18 years and older undergoing isolated coronary artery bypass (CABG) surgery who received a beta-blocker pre-operatively

34. **Perioperative Care: Discontinuation of Prophylactic Antibiotics (Cardiac Procedures)**

    Description: Percentage of cardiac surgical patients aged 18 years and older undergoing procedures with the indications for prophylactic antibiotics AND who received a prophylactic antibiotic, who have an order for discontinuation of prophylactic antibiotics within 48 hours of surgical end time

35. **Medication Reconciliation**

    Description: Percentage of patients aged 65 years and older discharged from any inpatient facility (e.g., hospital, skilled nursing facility, or rehabilitation facility) and seen within 60 days following discharge in the office by the physician providing on-going care who had a reconciliation of the discharge medications with the current medication list in the medical record documented

36. **Advance Care Plan**

    Description: Percentage of patients aged 65 years and older who have an advance care plan or surrogate decision maker documented in the medical record or documentation in the medical record that an advance care plan was discussed but the patient did not wish or was not able to name a surrogate decision maker or provide an advance care plan in the medical record

37. **Assessment of Presence or Absence of Urinary Incontinence in Women Aged 65 Years and Older**

    Description: Percentage of female patients aged 65 years and older who were assessed for the presence or absence of urinary incontinence within 12 months

38. **Characterization of Urinary Incontinence in Women Aged 65 Years and Older**

    Description: Percentage of female patients aged 65 years and older with a diagnosis of urinary incontinence whose urinary incontinence was characterized at least once within 12 months

39. **Plan of Care for Urinary Incontinence in Women Aged 65 Years and Older**

    Description: Percentage of female patients aged 65 years and older with a diagnosis of urinary incontinence with a documented plan of care for urinary incontinence at least once within 12 months

40. **Chronic Obstructive Pulmonary Disease (COPD): Spirometry Evaluation**

    Description: Percentage of patients aged 18 years and older with a diagnosis of COPD who had spirometry evaluation results documented

41. **Chronic Obstructive Pulmonary Disease (COPD): Bronchodilator Therapy**

    Description: Percentage of patients aged 18 years and older with a diagnosis of COPD and who have an FEV1/FVC less than 70% and have symptoms who were prescribed an inhaled bronchodilator

42. **Asthma: Pharmacologic Therapy**

Description: Percentage of patients aged 5 through 40 years with a diagnosis of mild, moderate, or severe persistent asthma who were prescribed either the preferred long-term control medication (inhaled corticosteroid) or an acceptable alternative treatment

43. **Electrocardiogram Performed for Non-Traumatic Chest Pain**

Description: Percentage of patients aged 40 years and older with an emergency department discharge diagnosis of non-traumatic chest pain who had a 12-lead electrocardiogram (ECG) performed

44. **Electrocardiogram Performed for Syncope**

Description: Percentage of patients aged 60 years and older with an emergency department discharge diagnosis of syncope who had a 12-lead ECG performed

45. **Vital Signs for Community-Acquired Bacterial Pneumonia**

Description: Percentage of patients aged 18 years and older with a diagnosis of community acquired bacterial pneumonia with vital signs documented and reviewed

46. **Assessment of Oxygen Saturation for Community-Acquired Bacterial Pneumonia**

Description: Percentage of patients aged 18 years and older with a diagnosis of community-acquired bacterial pneumonia with oxygen saturation documented and reviewed

47. **Assessment of Mental Status for Community-Acquired Bacterial Pneumonia**

Description: Percentage of patients aged 18 years and older with a diagnosis of community-acquired bacterial pneumonia with mental status assessed

48. **Empiric Antibiotic for Community-Acquired Bacterial Pneumonia**

Description: Percentage of patients aged 18 years and older with a diagnosis of community-acquired bacterial pneumonia with an appropriate empiric antibiotic prescribed

49. **Asthma Assessment**

Description: Percentage of patients aged 5 through 40 years with a diagnosis of asthma who were evaluated during at least one office visit within 12 months for the frequency (numeric) of daytime and nocturnal asthma symptoms

50. **Appropriate Treatment for Children with Upper Respiratory Infection (URI)**

Description: Percentage of children aged 3 months through 18 years with a diagnosis of upper respiratory infection (URI) who were not prescribed or dispensed an antibiotic prescription on or within 3 days of the initial date of service

51. **Appropriate Testing for Children with Pharyngitis**

    Description: Percentage of children aged 2 through 18 years with a diagnosis of pharyngitis, who were prescribed an antibiotic and who received a group A streptococcus (strep) test for the episode

52. **Myelodysplastic Syndrome (MDS) and Acute Leukemias: Baseline Cytogenetic Testing Performed on Bone Marrow**

    Description: Percentage of patients aged 18 years and older with a diagnosis of MDS or an acute leukemia who had baseline cytogenetic testing performed on bone marrow

53. **Myelodysplastic Syndrome (MDS): Documentation of Iron Stores in Patients Receiving Erythropoietin Therapy**

    Description: Percentage of patients aged 18 years and older with a diagnosis of MDS who are receiving erythropoietin therapy with documentation of iron stores prior to initiating erythropoietin therapy

54. **Multiple Myeloma: Treatment with Bisphosphonates**

    Description: Percentage of patients aged 18 years and older with a diagnosis of multiple myeloma, not in remission, who were prescribed or received intravenous bisphosphonate therapy within the 12-month reporting period

55. **Chronic Lymphocytic Leukemia (CLL): Baseline Flow Cytometry**

    Description: Percentage of patients aged 18 years and older with a diagnosis of CLL who had baseline flow cytometry studies performed

56. **Hormonal Therapy for Stage IC—III ER/PR Positive Breast Cancer**

    Description: Percentage of female patients aged 18 years and older with Stage IC through IIIC, estrogen receptor (ER) or progesterone receptor (PR) positive breast cancer who were prescribed tamoxifen or aromatase inhibitor (AI) during the 12-month reporting period

57. **Chemotherapy for Stage III Colon Cancer Patients**

    Description: Percentage of patients aged 18 years and older with Stage IIIA through IIIC colon cancer who are prescribed or who have received adjuvant chemotherapy during the 12-month reporting period

58. **Plan for Chemotherapy Documented Before Chemotherapy Administered**

    Description: Percentage of patients, regardless of age, with a diagnosis of breast, colon, or rectal cancer who are receiving intravenous chemotherapy for whom the planned chemotherapy regimen (which includes, at a minimum: drug(s) prescribed, dose, and duration) is documented prior to the initiation of a new treatment regimen

59. **Radiation Therapy Recommended for Invasive Breast Cancer Patients who have Undergone Breast Conserving Surgery**

    Description: Percentage of invasive female breast cancer patients aged 18 through 70 years old who have undergone breast conserving surgery and who have received recommendation for radiation therapy within 12 months of the first office visit

60. **Prevention of Ventilator-Associated Pneumonia—Head Elevation**

    Description: Percentage of ICU patients aged 18 years and older who receive mechanical ventilation and who had an order on the first ventilator day for head of bed elevation (30–45 degrees)

61. **Prevention of Catheter-Related Bloodstream Infections (CRBSI)—Central Venous Catheter Insertion Protocol**

    Description: Percentage of patients, regardless of age, who undergo central venous catheter (CVC) insertion for whom CVC was inserted with all elements of maximal sterile barrier technique (cap AND mask AND sterile gown AND sterile gloves AND a large sterile sheet AND hand hygiene AND 2% chlorhexidine for cutaneous antisepsis) followed

62. **Assessment of GERD Symptoms in Patients Receiving Chronic Medication for GERD**

    Description: Percentage of patients aged 18 years and older with the diagnosis of gastroesophageal reflux disease (GERD) who have been prescribed continuous proton pump inhibitor (PPI) or histamine H2 receptor antagonist (H2RA) therapy who received an annual assessment of their GERD symptoms after 12 months of therapy

63. **Vascular Access for Patients Undergoing Hemodialysis**

    Description: Percentage of patients aged 18 years and older with a diagnosis of end stage renal disease (ESRD) and receiving hemodialysis who have a functioning AV fistula OR patients who are referred for an AV fistula at least once during the 12-month reporting period

64. **Influenza Vaccination in Patients with End Stage Renal Disease (ESRD)**

    Description: Percentage of patients aged 18 years and older with a diagnosis of ESRD and receiving dialysis who received the influenza immunization during the flu season (September through February)

65. **Plan of Care for ESRD Patients with Anemia**

    Description: Percentage of patient calendar months during the 12-month reporting period in which patients aged 18 years and older with a diagnosis of end stage renal disease (ESRD) who are receiving dialysis have a Hgb ≥ 11g/dL OR have a Hgb < 11 g/dL with a documented plan of care for anemia

66. **Plan of Care for Inadequate Hemodialysis in ESRD Patients**

Description: Percentage of patient calendar months during the 12-month reporting period in which patients aged 18 years and older with a diagnosis of end stage renal disease (ESRD) receiving hemodialysis have a Kt/V ≥ 1.2 OR patients who have a Kt/V < 1.2 with a documented plan of care for inadequate hemodialysis

67. **Plan of Care for Inadequate Peritoneal Dialysis**

Description: Percentage of patients aged 18 years and older with a diagnosis of end stage renal disease (ESRD) receiving peritoneal dialysis who have a Kt/V ≥ 1.7 OR patients who have a Kt/V < 1.7 with a documented plan of care for inadequate peritoneal dialysis at least three times during the 12-month reporting period

68. **Testing of Patients with Chronic Hepatitis C (HCV) for Hepatitis C Viremia**

Description: Percentage of patients aged 18 years and older with a diagnosis of hepatitis C seen for an initial evaluation who had HCV RNA testing ordered or previously performed

69. **Initial Hepatitis C RNA Testing**

Description: Percentage of patients aged 18 years and older with a diagnosis of chronic hepatitis C who are receiving antiviral treatment for whom quantitative HCV RNA testing was performed within 6 months prior to initiation of treatment

70. **HCV Genotype Testing Prior to Therapy**

Description: Percentage of patients aged 18 years and older with a diagnosis of chronic hepatitis C who are receiving antiviral treatment for whom HCV genotype testing was performed prior to initiation of treatment

71. **Consideration for Antiviral Therapy in HCV Patients**

Description: Percentage of patients aged 18 years and older with a diagnosis of chronic hepatitis C who were considered for peginterferon and ribavirin therapy within the 12-month reporting period

72. **HCV RNA Testing at Week 12 of Therapy**

Description: Percentage of patients aged 18 years and older with a diagnosis of chronic hepatitis C who are receiving antiviral treatment for whom quantitative HCV RNA testing was performed at 12 weeks from the initiation of antiviral treatment

73. **Hepatitis A and B Vaccination in Patients with HCV**

Description: Percentage of patients aged 18 years and older with a diagnosis of hepatitis C who were recommended to receive or who have received hepatitis A vaccination or who have documented immunity to hepatitis A AND who were recommended to receive or have received hepatitis B vaccination or who have documented immunity to hepatitis B

74. **Counseling Patients with HCV Regarding Use of Alcohol**

Description: Percentage of patients aged 18 years and older with a diagnosis of hepatitis C who received education regarding the risk of alcohol consumption at least once within the 12-month reporting period

75. **Counseling of Patients Regarding Use of Contraception Prior to Starting Antiviral Therapy**

Description: Percentage of female patients aged 18 through 44 years and all men aged 18 years and older with a diagnosis of chronic hepatitis C who are receiving antiviral treatment who were counseled regarding contraception prior to the initiation of treatment

76. **Acute Otitis Externa (AOE): Topical Therapy**

Description: Percentage of patients aged 2 years and older with a diagnosis of AOE who were prescribed topical preparations

77. **Acute Otitis Externa (AOE): Pain Assessment**

Description: Percentage of patient visits for those patients aged 2 years and older with a diagnosis of AOE with assessment for auricular or periauricular pain

78. **Acute Otitis Externa (AOE): Systemic Antimicrobial Therapy—Avoidance of Inappropriate Use**

Description: Percentage of patients aged 2 years and older with a diagnosis of AOE who were not prescribed systemic antimicrobial therapy

79. **Otitis Media with Effusion (OME): Diagnostic Evaluation—Assessment of Tympanic Membrane Mobility**

Description: Percentage of patient visits for those patients aged 2 months through 12 years with a diagnosis of OME with assessment of tympanic membrane mobility with pneumatic otoscopy or tympanometry

80. **Otitis Media with Effusion (OME): Hearing Testing**

Description: Percentage of patients aged 2 months through 12 years with a diagnosis of OME who received tympanostomy tube insertion who had a hearing test performed within 6 months prior to tympanostomy tube insertion

81. **Otitis Media with Effusion (OME): Antihistamines or Decongestants—Avoidance of Inappropriate Use**

    Description: Percentage of patients aged 2 months through 12 years with a diagnosis of OME who were not prescribed/recommended either antihistamines or decongestants

82. **Otitis Media with Effusion (OME): Systemic Antimicrobials—Avoidance of Inappropriate Use**

    Description: Percentage of patients aged 2 months through 12 years with a diagnosis of OME who were not prescribed systemic antimicrobials

83. **Otitis Media with Effusion (OME): Systemic Corticosteroids—Avoidance of Inappropriate Use**

    Description: Percentage of patients aged 2 months through 12 years with a diagnosis of OME who were not prescribed systemic corticosteroids

84. **Breast Cancer Patients who have a pT and pN Category and Histologic Grade for Their Cancer**

    Description: Percentage of breast cancer resection pathology reports that include the pT category (primary tumor), the pN category (regional lymph nodes), and the histologic grade

85. **Colorectal Cancer Patients who have a pT and pN Category and Histologic Grade for Their Cancer**

    Description: Percentage of colon and rectum cancer resection pathology reports that include the pT category (primary tumor), the pN category (regional lymph nodes) and the histologic grade

86. **Appropriate Initial Evaluation of Patients with Prostate Cancer**

    Description: Percentage of patients, regardless of age, with prostate cancer receiving interstitial prostate brachytherapy, OR external beam radiotherapy to the prostate, OR radical prostatectomy, OR cryotherapy with documented evaluation of prostate-specific antigen (PSA), AND primary tumor (T) stage, AND Gleason score prior to initiation of treatment

87. **Inappropriate Use of Bone Scan for Staging Low-Risk Prostate Cancer Patients**

    Description: Percentage of patients, regardless of age, with a diagnosis of prostate cancer at low risk of recurrence receiving interstitial prostate brachytherapy, OR external beam radiotherapy to the prostate, OR radical prostatectomy, OR cryotherapy who did *not* have a bone scan performed at any time since diagnosis of prostate cancer

88. **Review of Treatment Options in Patients with Clinically Localized Prostate Cancer**

Description: Percentage of patients, regardless of age, with clinically localized prostate cancer AND receiving interstitial prostate brachytherapy, OR external beam radiotherapy to the prostate, OR radical prostatectomy, OR cryotherapy who received counseling prior to initiation of treatment on, at a minimum, the following treatment options for clinically localized disease: active surveillance, AND interstitial prostate brachytherapy, AND external beam radiotherapy, AND radical prostatectomy

89. **Adjuvant Hormonal Therapy for High-Risk Prostate Cancer Patients**

Description: Percentage of patients, regardless of age, with a diagnosis of prostate cancer at high risk of recurrence receiving external beam radiotherapy to the prostate who were prescribed adjuvant hormonal therapy (GnRH agonist or antagonist)

90. **Three-dimensional Radiotherapy for Patients with Prostate Cancer**

Description: Percentage of patients, regardless of age, with prostate cancer receiving external beam radiotherapy to the prostate *only* (no metastases) who receive 3D-CRT or IMRT

91. **Patients who have Major Depression Disorder who meet DSM IV Criteria**

Description: Percentage of patients aged 18 years and older with a new diagnosis or recurrent episode of major depressive disorder (MDD) who met the DSM-IV™ criteria during the visit in which the new diagnosis or recurrent episode was identified during the measurement period

92. **Patients who have Major Depression Disorder who are Assessed for Suicide Risks**

Description: Percentage of patients aged 18 years and older with a new diagnosis or recurrent episode of major depressive disorder (MDD) who had a suicide risk assessment completed at each visit during the measurement period

93. **Disease Modifying Anti-Rheumatic Drug Therapy in Rheumatoid Arthritis**

Description: Percentage of patients aged 18 years and older who were diagnosed with rheumatoid arthritis and were prescribed, dispensed, or administered at least one ambulatory prescription for a disease modifying anti-rheumatic drug (DMARD)

94. **Patients with Osteoarthritis who have an Assessment of Their Pain and Function**

Description: Percentage of patient visits for patients aged 21 years and older with a diagnosis of osteoarthritis (OA) with assessment for function and pain

95. **Influenza Vaccination for Patients > 50 Years Old**

Description: Percentage of patients aged 50 years and older who received an influenza immunization during the flu season (September through February)

96. **Pneumonia Vaccination for Patients 65 years and Older**

Description: Percentage of patients aged 65 years and older who have ever received a pneumococcal vaccine

97. **Screening Mammography**

Description: Percentage of women aged 40 through 69 years who had a mammogram to screen for breast cancer within 24 months

98. **Colorectal Cancer Screening**

Description: Percentage of patients aged 50 through 80 years who received the appropriate colorectal cancer screening

99. **Inquiry Regarding Tobacco Use**

Description: Percentage of patients aged 18 years or older who were queried about tobacco use one or more times within 24 months

100. **Advising Smokers to Quit**

Description: Percentage of patients aged 18 years and older and are smokers who received advice to quit smoking

101. **Inappropriate Antibiotic Treatment for Adults with Acute Bronchitis**

Description: Percentage of adults aged 18 through 64 years with a diagnosis of acute bronchitis who were not prescribed or dispensed an antibiotic prescription on or within 3 days of the initial date of service

102. **Dilated Eye Exam in Diabetic Patient**

Description: Percentage of patients aged 18 through 75 years with a diagnosis of diabetes mellitus who had a dilated eye exam

103. **Angiotensin Converting Enzyme Inhibitor (ACE) or Angiotensin Receptor Blocker (ARB) Therapy for Patients with Coronary Artery Disease and Diabetes and/or Left Ventricular Systolic Dysfunction (LVSD)**

Description: Percentage of patients aged 18 years and older with a diagnosis of coronary artery disease (CAD) who also have diabetes mellitus and/or left ventricular systolic dysfunction (LVSD) who were prescribed ACE Inhibitor or ARB therapy

104. **Urine Screening for Microalbumin or Medical Attention for Nephropathy in Diabetic Patients**

Description: Percentage of patients aged 18 through 75 years of age with diabetes mellitus who received urine protein screening or medical attention for nephropathy during at least one office visit within 12 months

105. **ACE Inhibitor or Angiotensin Receptor Blocker (ARB) Therapy in Patients with CKD**

Description: Percentage of patients aged 18 years and older with a diagnosis of advanced chronic kidney disease (CKD) (stage 4 or 5, not receiving Renal Replacement Therapy [RRT]), and hypertension and proteinuria who were prescribed angiotensin converting enzyme (ACE) inhibitor or angiotensin receptor blocker (ARB) therapy during the 12-month reporting period

106. **Chronic Kidney Disease (CKD): Laboratory Testing (Calcium, Phosphorus, Intact Parathyroid Hormone (iPTH) and Lipid Profile)**

Description: Percentage of patients aged 18 years and older with a diagnosis of advanced CKD (stage 4 or 5, not receiving Renal Replacement Therapy [RRT]), who had the following laboratory testing ordered at least once during the 12-month reporting period: serum levels of calcium, phosphorus and intact PTH, and lipid profile

107. **Chronic Kidney Disease (CKD): Blood Pressure Management**

Description: Percentage of patient visits for patients aged 18 years and older with a diagnosis of advanced CKD (stage 4 or 5, not receiving Renal Replacement Therapy [RRT]), with a blood pressure < 130/80 mmHg OR blood pressure ≥ 130/80 mmHg with a documented plan of care

108. **Chronic Kidney Disease (CKD): Plan of Care: Elevated Hemoglobin for Patients Receiving Erythropoiesis-Stimulating Agents (ESA)**

Description: Percentage of patient calendar months during the 12-month reporting period in which patients aged 18 years and older with a diagnosis of advanced CKD (stage 4 or 5, not receiving Renal Replacement Therapy [RRT]), receiving ESA therapy, have a hemoglobin < 13 g/dL OR patients whose hemoglobin is ≥ 13 g/dL and have a documented plan of care

109. **HIT—Adoption/Use of Health Information Technology (Electronic Health Records)**

Description: Documents whether provider has adopted and is using health information technology. To qualify, the provider must have adopted a qualified electronic medical record (EMR). For the purpose of this measure, a qualified EMR can either be a Certification Commission for Healthcare Information

Technology (CCHIT) certified EMR or, if not CCHIT certified, the system must be capable of all of the following:

- Generating a medication list
- Generating a problem list
- Entering laboratory tests as discrete searchable data elements

110. **HIT—Adoption/Use of e-Prescribing**

Description: Documents whether provider has adopted a qualified e-Prescribing system and the extent of use in the ambulatory setting. To qualify this system must be capable of **ALL** of the following:

- Generating a complete active medication list incorporating electronic data received from applicable pharmacy drug plan(s) if available
- Selecting medications, printing prescriptions, electronically transmitting prescriptions, and conducting all safety checks (defined below)
- Providing information related to the availability of lower cost, therapeutically appropriate alternatives (if any)
- Providing information on formulary or tiered formulary medications, patient eligibility, and authorization requirements received electronically from the patient's drug plan

111. **Diabetic Foot and Ankle Care, Peripheral Neuropathy: Neurological Evaluation**

Description: Percentage of patients aged 18 years and older with a diagnosis of diabetes mellitus who had a neurological examination of their lower extremities

112. **Diabetic Foot and Ankle Care, Ulcer Prevention: Evaluation of Footwear**

Description: Percentage of patients aged 18 years and older with a diagnosis of diabetes mellitus who were evaluated for proper footwear and sizing

113. **Universal Weight Screening and Follow-Up**

Description: Percentage of patients aged 65 years and older with a calculated Body Mass Index (BMI) within the past six months or during the current visit that is documented in the medical record and if the most recent BMI is ≥ 30 or < 22, a follow-up plan is documented

114. **Universal Influenza Vaccine Screening and Counseling**

Description: Percentage of patients aged 50 years and older who were screened and counseled about the influenza vaccine during the months of January, February, March, October, November, and December

115. **Universal Documentation and Verification of Current Medications in the Medical Record**

Description: Percentage of patients aged 18 years and older with written provider documentation that current medications with dosages (includes prescription, over-the-counter, herbals, vitamin/mineral/dietary [nutritional] supplements) were verified with the patient or authorized representative

116. **Pain Assessment Prior to Initiation of Patient Treatment**

Description: Percentage of patients aged 18 years and older with documentation of a pain assessment (if pain is present, including location, intensity and description) through discussion with the patient or through use of a standardized tool on each initial evaluation prior to initiation of therapy

117. **Patient Co-Development of Treatment Plan/Plan of Care**

Description: Percentage of patients aged 18 years and older identified as having actively participated in the development of the treatment plan/plan of care. Appropriate documentation includes signature of the practitioner and either co-signature of the patient or documented verbal agreement obtained from the patient or, when necessary, an authorized representative

118. **Screening for Cognitive Impairment**

Description: Percentage of patients aged 65 years and older who have documentation of results of a screening for cognitive impairment using a standardized tool

119. **Screening for Clinical Depression**

Description: Percentage of patients aged 18 years and older screened for clinical depression using a standardized tool

---

Retrieved April 2008 from http://www.cms.hhs.gov/PQRI/Downloads/ 2008PQRIMeasuresList.pdf

Teams in Healthcare Performance Improvement

■ Teamwork Is Key for Improving Performance

The healthcare industry has "discovered" the value of teamwork in improving performance in the past few years. Traditionally, the healthcare workplace has been organized hierarchically, with physicians at the apex and other workers supporting the "orders" given by the physician in the interest of the patient. This system seemingly worked well for decades, particularly as the medical knowledge base expanded exponentially, creating increasing specialization and highly esoteric medical practice. Subspecialties have allowed improved scientific understanding of disease entities, but at the same time the relatively arcane knowledge base required in each of the subspecialties has mandated that patient care become an interdisciplinary effort. Although the traditional method of having a single "captain of the ship," usually the physician, once prevailed in delivering care to patients, healthcare processes have become increasingly a matter of teamwork, with multiple staff members accountable for ensuring safe and high-quality care. Thus improvement initiatives must be interdisciplinary if they are to succeed, with each team member participating equally.

■ Choosing a Project

One of the concepts we discuss in this book is using work systems that involve lean process management and six sigma project measurement systems. Using these approaches entails consideration of several factors in project selection. It is conceivable that a project may make big improvements in quality and productivity that have absolutely no impact on net profit. A lean six sigma project often relies on the theory of constraints articulated by Goldratt[1] in the 1990s to determine which projects to pursue.

Every organization has constraints that usually come in many forms and may actually have a useful purpose. Goldratt proposed using the following rules when a process has a resource constraint:[1]

1. *Identify the system's constraint(s).* Review the process to determine if any bottlenecks are present. Managers often consider bottlenecks to be a negative

factor constraining a process, but a bottleneck may be a competitive advantage for a company. For example, an expensive piece of equipment, such as a positron emission tomograph, may be a bottleneck for a hospital, but the purchase and operational cost of the machine may make it a competitive advantage in a given market. Thus the bottleneck is actually a benefit for the organization, and upstream "push" and downstream "pull" are the areas in which efforts may be concentrated for improving the process.

2. *Decide how to exploit the system's constraint(s)*. Projects should minimize waste related to the constraints. For example, if the constraint is market demand, then the project may involve 100% on-time delivery to optimize customer satisfaction. If the constraint is a machine, as noted in step 1, the focus of the project is usually on reducing setup time, eliminating waste and rework, and optimizing run time.

3. *Subordinate everything else to the decision made in step 2*. Projects that maximize throughput of the constraint provide the greatest payback, and the selected project will eliminate waste from downstream processes and steps (i.e., once the constraint has been used to create something, wasting the output because of a process glitch is highly counterproductive). If downstream processes are already functioning efficiently, then upstream process steps that ensure an adequate supply of resources will be the next target for a project. Slack resources are often the issue for upstream process steps, whereas either slack resources or uniform output flow tends to create problems downstream.

4. *Elevate the system's constraint(s)*. Elevate the constraint means "lift the restriction." Often, the projects completed in steps 2 and 3 eliminate the constraint. If the constraint continues to exist after performing steps 2 and 3, then the next effective approach may try to identify projects that provide additional resources to the constraint, like purchasing additional equipment or hiring additional workers with particular skills.

5. *If, in the previous steps, a constraint has been broken, go back to step 1*. If the constraint has been elevated but process output remains suboptimal, the process may not have been properly characterized, and the next approach is to review and remap the entire process, with the goal of identifying steps that were left out of the initial evaluation. Thus the task of project selection begins again.

Another, more traditional, approach to project selection involves Pareto analysis, known to many as "the 80-20 rule." The basic principle states that 80% of the problems in a process are caused by 20% of the possible sources. Pareto analysis involves identifying all the possible causes of variation or problems in a process, quantifying the number of times each cause occurs, and then graphing the results or placing them in a table sorted by the largest number. A sample Pareto analysis is illustrated in EXAMPLE 2.1.

Example 2.1 Pareto Analysis

The laundry service at CleanCloth Hospital cycles bed linens once every 6 hours for the medical-surgical unit, using Machine C, which is dedicated to the medical-surgical linens. The linens need to be back on the floor 12 hours after they have been removed, that is, the laundry team must launder the linens within 6 hours so that they are dried, folded, and returned to the floor within 12 hours. The "upstream process" consists of environmental services removing the bed linens, putting them in the proper container, and transporting them in batches to the laundry, where they are sorted to ensure that the linens are matched with Machine C. The "downstream process" entails drying, folding, and delivering the linens to the appropriate closet on the medical-surgical unit. Over the past 6 months the manager of the laundry service noted that approximately 5.2% of the medical-surgical linens are late returning to the unit, which has required using supplemental linens at added cost. The manager studied the process through 300 cycles and collected the number of incidents of errors at each step upstream and downstream from the constraint (Machine C), with the following results.

Cause	Process Position	Frequency of Defects	Percent of Sample
Late collection of bed linens	Upstream	6	2.0%
Late transport to laundry	Upstream	3	1.0%
Sort time prolonged	Upstream	1	0.3%
Drying and folding delayed	Downstream	4	1.3%
Delivery to medical-surgical delayed	Downstream	3	1.0%
Total errors		17	5.6%

The traditional method of displaying these data is a bar chart, as follows:

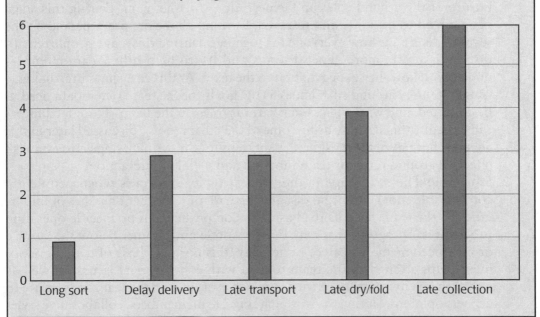

The Pareto analysis in EXAMPLE 2.1 clearly indicates that upstream processes are the most likely culprits for intervention, and both environmental services and laundry will initiate projects to improve that part of the process. As project parameters are being examined, several issues must be considered:

- Importance to the organization's stakeholders
- Impact on a specific performance measure or set of measures
- Regulatory requirements
- Alignment with the strategic plan
- Ability to perform the project in a reasonable time
- Technical feasibility of the project, given existing resources
- Reproducibility in other departments or divisions
- Available financial and material resources
- Human, financial, legal, and organizational risks
- Cultural readiness for dealing with results

Once projects are determined, the next step is to select an optimum team for developing improvement initiatives.

■ Team Development

Team formation and function tends to follow four specific stages:

1. *Forming:* The first stage of team development during which team members are unsure of the ground rules and expectations for the team. During this stage people tend to be polite and reserved, learning about the other people on the team to determine how everyone fits together. During this stage people tend to discuss issues in more general terms and try to help other team members understand how they expect to fit into the team. At this early juncture, dialogue usually centers around such issues as the goals for the team, what data need to be collected, and who will assume various roles on the team. Team facilitators can expedite this stage by using some of the "team tools" discussed later in this chapter, but one of the most important steps for the forming stage is to establish effective ground rules for team function and member interaction.

2. *Storming:* The next stage in the process typically occurs when people are comfortable enough to begin disagreeing with one another on issues of importance to the team, such as the basic mission of the team or specific operating procedures. Disagreements may be very subtle and simmer below the surface or may become more heated. Either way, this normal phase of team development helps strengthen the team to deal with controversial issues, as well as establish an environment of trust in which everyone on the team feels secure to express opinions. During the storming stage, team members' collaborative styles

become apparent, providing the team facilitator with important information about how to manage the group. Additionally, the team usually disagrees over some element of the team's structure or performance, often citing lack of progress as an indication that the team is dysfunctional. However, the critical need for this "shake out" phase becomes apparent as the team settles into the next stage of team evolution. Team leaders should bring disagreements to the surface for resolution, following the important ground rules of dealing with the issues rather than directing attacks at personalities. During the storming stage the team leader needs to continually reemphasize the team's purpose and charter to avoid letting the team wander off course.

3. *Norming:* After teams resolve the issues that surfaced during the storming stage, they enter the norming stage of team development. Team members begin to discuss constructive approaches to completing the group's work, using effective communication methods that were honed during the storming stage. With the emotional energy expenditures of storming behind them, members can focus on the purpose of the team and begin to develop effective processes for solving the problem at hand. At this point the ground rules established during the forming stage are easily applied and accepted by all team members, which accelerates resolution of conflicts that arise. The ideas that were generated in earlier stages are fleshed out, leading to decisions and action plans that help team members feel a sense of growth and accomplishment. Subgroups, based on mutual trust and respect, often predominate to help the team achieve goals faster. Team facilitators usually love this stage of the team's work, because harmony and progress characterize the effort and lead to realization of objectives. However, the team leader must remain engaged to ensure that the group remains on course, receives appropriate feedback on progress, and sticks to the timeline.

4. *Performing:* During this last stage of the team's evolution, the team has gelled into a highly effective, problem-solving unit that can come to consensus over useful solutions and predict problems before they become difficult to resolve. Teams often become proactive and seek other issues to attack, even before managers provide direction. These groups are highly cohesive, and members become loyal to one another, leading to respectful relationships that engender high performance and thrive on productive dissension. Team leaders become almost superfluous at this stage, because the group is capable of self-regulation; however, the leader frequently provides a focus for team bonding that creates the environment for high performance.

Although these stages are typical of team evolution, every team does not develop as neatly and sequentially as these four stages may suggest. Teams can progress from one stage to another relatively easily, or they may get stuck in one of the stages. If the team gets mired in the storming stage, for example, then it may end up disbanding because of lack of progress. Sometimes teams might actually regress to a prior stage, such as when an effective team leader is reassigned or a new member with a dominating personality joins the team. In those cases the team may need to retrace many of the steps that it completed successfully to reestablish team cohesiveness.

■ Application of the Team Approach

Teams are useful in a variety of circumstances, but not universally. The situations in which teams may be effective include the following:

- When a shared goal requires interdependencies or a project has complexities that require multiple skills and perspectives
- When the project crosses multiple processes or departments and coordinated effort is required to ensure success
- When project success depends on buy-in from multiple people
- When adequate time is available to allow a team to succeed
- When the issue or project is too complicated to be resolved in just a few meetings

On the other hand, some issues may not respond well to a team approach. These situations involve the following:

- Work that requires independent effort (e.g., writing a report) or involves only one person or department with no interdependencies with others (e.g., collecting data from a single source)
- Work that is more efficiently and effectively done by one individual
- Work that requires very specific expertise possessed by one person
- Projects that must be completed in a very short time
- Lack of willingness by managers to abrogate responsibility for a project to team members
- Lack of willingness of team members to assume accountability for the team's efforts

Organizational leaders must determine the suitability of a team approach, but it is important to remember that in some instances a team approach may be needed, even though one individual may want to solve a problem independently. In those situations, upper management intervention may be needed to ensure that a team functions properly.

In EXAMPLE 2.2A, which is not uncommon in healthcare organizations, the physician wishes to take charge of the renovation project and develop a plan that addresses the needs of the surgeons who operate at the facility. Dr. Davis is a highly respected surgeon, although more than a little overbearing and accustomed to issuing orders that are followed precisely in clinical situations. However, Terry knows that the project will require diverse viewpoints to succeed, with issues regarding supplies, regulations, bacteriological containment, finance, and many other items. Thus a team approach is the best method of ensuring that the renovation program will succeed, and EXAMPLE 2.2B reviews some approaches that might be helpful in this situation.

■ Steps in Creating Teams

A team charter serves as a roadmap for the team. The charter includes a statement of the mission of the team, objectives or statement of work, background of the project, authority or boundary conditions (scope, constraints, resources, and schedule), membership, requirements or specifications, and responsibilities for interactions with other

---

Example 2.2A The Issue

Dr. Davis is a widely respected surgeon at St. Change-Is-Now Hospital. His management style, which he learned in medical school and honed in his residency, is very directive, and the nursing staff knows that resistance is futile. Terry Thompson, the administrator at St. Change-Is-Now, has determined with his staff that the operating suites will require major overhaul in the next 3 years, and he now must determine what changes need to be made and develop a capital expenditure scenario to ensure that the program is affordable. Dr. Davis heard through the grapevine that the operating suites were about to be renovated, and he approached Terry to direct the planning and implementation of the program. He is confident that his extensive knowledge of the needs of surgeons will allow him to come up with an effective program for this project. How should Terry proceed?

Example 2.2B The Solution

Terry has a number of options, but, importantly, Dr. Davis needs to be involved in the project. Some approaches that Terry might take are as follow:

- Meet with Dr. Davis and explain the need for multiple viewpoints on the project, laying out the team design with a rationale for each team member (e.g., as in a team charter).
- Invite Dr. Davis to participate in the planning process, perhaps as a co-chair of the team or as the chair of a clinical subgroup that examines issues from a surgeon's standpoint.
- Keep Dr. Davis informed at each step of the process (e.g., through an "executive leadership team") so that any issues he might have may be either incorporated into the project or at least anticipated before a final report.

It should be self-evident that not taking a team approach in this situation could be very detrimental, but excluding Dr. Davis because he is not accustomed to being involved in teams would be equally damaging to the project. Additionally, exclusion of the other surgeons on staff would create major difficulties in gaining concurrence with the recommendations of the planning team.

groups and leaders. The charter should be specific enough to get the team started in the right direction but not so limiting as to presage the outcome of the team's work. Teams will establish more specific goals and plan once they comprehend the scope of their work, and the original charter is sometimes revised to better reflect the actual work of the group. Confusion, conflicts, or disagreements about the charter must be resolved before the onset of team activity because it will serve as the primary guide to focus the group and as a contract between the team and its sponsor.

Creation of a charter is usually a joint effort of the team leader and sponsor, and the document should consist of the following sections:

- **Section 1—Purpose:** The purpose introduces the charter and generally reviews how the team will use the document.
- **Section 2—Background:** The background describes the issues to be addressed, the evolution of a particular problem that is the subject of the team's work, and a summary of the products or services within the team's purview.
  - ○ **2.1—Program, project, or service description:** This section is a brief functional description of any required equipment or services that will be the subject of the project and how the product or service relates to the organization's strategic plan.
  - ○ **2.2—Organizational interfaces:** These interfaces describe where the team fits within the organization and with which other teams, groups, or outside organizations the team will interact during the project.
  - ○ **2.3—Users/customers:** The users and customers of the team's products, services, or output from the project are described here. Users are often other staff members and customers are usually external, but some companies consider all their staff members to be customers of one another.
  - ○ **2.4—Special or unique circumstances:** Any special or unique circumstances applicable to the team are mentioned (e.g., specific skills or urgency of the task), with a description of how these characteristics impact the team.
- **Section 3—Team mission and goals:** The mission statement establishes the team's purpose and direction. A well-written mission affirms the team's link to the organization's mission statement, vision, and values. Based on the mission statement, the team will identify approximately three to seven high-level goals that have a time horizon set by the project sponsor. If the team is formed to manage a process over time, the goals may be related to business processes and have a short-term time frame of 6 to 12 months and a longer term time frame of 3 to 5 years. However, if the team is constituted to perform a project, the sponsor usually sets the duration of the assignment.

    From these goals, the team will develop short- and long-term objectives to measure progress toward fulfilling its goals. Team objectives must be written so that they are measurable. In-process team metrics that measure progress to goals

Example 2.3 Team Mission Statement

The hospital's change team for improving the operating suites has formed a team that includes a mix of staff members with expertise in finance, construction, clinical issues, and support services. Terry Thompson and the Director of OR Services created the following mission statement for the group's work:

Mission: To create a plan for updating and modernizing the operating room suites that optimizes efficiency, reduces costs, and maximizes patient safety.

Goals: To ensure the highest quality pre-, intra-, and postoperative care at the lowest capital and operational costs.

through achievement of milestones and interim levels of improvement will be linked directly back to the team's objectives, as will longer term outcome measures (see EXAMPLE 2.3).

- **Section 4—Team composition:** A list is compiled of all cross-functional team members, including customers and suppliers, required for the team to achieve its mission. The listing should be specific with names or positions, contact information, and organizational unit represented. All high-performing teams develop a process for periodically reviewing and amending the list of team decision makers over the team's life cycle, and these changes must be reflected in updates to the team's charter. Sometimes there are so many potential team members that the size of the group may make it unworkable. In these situations the group may be subdivided into smaller units (e.g., core, extended, and support/advisory team members).
  - **4.1—Core team members:** Frequently, core team members are process owners and are required for conducting team business on a continuous basis, as well as being critical for team decision making. Core team members are listed by name, organization or unit, primary areas of responsibility, and contact information (phone number and e-mail).
  - **4.2—Extended team members:** These team members are involved in team activities on a part-time basis or specialize in particular phases of the project life cycle. Extended team members are free to participate in any team-based activities or decisions where they have expertise or their functional unit has an interest, including team decision making, particularly in their area of expertise or interest.
  - **4.3—Support/advisory team members:** Advisory team members provide support or specific expertise to other team members, much like consultants, but generally do not participate in team decisions. Typical advisory team members include customers, suppliers, consultants, and partners.

- **Section 5—Team membership roles:** Roles and responsibilities of both the organizations supporting the team and of each core and extended team member provide important information about the team's functions. If the team has chosen a different team membership division than "core, extended, and support/advisory," it will identify and explain how the team members are organized and which members are allowed to vote on recommendations and decisions. Definition of roles and responsibilities for both organizations and individual team members enables the team to identify required functional areas for team participation, to match these functions with specific team members, and to point out any gaps between in needed skills that may require adjusting membership. Each team member's supervisor must grant the member time and authority to represent the business unit on the team and vote on issues of importance.
- **Section 6—Team empowerment boundaries:** The team and sponsor will often work together to identify the specific empowerment needed by the team to achieve its goals, based on its mission, objectives, and the level of team member skills and capabilities. Empowerment allows the team to appropriately apply its expertise to the issues identified in the charter and devote team members' energies to resolving the issue, rather than struggling to find resources. With this level of empowerment comes an associated level of team accountability for the use of the resources to achieve the goals outlined in the charter. Empowerment boundaries provide a clear agreement between the team and the sponsor and remainder of the organization on those areas in which the team can exercise its discretion. Because the resources needed by a team must be justified, the team must assess its capabilities to ensure the sponsor that resources will be managed effectively. As the team performs its work effectively, the empowerment statement may be revised to allow greater flexibility and wider boundaries. EXAMPLE 2.4 shows an empowerment statement.

Example 2.4 Empowerment Statement

Terry understood that the team may need to access resources to create an effective renovation plan, and so he worked with the team leader to craft the following:
- **Renovation Program Empowerment:** Except as noted below, the OR Renovation Team is empowered to develop, approve, and update, as necessary, all operating room renovation plans and documentation including but not limited to:
  - Program planning documentation and architectural plans
  - System, equipment, and software specifications
  - Floor plan and supporting systems management requirements and plans
  - Acquisition management documentation
  - Contract deliverables for equipment and supplies
- **Limit:** The OR Renovation Team may not execute contracts without approval by the CEO or the Chairman of the Board of Trustees, nor may the Team create financial obligations for the corporation in excess of $1,000 (one thousand dollars).

- **Section 7—Team operations:** This section permits the team to describe the processes it plans to use in its operations and to identify required relationships with other teams, groups, or organizations crucial to its mission. The ability of a team to function properly may require new relationships and processes, and high-performing teams should address the following aspects of team operation:
  - **7.1—Closer proximity of team members:** To make team operations more effective, members may need to be located more closely together to enhance communications and interactions. As we discuss lean process management later in the book, the wisdom of "team pods" to facilitate effective team functions will become evident.
  - **7.2—Team shared accountability:** The accountability of team members should be explicit, with information about the percentage of time that team members will be expected to spend on team matters and the priority given team activity relative to the team members' usual duties.
  - **7.3—Decision-making processes:** The methods by which the team makes decisions will be important, particularly when the team consists of members from several departments at different levels on the organizational chart. Effective team operations generally require consensus decision making for all matters in which team stakeholders have interests, but at times other approaches, such as empowering an individual team member to decide and act, may be more appropriate. Those specific situations should be outlined in this section. Many times, teams may use flowcharts or other types of illustrations to describe these processes.
  - **7.4—Conflict resolution rules:** Internal conflicts are inevitable, and the team charter should have established rules for conflict resolution and an appeal process if the conflict deteriorates beyond the team's ability to resolve the issue. The inability to resolve conflicts may cause a team to lose focus and even disintegrate, and so this section is of particular importance.
  - **7.5—Problem-solving approaches:** Because most teams are devoted to resolving issues related to a new or existing process, the general approach to problem solving may be identified in the charter. For example, the team may be charged with using lean process management techniques or six sigma limits for resolving identified problems. To an extent, the problem-solving approaches may influence team composition, and so this section has implications beyond just providing the basis for improvement.
  - **7.6—Process improvement procedures:** High-performing teams understand that their own processes require continuous scrutiny for improvement, and so they constantly improve through monitoring, implementing, and tracking team processes. Opportunities for improvement should undergo the same analysis and implementation efforts as those for processes in the remainder of the organization.

○ **7.7—Changes in team membership:** Any team may need revision over time, as skill needs change, members leave the organization or are promoted to other positions, or to introduce new ideas into the mix. Procedures for identifying and then implementing changes in team membership should be codified at the beginning of the team's life so that these transitions are as smooth as possible.

○ **7.8—Leadership changes:** As team projects progress through various cycles, team leadership may need to be changed to better reflect the team's goals and objectives at each stage. Some teams may identify a succession plan to deal with changes expected as the team evolves, identifying criteria for change to new team leadership prospectively. Some criteria that may be used include the following:

- Leadership qualifications
- The point in the team life cycle
- Situations or issues encountered by the team
- Team maturity and operational dynamics

○ **7.9—Relationships with other teams:** Most teams must interact with other groups or teams in the organization or with partners and suppliers, and any specific relationships should be delineated. However, this section should also include proposed relationships as the team matures, so that these interactions can be developed without delay. For each organization identified, methods should be outlined to ensure the proper interface, interaction, and integration of activities.

○ **7.10—Other relationships:** Any other relationships, such as with user or customer organizations, suppliers, or other groups that the team needs to interact with to effectively carry out its mission, goals, and objectives, should be acknowledged, with methods described for how the team will ensure the proper interface, interaction, and integration of activities.

- **Section 8—Team performance assessment:** To identify opportunities for improvement that must be recognized to ensure high performance, teams must have methods of assessing performance. Metrics should include "in-process" measures that determine the efficiency of team processes and "outcome" measures that determine the effectiveness of the team's operational processes. The team and sponsor should work together to define key areas of performance that need to be measured and assessed to continuously improve. Often, these measures are labeled "Candidates for Internal Team Metrics" in the charter and address both how the team functions and how well it progresses toward meeting the team goals and objectives stated in Section 3. The candidates for the metrics list should be comprehensive and include measures that the team is already using or that might be required because of internal or external regulations. These metrics are usually confidential for the team's use only, but in some cases the measures might be used by senior managers to determine team progress.

- **Section 9—Team support requirements:** Many teams require outside assistance to succeed (e.g., consultants for specific tasks that are not available within the organization), and this section is used to document these needs. In addition to delineating these requirements, any shortfalls identified here should include proposed solutions (e.g., the name of a consultant or outside vendor, facility, educational program, or other resource needed to supply specific services). The team sponsor should be prepared to deal with any deficiency to ensure success of the project.
- **Section 10—Appendices:** Often used to amplify specific sections, appendices may be useful to delineate complex areas of the team's work that might not be immediately germane for all stakeholders who review the charter. For example, intricate data collection or analysis details may not be of interest to managers but may be of utmost importance in describing the team's work, and the appendices can serve as the location in the charter to provide these details. Additionally, many charters use appendices to outline any content that is likely to change on a recurring basis to prevent numerous revisions to the body of the charter. Additionally, the budget for the project is often placed in one of the appendices, and the detailed project timeline can be detailed in another of these attachments.

As part of the finalized charter, the team usually prepares an executive summary that allows senior managers to quickly understand the plan. These summaries are usually three to five pages, with the following components:

1. Team name
2. Mission statement and list of major products and/or services—with references to specific sections and page numbers in the charter
3. Team leader name and organizational chart
4. Empowerments—the title and one sentence summary of each requested empowerment accompanied by its location in the charter by section and page numbers
5. Team operations concepts—summarize how the team will address each of the following items with the section and page number:
   a. Team decision-making process
   b. Team conflict resolution approach
   c. Relationships with other teams
   d. Plan for leadership transition and member replacement
6. Support requirements—provide a list of needed resources, with section and page numbers
7. Special considerations—any other items in the charter that require special review by senior leaders, along with section and page references

Approval of the charter is the last step before creating the team. Team plan/charter preparation is complete when all decision-making members of the team demonstrate their concurrence by signing the plan/charter and supporting executives conduct a final review and sanction the effort. In some cases the plan may become part of the organization's strategic planning process and gain final acceptance as one of the primary initiatives for the company.

■ Team Selection

Most organizations use quality improvement teams in two situations: for specific projects (e.g., for improvement of throughput in the emergency department) and for ongoing process management (e.g., patient care in a clinical unit or for management of a specific business function). In both situations the team's task dictates the composition of the group.

Some organizations develop the team charter before the team is chosen, whereas others may select a team and have the group create the charter. In the former case senior management often has objectives for the team, whereas in the latter situation senior managers may defer to the team's expertise to define and address the issue by first creating the charter. A few principles apply to selecting a team.

Team Composition

A well-rounded team includes a mix of people and skills:

- *Content experts:* People who have a deep understanding of the processes to be examined; these individuals may come from any area in the organization and may be at any level of the organizational chart.
- *Process users:* Staff members who use the process on a regular basis and work closely with customers of the process; these individuals bring a wealth of knowledge of the practical aspects of the process. In some cases labor union representation may also add value to the team.
- *Technical support staff:* These important members often provide support for the process through information services, technical maintenance, and repair of equipment that is vital to the process or have in-depth knowledge of a highly technical engineering aspect of the process.
- *Customers and suppliers of the process:* When possible these team members are added so that inputs and outputs from the process may be properly assessed.

The team may occasionally add new members to bring a fresh perspective to the process review. For example, consultants may serve on teams to bring a broader perspective and, perhaps, a level of objectivity to the team. In this role the consultant can enhance the team's work by widening the scope of potential solutions to process problems. Teams may also find other types of members helpful at times, such as staff members who operate parallel processes in other departments who may be able to help integrate the team's work with other initiatives in the organization.

Team Selection Criteria

Every team should strive to have the "best and brightest" as members, but these people also need to also be able to work together. Desirable team member characteristics include:

- Creativity and open-mindedness
- Ability to work with others in a collaborative mode
- Respected among peers and organizational leaders

By finding team members with these qualities, the team leader can optimize the team's work environment as well as expedite the work of the group.

Team Size Considerations

The recommended size of the team varies depending on the team's scope of work. Process reengineering teams, for example, generally have between 3 and 12 members. Teams with three or four members tend to work faster and produce results quickly. Teams with greater than seven or eight members usually require additional facilitation and often require subgroups to allow the team to operate efficiently. Larger teams of more than eight members often have an "executive group" or core leadership subgroup of three to four people who manage the overall project and oversee subgroups consisting of between two and four people each.

Larger teams are sometimes necessary to attain broader functional representation to bring different business perspectives and a greater knowledge base to the project. The price of this larger size is usually a slower pace of the team's progress due to such issues as scheduling conflicts and longer times to reach consensus on complex issues.

The number of people on a team is always a consideration from a cost standpoint as well. Larger teams cost more to run, because the time taken from the team members' regular work creates costs in the affected departments.

Core Team Roles

Each team must have a certain number of defined roles for the team to function properly:

- Team leader
  - Coach team members in their roles in the group
  - Assume accountability for the team's actions and outcomes
  - Work with team members to define methods and approaches
  - Liaison with other organizational resources to ensure team effectiveness
  - Interact with the steering committee, oversight group, or executive champion

- Manage the budget
- Resolve disputes and manage conflict
- Project manager (may be the team leader for small teams)
  - Develop the project schedule and milestones, with tracking
  - Manage all subgroup meetings and projects
  - Monitor progress and focus on timelines and deadlines
- Facilitator (not always required for small teams)
  - Plan and lead team meetings
  - Utilize team-building and management approaches to ensure team effectiveness
  - Coordinate meeting records and follow-up
- Team members
  - Carry out assigned tasks and contribute to team progress
  - Assume responsibility for team progress and meeting deadlines

See EXHIBIT 2.1 for an example of a case of team development. Once team roles are established and the charter is created, the team is ready for action!

| Exhibit 2.1 | Crew Resource Management—A Special Case of Team Development |

Many healthcare organizations have taken a technique used by the aviation industry since 1979 that was designed to use all available resources, such as information, equipment, and people, to achieve safe and efficient flight operations. Many patient safety initiatives are designed around this approach, which empowers team members to interrupt a process when an error is detected. Crew resource management (CRM) programs usually involve three error elimination approaches: (1) avoidance of errors, (2) trapping potential errors before they occur, and (3) alleviation of error consequences after they have occurred. Effective CRM programs involve training teams in each of these three errors, but, even more fundamentally, the training is about empowering team workers to identify and deal with potential errors and creating a blame-free environment in which team members can be assured of being respected for their views and observations. Educational programs teach teams that fatigue, work overload, and emergency situations can create the situations in which errors become difficult to avoid. The ability to assess personal and team member behavior is important to effective CRM, and so team training includes curricula providing insight into behavioral aspects of team effectiveness. Additionally, team members are instructed in how to find relevant operational information and then how to advocate for correct processes, communicate appropriate actions, and resolve conflict productively.

■ Teamwork Tools

Getting teams to work together may be easy or it can present a real challenge for the team leader. Many teams are selected for compatibility, but in some cases team members have no prior relationship, which creates a need for team building early in the process. Additionally, teams have a toolbox of approaches to help stimulate creativity and expedite the process of achieving the goals set out in the charter. These tools include:

- Brainstorming and its variants, like brainwriting and nominal group technique (NGT)
- Benefits and barriers exercises (BBEs)
- Multivoting and list reduction

All these approaches are designed to help teams explode with new ideas and then gradually winnow the list of ideas down to the critical few for the team to pursue.

Brainstorming
When To Use This Approach
Brainstorming's benefits arise from the group interaction and rapid generation of ideas. One of the major advantages of the approach may be the improved morale that it generates in the group, because a well-conducted session usually energizes the group and can enhance team cohesiveness.

Principles for Use
The brainstorming process is designed to help each team member feel empowered to contribute to the group effort. The basic framework of the procedures includes the following:

- *Strive for quantity:* Don't worry about the "quality" of ideas but rather work to generate the largest number possible, with the precept that within the large number of concepts generated will reside the nub of an innovation.
- *No criticism allowed:* Any ideas generated during the session are recorded without any critique offered. Group members should try to expand on a relatively weak concept rather than dismiss it. The atmosphere during the brainstorming session should remain completely supportive.
- *Go for the unusual:* One sign that the process is effective is the appearance of unusual or even bizarre ideas that may not have much chance to make the cut later, but often these thoughts stimulate variants that can be implemented.
- *Combine and improve ideas:* Group members should be encouraged to amplify, modify, or combine suggestions generated during brainstorming. Some facilitators

like to put the equation "$1 + 1 = 3$" in plain sight during the exercise to emphasize this concept.

Procedure

The steps in the brainstorming process include the following:

1. Definition of the problem with a problem statement that is clear, focused, and usually formulated as a question like, "How can we move patients through the outpatient clinic faster?" If the question is too broad, then it should be divided into smaller, more manageable components like, "How can we ensure that the patient chart is available to avoid delays in outpatient?"
2. Provide background on the issue through a short summary sheet or informational handout for the group. Sent with the invitation to participate, the summary should provide a quick review of the issue so that potential participants can determine their interest and ability to contribute. The background sheet may include some example ideas, so that when the session slows down or goes off track, the suggestions may help stimulate thought and bring the group back into a focused framework. Participants should have a few days to consider the issue, and so the background information should be distributed several days in advance.
3. Select participants according to expertise and interest, much as the selection process for any other team. In most cases groups of 5 to 10 provide the best possibility of coming to some conclusions in a timely manner. In most cases participants come from the team responsible for the overall project or operational area, but in many cases group members from other departments or outside the organization may add new ideas or a different perspective to the process. One person should be designated the facilitator and one the recorder.
4. Prepare for lapses in creativity by having some motivational questions ready. For example, the facilitator might ask if some of the ideas may be combined, or if the problem might be viewed from another perspective (e.g., outpatient throughput from the nurse's standpoint).
5. Conduct the session with the facilitator leading and recording, ensuring that ideas and discussion are captured. Key to success of the exercise, however, is observance of the rules for equal participation and no criticism. In some cases new participants may need a short practice session to learn how to function in a criticism-free zone, and a mock session using a relatively easy question may be beneficial. When the session begins, the facilitator presents the question and brief background, with the assumption that everyone has already read the background information. As each participant provides an idea, the recorder puts it on a flip chart, marker board, or computer screen so that everyone can see. Occasionally, an idea may not be clear, and the facilitator may ask for further information before moving on to the next thought, but no idea should be vetted until the exercise has been completed. Once all ideas have been

presented, the group might take a short break so that the facilitator can organize the ideas into logical subsets for the group to review. At this point, the list can be reduced by one or more of the techniques discussed later in this chapter.

Tips for Improving the Brainstorming Process

- Provide paper and pencil to allow team members to write down ideas if they find it hard to speak. The group member can then present it later when the rate of idea generation slows.
- Have the recorder number the ideas to help the team identify each thought but also as a running tally for stimulating productivity.
- Do not invite managers and superiors to reduce the likelihood that the team may be inhibited in creative thought.

Nominal Group Technique

When To Use This Approach

The NGT is a type of brainstorming that encourages all participants to have an equal say in the process and is often used when group members find it difficult to speak openly. It can also be used to narrow a list of brainstormed ideas.

Principles for Use

NGT is very useful in a large group that is subdivided into smaller subgroups to work on specific parts of the project. For example, to determine the parameters of a new service, like a new outpatient clinic, a large group may be formed with experts in a number of areas. One subgroup may work on the hours of the clinic, whereas another subgroup may work on staffing, and still another on the equipment needed in the clinic. Each subgroup returns to the larger group to gain help in ranking the listed ideas. In some cases ideas that were previously dropped may be brought forward again once the group has had an opportunity to provide input.

Procedure

Preparation involves ensuring that everyone on the team starts with the same information about the issue at hand. Participants are provided with background information, much as in brainstorming, and the work area is prepared for the session. Generally, the materials involve only pencil and paper, but more sophisticated systems may be used that allow for collaboratively entering ideas into a computer file that is shared via a whiteboard on an interactive system, for example, when participants are at different sites and must communicate via webinar.

Participants are asked to write down their ideas anonymously, and then each group member's work is collected by the facilitator and arranged for voting either by secret ballot or by show of hands in a process known as "distillation." After distillation, the top-ranked ideas may be sent back to the group or to subgroups for further brainstorming. After a few cycles, the NGT process usually yields a short list of ideas.

Brainwriting

When To Use This Approach

Also known as the "group passing technique," brainwriting is an approach that stimulates a group of reticent individuals to contribute to the brainstorming process. When the facilitator is having trouble gaining input from all participants, the brainwriting technique provides an approach that all but requires people to participate.

Procedure

The group is seated in a circle so that sheets of paper can be passed easily. Following a process similar to brainstorming, each person in the circle writes down one idea on a form, such as that shown in TABLE 2.1, and then passes the piece of paper to the next person in a clockwise direction. Each person in turn adds thoughts to the form and passes it to the next person, who also adds some thoughts. This procedure repeats until everyone gets his or her original piece of paper back. By the time the paper makes its rounds, a wealth of new ideas should be generated by the group.

A popular variant to brainwriting mimics the NGT. This alternate approach uses an "idea book" with a distribution list. Each person on the list receives the book and posts one or more ideas in the book. The book contains forms like in TABLE 2.1 and may address multiple problems rather than just a single issue as in a typical brainstorming or brainwriting exercise. Each individual can add new ideas or expand on any of the thoughts already in the book. The process continues until the distribution list is exhausted, and then a facilitator conducts a follow-up meeting to discuss the ideas logged in the book. Although the idea book technique takes longer, it allows individuals to spend more time to think more extensively about the problem(s). If time is not

Table 2.1	Example of a Brainwriting Form			
Issue: Get to work on time				
Owner: John Administration				
Use alarm clock	Take a cab	Drive fast	Take a shortcut	Don't stay out too late the night before
Get a wake-up call	Get someone to drive	Have a taxi waiting when you're ready to go	Use alternative, like train or bus	Change expectations of work hours

constrained in the search for a solution, the idea book approach may actually yield higher quality results.

Benefits and Barriers Exercise (BBE)

When To Use This Approach

The goal of this exercise is to help individuals or a group to identify the benefits of a particular change and to determine any obstacles to implementation of the change. Using this approach, a team can gain buy-in from its own members and from leaders who need to support the project. Additionally, the exercise can pinpoint issues that may interfere with the change process. The BBE is usually applied when a significant change is to be implemented and the extent of buy-in is unclear, or when the change is encountering resistance from one or individuals or groups in the organization. A BBE is often useful when the team has identified the need for a new initiative through brainstorming or other methods of idea creation, because the barriers portion of the exercise can help define some of the approaches that the group may consider to ensure effective implementation. Particularly important is the need to recognize who might raise the greatest resistance to the new proposal and ensure that those individuals or groups are represented in the deliberations of the exercise.

Procedure

The exercise uses one of the brainstorming approaches described earlier to generate ideas regarding the benefits of a particular change and the barriers to reaching the desired outcome.

1. Groups of interested staff members and customers are selected based on their interest or involvement in a proposed change. Larger groups should be subdivided into smaller subgroups of four to seven individuals, preferably mixed among departments or divisions to ensure diversity on each team and to gain a broad range of input.
2. Each subgroup, or "BBE team," includes a facilitator to organize and lead the discussion. The tools required are minimal, consisting only of a flip chart or a pad of paper on which ideas are recorded, although some teams now use an electronic "whiteboard" projected on a screen to record ideas and changes quickly.
3. Each subgroup then receives a complete briefing on the proposed change, including data where applicable, so that everyone understands the issue well. Facilitators for each BBE team lead a discussion of benefits for team members' individual situations, as well as those for external customers, suppliers, and internal customers, such as the board or executive managers. The facilitator may record these ideas or a recorder may be appointed to free the facilitator to lead the discussion.
4. The full group should reassemble at this point to share the lists of benefits from all the teams and begin the process of narrowing the list using list reduction

approaches described in the next section. Once the list has been revised to a manageable level (usually 5–10 highest priority thoughts), the group often breaks for a period of time before beginning the challenging barriers portion of the exercise.

5. After the break, subgroups reconvene to discuss organizational barriers to the proposed change. In almost a reverse to the prior approach, organizational barriers are considered first, and then each barrier may be dissected further to a department, division, and even individual level. Thoughts are again recorded for presentation and discussion in the larger group.

6. As the larger group meets again, the similarities between the groups are highlighted and used to prioritize the list of barriers to be surmounted by the implementation process. Additionally, the group should spend time strategizing the ways that the benefits may be used to address the barriers during the period of change. At the conclusion of this portion of the meeting, the larger group will have identified the highest priorities for both emphasizing benefits and dealing with barriers during the change process.

7. The group leader will create a final report from the BBE that includes (1) a brief description of the issue, (2) a description of the proposed change, (3) benefits to all stakeholders, (4) prioritization of barriers, and (5) implementation strategies for overcoming barriers. Many groups share the report with group members for final ratification before submitting it to senior managers.

Tips for Improving This Approach

- It is usually best to begin with individual benefits before extending to more "macro" situations, because people can most readily define the benefits for themselves first and then combine and build on those benefits for other stakeholders.
- During the barriers portion of the BBE, the facilitator must use care to keep the issue in focus and avoid letting the discussion move to a personal level that may threaten group members and diminish effectiveness of the BBE.
- The break between the discussions of benefits and barriers may be of value in allowing group members to better understand the advantages of the proposed change before discussing the problems with implementation. Often, it allows group members to reflect on how these advantages may be leveraged to better address the potential detriments from the change.

List Reduction and Multivoting

When To Use This Approach

After one of the brainstorming approaches is completed, a team often ends up with a long list of alternative ideas to examine, but the list usually has duplicate or very similar ideas that need to be combined or eliminated to make the list more useful. The list-reduction process provides a method of making a long list of alternatives more useful by removing duplicates and combining similar ideas.

Procedure

List reduction and multivoting follows a process similar to brainstorming, but the goal is not to increase the number of ideas under consideration but rather to bring the list under control. The procedure that follows is designed to systematically pare the list to a manageable level:

1. Display the complete list of items for everyone involved and review the process with team members.
2. Review all items on the list to ensure full understanding by all team members of all items to be considered. Some items may be combined in this early phase if the combination does not reduce the impact of either of the items.
3. **First vote:** During the first round of voting, everyone is allowed to vote for the items on the list that they consider most significant, and the votes are not weighted in any way. Group members may only vote once for an item but may vote for any number of items that seem most significant. During this phase group members do not discuss or negotiate any of the items.
   ○ After the first round votes are counted, items with the larger number of votes are circled, with the team deciding how many votes are necessary to circle an item.
4. **Second vote:** All members vote a second time on the smaller list. This time each team member is allowed only the number of votes equal to half the remaining list, so if there are six items remaining, each team member may vote only for the three items they consider most important. Again, no lobbying or negotiation of voting is permitted.
   ○ The second vote process is repeated to continue reducing the list until there are only from three to five items remaining for consideration.

Tips for Improving This Approach

- Never reduce the list to one remaining item. Voting down to one item creates a win/lose situation not desired for team dynamics.
- Ensure that everyone clearly understands the process in the beginning. Distribution of a one-page summary of the rules at the outset of the exercise may provide the needed information to ensure the process works according to plan.
- Although this process reduces a list of ideas to a critical few, it may still be necessary to finalize a decision on just one item. In that case, other methods may be used (e.g., statistical analysis of critical variables).
- Multivoting works best when done quickly and with no discussion of alternatives. Discussion is allowed only if an item is unclear to the group.

■ Discussion Questions

1. How do teams improve the performance of healthcare organizations? Give examples of team approaches in your organization.
2. How should senior managers and team leaders determine which projects are most important to the organization? Describe use of the approach in a healthcare organization.
3. Describe Goldratt's theory of constraints. How will the theory ensure appropriate team alignment with process improvement?
4. What is the basis of the "80–20 rule"? Compare this principle to Goldratt's theory of constraints.
5. What are the four stages of team performance? How does effective management of each stage ensure team success?
6. What situations make the team approach most likely to succeed? When is the team approach not as likely to produce the best results?
7. How can managers and leaders ensure success in situations when physicians are involved?
8. What are the major elements of a team charter? How does a charter contribute to team effectiveness and success?
9. Name the two situations in which most organizations deploy quality improvement teams. Provide an example of each from your experience.
10. What criteria should be used for selecting team members? What considerations should be given to determining team composition?
11. List the core team roles in a typical team. How does each one contribute to the team's function and success?
12. Describe crew resource management. Discuss the origins and advantages of this approach.
13. What are the most common methods of generating ideas in a group? Describe each approach with necessary caveats.
14. Why do groups use a benefits and barriers exercise? Describe the process and desired outcome.
15. How do groups create manageable lists of tasks from a brainstorming exercise? Describe the process and expected outcome.

■ Reference

1. Goldratt MV. "Theory of constraints" thinking processes: A systems methodology linking soft with hard. Retrieved July 2008 from http://www.systemdynamics.org/conferences/1999/PAPERS/PARA104.PDF

■ Additional Resources

Allen J, Rogelberg S, Scott J. Mind your meetings. *Quality Progress*. 2008;April:49–53. Retrieved September 2008 from http://www.asq.org/quality-progress/2008/04/full-issue.pdf

Coppola N. Leveraging team building strategies. *Healthcare Executive*. 2008;May/June:70–73.

Institute for Healthcare Improvement. Engaging physicians: How the team can incorporate quality and safety. *Healthcare Executive*. 2008;May/June:78–81.

Joint Commission on Accreditation of Healthcare Organizations. *Using Performance Improvement Tools in Ambulatory Care*. Oakbrook Terrace, IL: Joint Commission on Accreditation of Healthcare Organizations; 1998.

Laman S. Testing the limits of team development. *Quality Progress*. 2008;April:35–38. Retrieved September 2008 from http://www.asq.org/quality-progress/2008/04/full-issue.pdf

Tague N. *The Quality Toolbox*. Milwaukee, WI: American Society for Quality; 2005.

Thiraviam A. Simple tools for complex systems. *Quality Progress*. 2006;June:40–44. Retrieved September 2008 from http://www.asq.org/pub/qualityprogress/past/0606/qp0606thiraviam.html

Process Tools

■ All Work Consists of Processes

Although it may seem intuitive for a quality professional, healthcare practitioners often have a hard time recognizing that all work in health care can be evaluated using the same process analysis tools that have been applied in the industrial sector for decades. Healthcare workers often surmise that the sanctity of the "patient relationship" makes analysis of the related processes difficult or impossible. However, society is showing us just how wrong that philosophy can be, through payers that are now demanding data on operational effectiveness, consumer groups demanding higher quality, federal agencies providing incentives for reporting and improved performance, and the ever-present medical malpractice industry nipping at the heels of healthcare providers who provide substandard care. The quality management and performance excellence movement in health care has hit full stride, and organizations that fail to recognize the importance of demonstrating quality in the work they do will become as extinct as the allosaurus.

An important aspect of this recognition is the need to concede that all work in health care is based on processes, all of which are subject to the tools of process analysis applied daily in industries throughout the world. Even though U.S. manufacturers took time to adopt some of these approaches, Japanese producers exploited quality improvement methods to change perception of their products from "never buy Japanese" in the 1940s and 1950s to world standard setting products in the 1980s and beyond. Pioneering approaches like lean six sigma helped the Japanese make quantum leaps in the latter decades of the 20th century to become fierce competitors and world leaders in automobiles and electronics, as well as a number of other industries. As U.S. companies watched the transformation, they gradually changed their operational approaches to adopt these new methods and at least remain competitive, but innovation in process management has kept Japanese industry at the forefront in a number of areas. Health care has lagged behind American industry in adopting the new philosophy, but as the world becomes more competitive and healthcare costs rise to greater percentages of the U.S. gross domestic product, manufacturers are demanding that the healthcare industry become more efficient and effective. Thus the need to understand and improve processes in healthcare organizations has never been greater. American industry is demanding value from healthcare services.

■ What Is the Value Proposition?

In today's economic climate, the key word is *value*. From a business standpoint, value has a specific definition:

$$Value = \frac{Quality}{Cost}$$

This equation is often used to define the "value proposition," and regardless of the industry, value for a consumer equates to the highest quality product or service purchased at the lowest cost. For example, when buying a new car the goal is to find the best automobile possible (air conditioning? gas mileage? power steering? etc.) at the lowest cost. For most people, buying a car is easier than finding the best value in health care. However, just as with a car, value may mean different things to different people. For example, some will feel that they had a valuable experience if the food in the hospital is above average, whereas others may just want a "pretty scar" after surgery. Healthcare organizations have evolved a number of ways to demonstrate value for customers, and society has dictated value in many cases. Federal and state governments have developed a number of different types of measures, and payers of all types have created metrics to ensure that customers are realizing value when they have a healthcare encounter. To encourage providers to use these metrics, agencies like the Centers for Medicare and Medicaid Services (CMS) have developed programs like pay for reporting that remit financial rewards for practitioners who submit data for certain metrics considered important for patient care quality and safety. Use of the data for determining reimbursement rates was not implemented in 2008, but CMS has begun to tighten rules for paying providers for certain "never events," complications that should never occur, like pressure ulcers and catheter-related bloodstream infections. These changes in payment practices have made the need for process review and improvement greater than in the past.

As part of the value proposition, quality professionals determine the *value stream*, those steps in the processes of care that provide customer value. Taken from the Toyota Production System, or lean process management, the value stream concept helps focus efforts on those process stages that contribute to producing a high-quality service or product for which a customer is willing to pay. Process analysis tools help identify those steps that do not add value to the process and can be modified or eliminated without hurting the end product or service. Elimination of these *non–value added* steps usually improves efficiency of the process, reduces costs, and enhances quality. The tools in this chapter have been applied for decades in the industrial sector around the world and in the recent past are being quickly adapted for medical process analysis.

■ Process Analysis Toolkit

The process analysis toolkit consists of four basic approaches and their variations:

1. Flowcharts
2. Matrices
3. Decision trees
4. Special diagrams

Flowcharts: Blueprint in the Quality Improvement Professional's Toolbox

Just like a blueprint, flowcharts help performance improvement teams understand a process in exquisite detail. Basic and specialized flowcharts help define steps in the process as well as sequence events to determine requirements at each step. The basic flowchart is most commonly used to describe process flow, but many other specific types of flowcharts can be used to help define detailed attributes of a particular process. Three types of flowcharts that are helpful for understanding some of the more salient process characteristics are:

1. Basic flowchart
2. PERT chart
3. Deployment flowchart

Basic Flowcharts

As mentioned previously, basic flowcharts are most frequently used as a starting point to understanding process flow. The basic flowchart provides a graphic representation of the path that the process follows from input(s) to output(s) and can be easily constructed using an inexpensive template purchased at a business supply store or, as is done more frequently, using a computer program like Microsoft Visio. All examples in this chapter were created using Microsoft Visio unless otherwise noted. Many quality improvement professionals quickly become facile with computer programs to create spreadsheets, because the diagrams can be created quickly and edited readily.

When To Use
Basic flowcharts are used in several situations:

- During initial analysis of a process being studied for potential improvements
- When process measures are being identified
- As a starting point for problem analysis (e.g., root-cause analysis [RCA])
- For planning solutions to issues identified during any type of problem analysis, like RCA or failure mode and effects criticality analysis (FMECA)
- To demonstrate to others how a process is performed

The old saying, "a picture is worth a thousand words," is truly applicable to the basic flowchart, because the diagram often reduces the need for long written descriptions of the process. The basic flowchart can be key to identifying a number of process issues:

- *Redundancies:* Excess steps in the process that lengthen the time for completion without adding any other value
- *Inefficiencies:* Points in the process that have built in or de facto waiting times that delay output without improving the process

Shape	Use
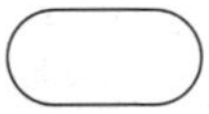	**Terminator –** The terminator symbol marks the starting or ending point of the system. It usually contains the word "Start" or "End"
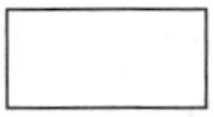	**Action or Process –** A box can represent a single step ("draw blood"), or an entire sub-process ("take chest x-ray") within a larger process
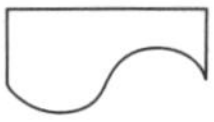	**Hardcopy –** A printed document or report
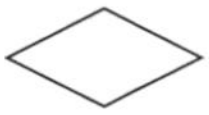	**Decision point –** Lines representing different decisions emerge from different points of the diamond
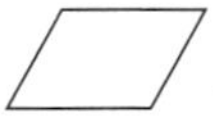	**Input/Output –** Represents material or information entering or leaving the system, such as physician order (input) or a completed service or product (output)
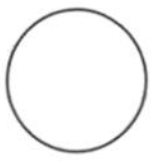	**Connector –** used to show that process flow continues where a matching symbol (containing the same letter or number) has been put into the flowchart
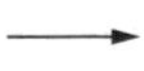	**Arrow –** Arrows indicate the sequence of steps and the direction of flow and connect the shapes in the flowchart
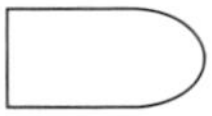	**Delay –** a stopping point or delay in the process, e.g. the hard stop prior to surgery to review all pertinent information
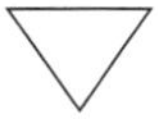	**Merge –** two or more sub-lists or sub-processes become one
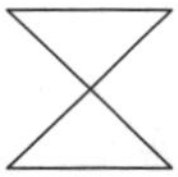	**Collate –** formatting step that puts information into a standard format for reporting or display

FIGURE 3.1 Flowchart Shapes

Shape	Use
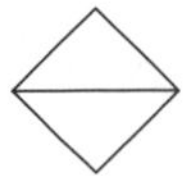	**Sort –** sequencing step that organizes a list of items based on some pre-determined criteria, e.g. alphabetic or numeric order
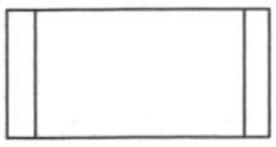	**Subroutine –** connotes a sequence of actions that perform a specific task embedded within a larger process; may refer to a sequence described in greater detail on a separate flowchart
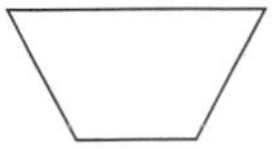	**Manual Loop –** a sequence of steps or commands that will continue to repeat until stopped by external intervention
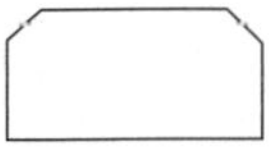	**Loop Limit –** point at which a loop should stop
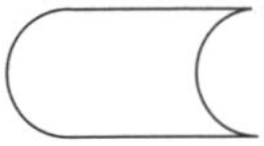	**Data storage –** step in which data is stored
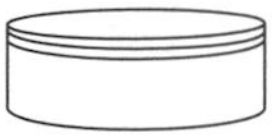	**Database –** usually used to indicate an electronic storage system with a standard structure that allows for editing, searching, sorting, and reporting
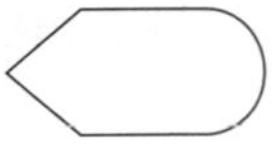	**Display –** often used to represent a real time display or a process step that displays information
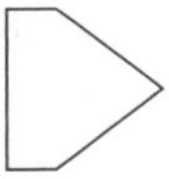	**Off Page Indicator –** process continues off page; used when flowchart needs to extend over more than one page

FIGURE 3.1 Flowchart Shapes (*continued*)

- *Misunderstandings:* Process steps that some on an improvement team may have thought were being performed or vice versa
- *Loops:* Repetitive steps in the process that require rework or additional non–value added time

The use of a flowchart expedites analysis of these problems and can lead to "aha" moments during team sessions focused on improvement.

Procedure

Flowcharts use standard shapes such as those listed in FIGURE 3.1. Although not *absolutely* necessary, using these shapes makes interpretation of the flowchart easier for those who have experience using this tool.

The flowchart process may be done by an individual or with a team. Here are the steps to creating a basic flowchart using a team:

1. Gather the needed materials, such as sticky notes or cards, a large piece of flip chart paper or an empty area of wall, and marking pens.
2. Define the process to be diagrammed and put the title on the worksheet.
3. Discuss and decide on the boundaries of your process:
   a. Where, when, why, and how does the process start? Who initiates the process?
   b. Where, when, why, and how does the process end? Who stops the process? What conditions stop the process?
   c. What level of detail needs to be included in the diagram?
4. Brainstorm the steps in the process:
   a. Write each activity, event, or step on one of the sticky notes or cards. Do not be concerned about the order of the steps at this stage.
   b. Different colors of sticky notes may be used to designate subprocesses or phases of the process.
5. Arrange the activities/events/steps in the correct sequence, and once consensus has been reached in the group on the sequence, connect the shapes with arrows.
6. Share the flowchart with others who either use the process or are customers of the process (e.g., coworkers, managers, suppliers, and customers). Use their input to revise the flowchart to reflect the process accurately.

Although programs like Microsoft Visio or SmartDraw can expedite creation of the final flowchart, the brainstorming process outlined above generally is more effective for developing the chart than trying to use these programs. An example of a computer-generated flowchart is shown in FIGURE 3.2.

Tips and Tricks

- Be sure to clearly label the flowchart with a title identifying the process that it illustrates (e.g., "patient registration process"). Labels help people using the charts to quickly put it into context.
- Plainly indicate the starting and ending points of the process by using the standard terminator symbols. This approach ensures that process boundaries are clear.
- Keep the direction of flow moving from top to bottom and left to right. Because flow reversals are rare in most processes, putting such a reversal in the diagram could be misleading, or at least confusing.
- Be consistent in level of detail of process steps. Avoid providing excessive details in one part of the diagram and insufficient detail in other parts. If one step or task needs to be displayed in more detail, then a separate chart should be used to illustrate the subprocess. Some computer programs allow creating a hyperlink between process points to another flowchart to allow quick access to details.

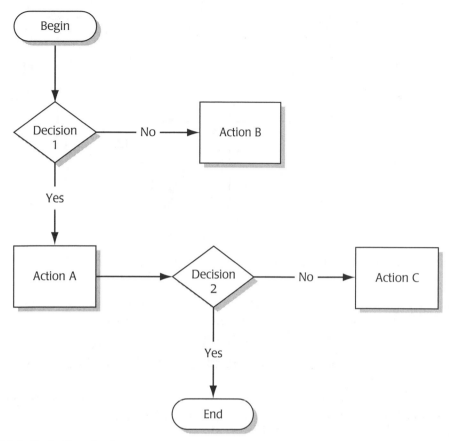

FIGURE 3.2 Basic Flowchart

- In a well-designed flowchart, arrows and connectors should not cross each other. By rearranging a chart you can usually get rid of crossed lines. If two lines must cross, use a "bridge" (also known as a "line hop") to show that the lines do not intersect (see FIGURE 3.3).
- Label flowchart components (e.g., apply active verbs to activity steps and questions for decision steps). Ensure that outcomes from a decision diamond answer the question in the diamond.
- Flowcharts can be created either by a process expert or by a team of people who participate in the process. Some teams even include customers of the process to gain insight into the use of outputs to better refine the work system.
- Ensure that all key people involved with the process are on the team, including suppliers, customers, and supervisors. If these stakeholders cannot attend meetings to create the flowchart, involve them through interviews before the sessions and show them the evolving flowchart between meetings for their feedback.

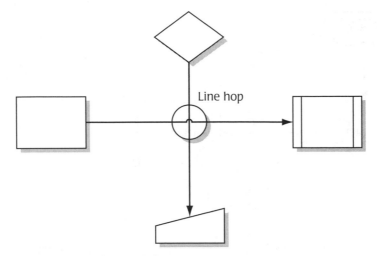

FIGURE 3.3 Bridged Connector ("line hop")

- When teams have trouble creating a flowchart, the issue often relates to ambiguities in the design and execution of the underlying policies and/or procedures. A few tricks might help resolve the situation:
  - Use the brainstorming techniques in Chapter 2 to refine the process and clear any ambiguities.
  - Break the process down into smaller parts to focus on areas that are nebulous. Smaller "bites" at the process may help clarify the issues.
  - Collect more data to elucidate the problem areas.
  - Expand the team to include experts in the areas of the process that are unclear.
- People who actually perform the process should create the flowchart as a way of ensuring the chart is correct. Although others may be more facile with the diagram creation software, the overarching goal should be to have a flowchart that reflects the actual process.

Basic flowcharts comprise the basis for much of what quality professionals do to analyze and improve processes. A little experience using programs like Visio or SmartDraw can be leveraged to produce diagrams that convey a wealth of information. In addition to basic flowcharts, though, a few other flowcharts can help with analysis of processes, identify waste, and produce the information needed to achieve improved performance.

PERT Charts (Network Diagrams)

Program evaluation and review technique (PERT) is an approach to process analysis that identifies not just the steps in the process, but also the time required to complete each task, slack times, and minimum and maximum times for process completion.

The approach was developed by Booz Allen Hamilton, Inc. in 1958 under contract to the U.S. Navy as part of the Polaris submarine ballistic missile project and was so successful in coordinating that project that some U.S. government contracts require that PERT be used as part of management supervision. PERT charts are often called network diagrams because they are used to describe networks of tasks that are related.

PERT was developed primarily to organize planning and scheduling of complex projects. The approach addresses uncertainty by including slack times in the analysis to account for process variation as well as steps in which times are unmeasured. One important feature of the PERT chart is identification of the "critical path," which connotes the essential steps in the process leading from inputs to outputs. Although PERT was originally intended for very large scale, complex projects, it is also a powerful tool to analyze processes for slack time and non–value added work.

Although there are several templates for the PERT chart, one that provides the greatest information in each cell is shown in TABLE 3.1. An example PERT cell with times in each section of the cell is demonstrated in TABLE 3.2. The definition of each of the components and relationships between the various times are as follows:

1. *Earliest start*: The earliest time that the process step can start. If time is being measured in "elapsed time," then this value is zero (0:00).
2. *Duration*: The most efficient or shortest time for this step in the process.
3. *Earliest finish*: The earliest time that this step in the process can end. It is calculated as:

$$\text{Earliest finish} = \text{earliest start} + \text{duration}$$

4. *Latest start*: The latest time that the process step can start.
5. *Slack time:* The time that is consumed by non–value added work, such as waiting, transit time, wasted motion, and rework.

Table 3.1	PERT Chart Cell	
Early Start	Duration	Early Finish
	Task Name	
Late Start	Slack	Late Finish

Table 3.2	PERT Chart Cell with Example Times	
0:00	1:45	1:45
	Task 1 in Sequence	
2:00	1:15	5:00

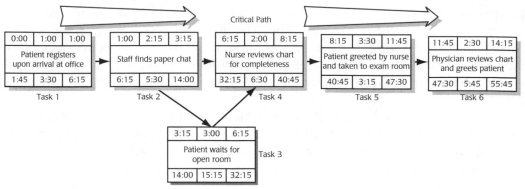

Critical Path

Task 1 — Patient registers upon arrival at office: 0:00 | 1:00 | 1:00 / 1:45 | 3:30 | 6:15

Task 2 — Staff finds paper chat: 1:00 | 2:15 | 3:15 / 6:15 | 5:30 | 14:00

Task 4 — Nurse reviews chart for completeness: 6:15 | 2:00 | 8:15 / 32:15 | 6:30 | 40:45

Task 5 — Patient greeted by nurse and taken to exam room: 8:15 | 3:30 | 11:45 / 40:45 | 3:15 | 47:30

Task 6 — Physician reviews chart and greets patient: 11:45 | 2:30 | 14:15 / 47:30 | 5:45 | 55:45

Task 3 — Patient waits for open room: 3:15 | 3:00 | 6:15 / 14:00 | 15:15 | 32:15

FIGURE 3.4 **Example PERT Chart**

6. *Latest finish*: The latest time that this step in the process can end, calculated according to the equation:

$$\text{Latest finish} = \text{latest start} + \text{duration} + \text{slack time}$$

This configuration of a PERT chart cell provides a complete picture of the important parameters of the PERT analysis. A simple but complete example of a PERT chart is shown in FIGURE 3.4. Note that the critical path (i.e., the longest path for the process that must be completed to move from inputs to outputs) is denoted by the steps along the top of the chart. Steps that are not critical to completion of the process are placed on a different level from the critical path.

When To Use
The PERT chart can be applied in a number of situations, but the following conditions usually apply:

- There is a need for scheduling and monitoring tasks within a complex project or process with interrelated tasks and resources, and
- When the steps, sequence, and timing of the project or process are known, and
- When time for the process is a critical factor for the project and customer satisfaction, with serious consequences for lateness or advantages for improved throughput.

PERT charts can help teams define the critical path and find ways of improving a process or project by reducing slack time and removing non–value added steps.

Procedure

1. Gather the needed materials, such as sticky notes or cards, marking pens, large writing surface (flip chart pages or a large section of a wall). Create the PERT cell diagram on the sticky notes or cards to enter the PERT statistics. Unlike creation of the basic flowchart, in some cases it might be easier to perform this exercise using a computer program like Visio or SmartDraw with a projector to

create the PERT chart electronically. One person can manipulate the shapes and enter data, while the remainder of the team provides input into the process.

2. List all the necessary tasks in the project or process on the sticky notes or cards, much like the basic flowchart.
3. Determine the correct sequence of the tasks by asking three questions for each cell:
   a. Which task(s) must happen before this one can begin?
   b. Which task(s) can be done at the same time as this one?
   c. Which task(s) should happen immediately after this one?
4. Create a diagram of the network of tasks by arranging the PERT cells in sequence on a large piece of paper or using a software program like Microsoft Visio. The process should flow from left to right, and concurrent tasks should be aligned vertically, as in FIGURE 3.4. Some space should be left between the cells for insertion of other subtasks if the need arises, and the computer software makes this task very easy.
5. Determine the PERT times for each cell and fill in the boxes in the cells. Use the equations for the times to calculate start and stop times for each cell and to compute the critical path time.

If the exercise is performed using note cards or sticky notes, then the information can be entered into the PERT template in the diagram program.

Tips and Tricks

- As with other such exercises, this approach is most effective if it includes stakeholders of the process or project, including customers, managers, staff members, and suppliers.
- If the manual approach is used, it may be useful to create a table with four columns to organize the sequence of tasks with one column each for prior tasks, this task, simultaneous tasks, and following tasks. An example of a table based on the PERT chart in FIGURE 3.4 is shown in TABLE 3.3.

Table 3.3	PERT Sequencing Table for PERT Chart in Figure 3.4		
This Task	Prior Tasks	Simultaneous Tasks	Following Tasks
1	0	0	2, 3, 4, 5, 6
2	1	3	4, 5, 6
3	1	2, 4	5, 6
4	1, 2	3	5, 6
5	1, 2, 3, 4	0	6
6	1, 2, 3, 4, 5	0	0

- Although diagram-producing software like Microsoft Visio and SmartDraw is often used to create PERT charts, these programs require the chart designer to calculate the time parameters. Programs like Microsoft Project have templates that calculate times while producing the PERT chart.
- Data for the PERT cells can come from a number of sources:
  - Estimates by team members of each of the time parameters
  - Short-term time-motion studies to find each of the parameters within experimental error
  - Determination of times from benchmarked processes in other organizations

- When PERT is used to plan a project, the time frame is often days or months. When making such a plan, ensure that the times account for time off, such as weekends, holidays, and vacations. Allocation of slack time should try to take into consideration such imponderables as support system downtime, unexpected iterations of processes to pilot certain parts of the project, and overhead time for meetings and interim report creation.
- Ensure that any constraints or assumptions are documented. For example, if a critical element of the process must be fabricated before use, the process might be constrained by on time delivery of the element.
- The goal of a PERT analysis is to identify opportunities for streamlining the process. These potential opportunities are usually found in three places:
  - The largest slack times in the process steps that can be reduced by such interventions as reducing waiting, putting process stations closer together to reduce transit time, etc.
  - Redundant or sequential tasks that can be either eliminated or made simultaneous with other steps.
  - Duration times that are excessive and may be reduced by improving efficiency or adding resources to a step.

PERT charts were originally designed to organize and optimize projects during the planning phase, but they are also indispensable for finding process inefficiencies and opportunities for streamlining systems.

Deployment Flowcharts

A deployment flowchart, sometimes referred to as a cross-functional flowchart, is a process mapping tool used to articulate the steps and stakeholders of a given process. Deployment flowcharts consist of a sequence of activity steps arranged in a way that allows assignment to specific individuals or groups accountable for making the step happen. Each participant in the process is displayed on the process map, which looks similar to the basic flowchart in use of symbols and connectors, but process steps assigned to that individual are diagrammed below that individual's name on the chart. In some ways a deployment flowchart is a cross between a flowchart and a matrix.

Because deployment flowcharts highlight the relationships between stakeholders in addition to the process flow, they are especially useful in highlighting areas of inefficiency, duplication, or unnecessary processing. This type of flowchart is frequently helpful as organizations implement six sigma programs, because they help narrow down the areas for improving productivity and reducing waste due to dysfunctional interfaces between "participants" that cause delays and other associated issues. As with the other types of flowcharts, software programs like Microsoft Visio and SmartDraw make the creation of these diagrams relatively painless.

As with other process mapping approaches, deployment flowcharts require detail, but the detail is focused on assignment of tasks and accountability as well as on process sequencing. Because of the importance of assigning responsibility, care must be taken to ensure that the correct stakeholder is attributed to the correct step of the process. Additionally, these diagrams can appear more complex to the unfamiliar eye, and so additional explanation is often included to clarify any ambiguities, especially where a flow is unclear or many stakeholders are assigned to a specific step. An example deployment flowchart is shown as FIGURE 3.5. The procedure described in the diagram

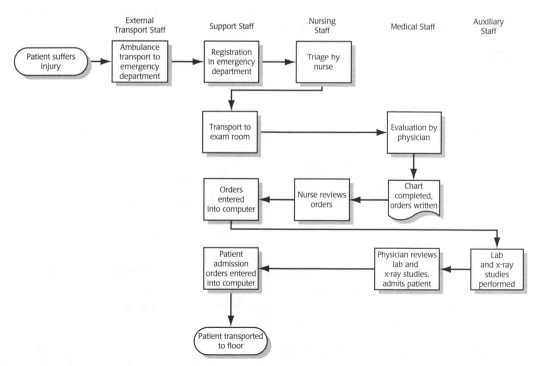

FIGURE 3.5 Deployment Flowchart

is that of a person being injured through admission to the hospital. The process includes the following steps:

1. Person is injured outside the hospital.
2. Ambulance transporters bring the patient to the hospital.
3. The patient is triaged by the nursing staff.
4. Following triage, the support staff transfers the patient to an exam room.
5. Once in the exam room, the patient is examined by the physician.
6. The physician completes her entry into the chart and writes orders.
7. The nurse reviews the orders to determine if there are any immediate issues to be managed.
8. The orders are entered into the computer by the support staff.
9. Lab and x-ray studies are performed by the appropriate auxiliary staff members.
10. Lab and x-ray results are reviewed by the physician and an admission order is issued.
11. Admission orders are entered into the computer system by support staff.
12. The support staff transports the patient to the hospital ward.

The flowchart is embellished a bit with symbols for each of the staff categories, but the basic format of the chart is clearly a cross between a matrix (table) of staffing and the flowchart to demonstrate the process path.

Procedure

The basic steps in creating a deployment flowchart are designing a basic flowchart and assigning responsibility to each step in the process. The procedure for making a deployment flow diagram is as follows:

1. Define the steps in the process in the same way as for the basic flowchart. It is sometimes helpful to construct a table such as that in TABLE 3.4, which was constructed for the process displayed in FIGURE 3.5.
2. Determine all individuals or groups (e.g., medical staff, nursing staff, etc.) who are responsible for each step in the process, and match the accountabilities with the step in the process.
3. Place the individual or group identifiers across the top of the page on which the flowchart will be placed.
4. Put the tasks related to each individual or group in a column below the appropriate identifier. The tasks should be arranged in sequential order to make creation of the flowchart and connection of the shapes easier.
5. Connect the tasks with arrows indicating the process flow.

Thoughtful arrangement of the tasks on the template makes connection of the shapes easier, and computer programs provide the ability to readily move the shapes to accommodate the connections.

Table 3.4	Deployment Flowchart Worksheet Table	
Step	Description	Accountability
1	Person is injured outside the hospital.	None
2	Ambulance transporters bring the patient to the hospital.	External transport staff
3	The patient is triaged by the nursing staff.	Nursing staff
4	After triage, the support staff transfers the patient to an exam room.	Support staff
5	Once in the exam room, the patient is examined by the physician.	Medical staff
6	The physician completes her entry into the chart and writes orders.	Medical staff
7	The nurse reviews the orders to determine if there are any immediate issues to be managed.	Nursing staff
8	The orders are entered into the computer by the support staff.	Support staff
9	Lab and x-ray studies are performed by the appropriate auxiliary staff members.	Auxiliary services staff
10	Lab and x-ray results are reviewed by the physician and an admission order is issued.	Medical staff
11	Admission orders are entered into the computer system by support staff.	Support staff
12	The support staff transports the patient to the hospital ward.	Support staff

Tips and Tricks

- Deployment flowcharts are sometimes called "swim lane" flowcharts, because they line up resources in the columns of the chart, much like swim lanes.
- Review the flowchart with all stakeholders to ensure that it reflects the correct accountabilities. Remind each stakeholder that the assignment of responsibility on the deployment flowchart entails accountability for that step in the process. Each stakeholder must be aware and willing to accept that accountability.
- After the flowchart has been verified by all stakeholders, it is often useful to perform a walkthrough of the process with one or more of the stakeholders to validate the conclusions made in the diagram.
- In some cases two people or groups may be involved with the same step, as in steps 6 and 7 in TABLE 3.4 (physician writes orders, nurse reviews orders). If the step has not been divided into two parts, changing a single step into two steps, like steps 6 and 7, allows proper assignment of responsibilities.
- The computer programs used for creating these flowcharts allow for color coding. Colors may be useful in identifying responsible individuals and groups. Additionally, if specific individuals are identified in the chart, including pictures of the individuals at the top of the column(s) personalizes the diagram and makes it more appealing.

Deployment flowcharts provide another approach to honing in on opportunities for improvement. By identifying accountabilities for each step in a process, formulating teams for developing interventions can focus on those individuals and groups who can add the most to the improvement process.

Matrices

Matrices present the relationship between groups of information. Depending on how many data sets are to be compared, matrices can be relatively simple (e.g., the L-shaped matrix for relating two groups of data or complex, such as the X-shaped matrix that compares four groups of data). However, the essential matrices are those that compare two or three variables, and those are described in more detail.

The type of matrix with number of variables is shown in TABLE 3.5, which, by the way, is an L-shaped matrix. Several of the figures in this chapter are examples of the most common type of matrix, the L-shaped matrix. The T- and Y-shaped matrices are also discussed in this section.

L-Shaped Matrix

L-matrices are the most commonly used and produce tables of information that relate two variables to each other. TABLE 3.6 shows a matrix of this type that relates managed care customers with the type of plan they have chosen for their employees. The relationship between company and type of plan is indicated by an X in the appropriate cell of the table.

When To Use

L-matrices are used when relating two parameters to each other. The relationship can be either an association, as in TABLE 3.6, or numeric, as in TABLE 3.7, which relates the same two parameters in TABLE 3.6 but uses the number of enrollees in each type of plan. Clearly, relationships are readily apparent using this type of matrix.

The elements being compared in a matrix may be in the form of information, concepts, conditions, activities, or other elements like people, equipment, tools, and materials. The matrix diagram can be used in almost all types of decision making that

Table 3.5	Matrix Selection Based on Numbers of Variables	
Matrix	Number of Groups	Comparison Type
L-shaped	2	Group 1 to Group 2
T-shaped	3	Group 1 to Group 2, and Group 2 to Group 3, but NOT Group 1 to Group 3
Y-shaped	3	Group 1 to Group 2, and Group 2 to Group 3, and Group 1 to Group 3

Table 3.6	Example of L-Matrix for Managed Care Plan Assignment			
Company	HMO 1	HMO 2	PPO 1	PPO 2
XYZ Corp.	X		X	X
Bob's Manufacturing	X	X		X
Mary's Diner	X		X	X
International Info, Corp.		X	X	
Areawide Banking, Inc.	X	X	X	X
HMO, health maintenance organization; PPO, preferred provider organization				

Table 3.7	Example of L-Matrix with Numeric Association			
Company	HMO 1	HMO 2	PPO 1	PPO 2
XYZ Corp.	522		283	191
Bob's Manufacturing	15	28		67
Mary's Diner	3		8	15
International Info, Corp.		294	124	
Areawide Banking, Inc.	108	112	119	94
HMO, health maintenance organization; PPO, preferred provider organization				

involve multiple alternatives, such as multiple clinical conditions in a patient population, selection among several marketing alternatives for a new service line, and evaluation of a capital purchase for a new piece of equipment.

Procedure

1. Select two data sets that have a relationship and determine if the matrix will demonstrate an association (as in TABLE 3.6) or a numeric relationship (as in TABLE 3.7).
2. Choose one data group to be in the rows and one to be in the columns.
3. Complete the matrix with the information relating the two parameters.

L-matrices are relatively easy to create but can provide a wealth of information about a relationship between two variables. Additionally, these matrices serve as the starting point for graphic representation of the data as well as some types of statistical analyses.

Tips and Tricks

- Use of color, bolded, or italic text can draw attention to specific relationships in the matrix. This approach is often used in "dashboards" like that shown in

Table 3.8	Example Dashboard	Rates				
Metric		Q1	Q2	Q3	Q4	Target
Beta-blocker utilization		*45%*	*62%*	*75%*	80%	80%
ACE inhibitors for CHF		**81%**	*79%*	*69%*	*72%*	80%
Antibiotics for pneumonia		*29%*	*34%*	*28%*	*41%*	60%
Flu vaccine rates		*80%*	*79%*	*84%*	**89%**	85%

Numbers in bold exceed the target, whereas numbers in italic are below the target. ACE, angiotensin-converting enzyme; CHF, congestive heart failure

Table 3.9	T-Matrix for Adult and Pediatric Data					
	Antibiotics for pneumonia	38%	41%	32%	46%	50%
Pediatrics	Influenza vaccination	75%	72%	81%	79%	80%
	Recommended preventive visits	78%	74%	79%	84%	85%
	Quarter	Q1	Q2	Q3	Q4	Target
	Antibiotics for pneumonia	53%	48%	64%	72%	80%
Adult	Influenza vaccination	90%	81%	74%	68%	90%
	Recommended preventive visits	51%	57%	43%	56%	50%

TABLE 3.8, which has high and low values represented as bold or italic. Commonly used dashboards use red, yellow, and green colors to indicate out of spec, borderline, and within specification values in the table. These dashboards are often called "Christmas tree tables."

- Many different applications of the L-matrix have specialized purposes and names (e.g., the decision matrix, which places a number of values in the matrix with weights for each one that provides an index value that is easily determined using mathematical formulas). These matrices provide a quick and complete picture of a data set to facilitate a decision.

T-Matrix

Another variant of the matrix tool is the T-matrix, which compares two groups of variables with one other data set (see TABLE 3.9). Creation of the T-matrix follows the same procedure as for the L-matrix, except that another set of data is added to the "top" of the L-matrix. As seen in TABLE 3.9, adult and pediatric measures are compared in the same table but are separated so that they are clearly differentiated for the reviewer. The ability to make rapid comparisons of data sets that are similar, but not quite the same, makes the T-matrix particularly useful.

Table 3.10	Decision Matrix				
Parameter	Market Penetration	Population Of Women	Cost Of Implementation	Staff Capability	
Weight	15%	40%	30%	15%	
Clinic	Weighted Scores				Total Score
1	0.75	0.4	0.9	0.45	2.50
2	0.6	2	0.6	0.6	3.80
3	0.15	0.4	1.2	0.15	1.90
4	0.45	0.4	1.5	0.45	2.80
5	0.15	0.8	1.2	0.45	2.60
6	0.15	0.8	1.5	0.15	2.60

Decision Matrix

As mentioned previously, the decision matrix is a variant of the L-matrix that helps support decisions where several complex alternatives exist. The decision matrix uses the L-matrix format, but it includes rows for weights so that several options may be evaluated simultaneously using weights established in a number of ways. TABLE 3.10 provides an example of a decision matrix. EXHIBIT 3.1 presents a scenario for TABLE 3.10.

Exhibit 3.1   Application of a Decision Matrix

The corporate board plans to implement a new service that will provide customized women's services at some of the organization's sites, and a decision must be made regarding which sites to include in the project. Six of the organization's outpatient facilities indicated an interest in the project, and each one was evaluated on the following characteristics:

- Market penetration
- Population of women in the area
- Cost of implementation of the project
- Existing staff capability for the project (to reduce the need to hire new staff)

A consultant was asked to gather data for each of these four parameters, and senior staff then reviewed the data and scored each facility on its ability to meet the criteria. The board believed that the selected factors were not equally important in influencing a decision, and so weights were assigned to each of the parameters, as indicated in Table 3.10. The scores were averaged for each candidate facility and then each score was multiplied by the appropriate weight to create the scores in each cell of the table. The scores were totaled by facility, then the scores were sorted in descending order as shown in Table 3.11, and the four top scoring facilities were selected.

Table 3.11	Decision Tree Results in Sorted Order
Clinic	Score
2	3.80
4	2.80
5	2.60
6	2.60
1	2.50
3	1.90

When To Use

As shown in TABLES 3.10 and 3.11, the decision matrix can help provide a more quantitative approach to arriving at a conclusion when the choices may be complex. As a decision support tool, this matrix can help teams make decisions more rationally. Specifically, the matrix is used:

- During quality planning activities to select product or service features and goals,
- To develop process steps and weigh alternatives,
- To select a project during the quality planning phase, or
- To evaluate alternative solutions to problems or designing remedies.

Procedure

1. Identify alternatives: Depending on the team's needs in the usage categories above, alternatives can be product or service features, process steps, projects, or potential solutions (as in EXHIBIT 3.1). These alternatives comprise the columns of the matrix.
2. Design scoring system: Each alternative must be scored so that the decision criteria can be assessed quantitatively. Many rating systems are based on Likert scales (e.g., 1 to 5 for least to most), and it is important to select the scale so that people doing scoring can appropriately differentiate between subtle degrees of difference in each alternative. In most cases a description of each of the scoring levels is helpful in ensuring that scorers understand the various levels on the scale as they score the alternatives.
3. Identify decision and selection criteria: Key criteria become the rows of the matrix and may come from brainstorming or from criteria established by customer demand or senior management. Everyone involved in the project must have a clear understanding of what the criteria mean. It is also a generally good practice to ensure that the criteria are written so that a high score for each criterion represents a favorable result and a low score represents an unfavorable result. The criteria become the rows of the matrix. In the case of EXHIBIT 3.1,

the decision criteria were represented by the six clinics being screened for the new service.

4. Assign weights: The greatest value of the decision matrix is the ability to weight the alternatives to reflect the relative importance of each alternative. In EXHIBIT 3.1 the weights assigned to each of the alternatives (market penetration 15%, population of women 40%, cost of implementation 30%, staff capability 15%) were assigned by the board of directors working with senior management. Weights may be provided from many different sources but are often determined by senior leaders. However, weights may also be assigned based on regulatory factors (e.g., satisfaction of Joint Commission or National Committee on Quality Assurance standards) or constrained by legal issues.

5. Rate the alternatives: This part of the process may be done in a variety of ways, from having senior managers rate the various alternatives for each of the criteria selections to recruiting outside experts to perform the ratings. For example, in our scenario staff may have had senior managers perform the ratings but also have included the consultant and experts in women's services from other organizations. Having a diverse group performing ratings helps in a number of ways. First, multiple opinions are usually valuable to gain the best possible decision. Second, larger numbers of ratings tend to remove some of the bias factor that may exist if only one group is involved in the ratings. Finally, more ratings make the analysis more valid by providing more data for analysis and remove any statistical discrepancies that occur because of small numbers. After the data are gathered, in most cases, the data for each alternative and criterion combination are averaged and used for the final calculations.

6. Apply the weights to the scores: Once the individual scores for each alternative are collected, they are averaged and multiplied by the weights determined in step 4 to produce the decision matrix like that shown in TABLE 3.10. Each cell in the matrix contains the average score for each alternative and criterion combination multiplied by the corresponding weight (indicated in the row labeled "Weight").

7. Total the scores: Each criterion row is then totaled to arrive at the overall score for that criterion based on all the alternatives. The final column in TABLE 3.10 provides the totals for all of the criteria (in this case clinics), and the data can then be presented to the team and senior managers in a format as in TABLE 3.11, which sorts the data in descending fashion and makes it easier to interpret.

Tips and Tricks

- In some cases, presenting the entire weighted decision matrix is valuable, because the scores for each of the alternatives may be of interest to decision makers. In many cases a final report to senior managers or the board may include a description of the approach to the analysis to ensure the process was as rigorous as possible.

- Decision matrices have a number of uses, but one caveat is important: Data are often based on opinion surveys and could be biased based on selection of the surveyed group. Thus a more diverse survey group can add to the value of the analysis by reducing this selection bias.
- The decisions supported by this approach should be manageable by the group, but in those cases where the decision is quite broad, it sometimes helps to break the larger group into subgroups to deal with specific aspects of an issue. For example, in EXHIBIT 3.1 the group may have been subdivided with each subgroup reviewing a single clinic or, conversely, subdivided so that each subgroup deals with a single alternative (e.g., the population of women). The subgroups then provide a report or presentation to the assembled group to help better understand the specifics of each category or alternative.

Four-Quadrant Matrices

Some matrices are presented as four quadrants, with each quadrant representing a category or combination of variables. A classic example of this type of matrix is represented by the Boston Consulting Group matrix shown in FIGURE 3.6. This four-quadrant matrix is intended to describe product or service lines in an organization

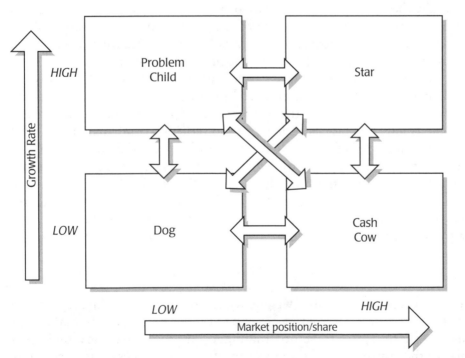

FIGURE 3.6 BCG Matrix

in a visually appealing and easily understandable format. Each of the four quadrants has a definition:

- *Star*: A most desirable situation in which the product or service has a high market share and prospects for growth. Usually, these services have good cash flow but often require more capital to sustain, so the margin may not be the highest of the four categories. Just like in Hollywood, though, stars represent a small number of the panoply of actors. The problem child described below is often nurtured to become a star.
- *Cash cow*: The next most desirable condition where the product or service has a high market share and/or excellent cash flow; these products often are late in their life cycles (i.e., they are about ready to become obsolete), but they still command an excellent market share and excellent income. Cash cows are "milked" for as long as possible but usually require relatively little capital investment to sustain. Stars often become cash cows near the end of their business lives.
- *Problem child*: These services or products are on the edge between becoming a dog or a star. In many cases these are services that have shown promise but have a number of difficulties in execution or uncontrolled costs. Managers (like parents) usually spend an inordinate amount of time with their problem children, and proper attention often can develop a problem child into a star.
- *Dog*: Although most people are dog lovers, this category represents the least desirable situation. Dogs are those services or products that have little or no prospect of ever becoming a star or a cash cow and typically are eliminated from the product mix offered by the company. Like it or not, some problem children morph into dogs rather than stars, and business acumen helps to determine which direction the problem child is taking.

The Boston Consulting Group matrix is an example of a diagram that explains a complex analysis in a relatively straightforward (and rather entertaining) manner. Any combination of variables can be put into this format to make a relationship clearer.

When To Use

Four quadrant matrices are used in a number of situations:

- To focus attention on a particular relationship between two variables in a way that illustrates the association graphically
- To represent data in a manner that clarifies positions of specific variables to some standard or benchmark

Procedure

1. Choose two variables to compare that have some relationship to each other.
2. Starting with a table (L-matrix), enter the data into two columns.

Table 3.12	Table of Data for Bubble Chart in Figure 3.7		
	Staff	Customer	Effect Magnitude
Service 1	−20	−10	200
Service 2	−30	6.5	195
Service 3	7	8	56
Service 4	16	−2	32
Service 5	4	−20	80
Service 6	18	9	162
Service 7	−5	14	70
Service 8	6	−9	54

3. Choose a graph type that allows all four quadrants to be shown (i.e., that can take negative numbers for both *x* and *y* values).
4. The bubble graph function in Microsoft Excel is useful for this purpose. The bubble graph requires three parameters, however, and so for a matrix like this, a third column must be added to determine the size of the bubble. TABLE 3.12 shows the table used to create the matrix in FIGURE 3.7, which demonstrates the need for the third variable to create the bubble graph. The last column in the table represents the "size" of the bubble. In this particular situation the effect magnitude column was calculated as the absolute value of the product of the staff and customer scores.
5. In many cases it is helpful to label the axes with the appropriate levels of the parameters (e.g., "Low" and "High" in FIGURE 3.7) so that the reader knows how to interpret the various positions on the matrix.

Tips and Tricks

- Interpretation of the four-quadrant matrix is pretty straightforward with a little practice and familiarity. Each quadrant represents a combination of the two variables. In FIGURE 3.7 there are four combinations:
  ○ Low staff/low customer (lower left quadrant): The service has low value for both customers and staff.
  ○ Low staff/high customer (upper left quadrant): The service is valued low by staff but high by customers.
  ○ High staff/low customer (lower right quadrant): The service is valued highly by staff but low by customers.
  ○ High staff/high customer (upper right quadrant): Both staff and customers value the service highly.

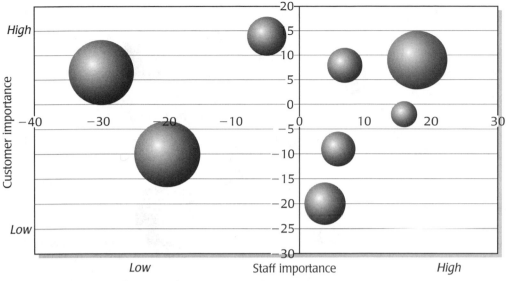

FIGURE 3.7 Four Quadrant Matrix–Importance/Importance

- Several possible combinations of variables can be used to create one of these matrices. For example, the graph in FIGURE 3.7 is termed an "Importance/Importance" matrix, because an importance metric is on each axis. Another example is the "Importance/ Performance" matrix, as shown in FIGURE 3.8, which compares an importance factor (e.g., how important a product or service is to staff) with performance on delivering that product or service to the customer using satisfaction data.

Decision Trees

A decision tree, sometimes also called a "tree diagram," uses a graphic representation to model a set of criteria leading to a decision or the consequences of a specific decision. Decision trees can incorporate probabilities in each branch to help establish the likelihood for that particular decision. By including probabilities, the decision tree can be used to calculate conditional probabilities for each branch (i.e., the probability that given the preceding conditions in the tree, the indicated node will occur). This approach has a number of advantages in a decision support scenario:

- *Simple to understand and interpret*: The decision tree is generally easy to understand and explain. Generally, users can understand the flow of the decision support model after a relatively short discussion.
- *Can be used when only expert opinion is available*: Many quality improvement activities rely on data, and even the decision tree benefits from data; however, decision trees can be created by experts who have in-depth understanding of a situation and preferred outcomes.

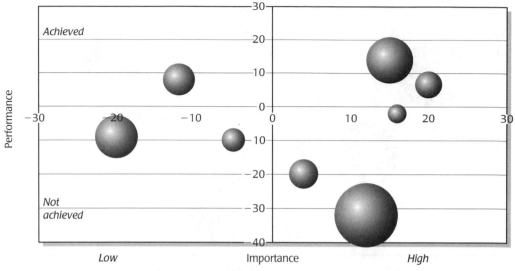

FIGURE 3.8 Importance/Performance Matrix

When To Use

- To identify the strategy most likely to reach a goal
- As a graphic approach for calculating and displaying conditional probabilities
- As a predictive model for data mining (i.e., a mapping from observations about an item to conclusions about its target level or value)

Procedure

EXHIBIT 3.2 is used to create a decision tree.

Decision tree construction uses three types of nodes as shown in FIGURE 3.9. The process for creating a decision tree is as follows:

1. Identify the objective of the decision-making process.

    a. Optimization of a favorable outcome like profit, sales, satisfaction, or throughput, or

    b. Elimination of a problem (e.g., defects, excess time, or waste)

2. Identify constraints on the decision-making process: Constraints may become additional subobjectives and could prevent the goal from being accomplished at the expense of other goals. For example, an objective to increase patient volume could be achieved at the expense of short-term margins because of lag in payments of insurers' bills unless some constraints are used, such as phasing in marketing programs to cause incremental increases in patient visits.

Use of a Decision Tree

Tony, the COO of the Super Docs Health System, is trying to improve revenues and profits by either increasing radiology services or laboratory tests. The staff has done a great job of identifying the effect on net profits of a number of activities, leading to increases in volume for each of the service lines. The outcomes table shown in Table 3.13 associates activities and events with outcomes measured in relative increases in expected profits based on increased revenue. Table 3.13 was converted into the decision tree shown in Figure 3.10 to provide senior management with a rapid method of identifying the various alternatives and their associated outcomes. From the decision tree the board could prioritize the direction of the initiative to the following combinations in descending order, A1/E1, A3/E2, and A2/E1, which translates to increasing patient volume and prices, increasing radiology volume and decreasing prices for that service, and increasing laboratory volume and increasing prices for that service line. Because the first combination is obvious, the other two alternatives were chosen as a method of achieving the goal of increased profits.

Node	Shape
Decision	Square
Chance	Circle
End	Triangle

FIGURE 3.9 Decision Tree Shapes

3. List the set of possible actions to be considered: These actions become the decision nodes in the tree. For example, if increases in clinical productivity are targeted, then improved workflows and work practices may become potential actions. The list of options should be relatively short, usually two to four actions, to minimize the complexity of the final diagram. The group may start with a longer list and then use some of the list reduction techniques described earlier to shorten the list to a manageable few.

4. List possible events that may follow each action: Try to include all possible events for each action, but avoid extremely low probability events. Events may be dependent or independent:

    a. Dependent events are a direct consequence of an individual action and are different for each action. For example, the action of increasing laboratory test volume time may cause an increase in error rates.

    b. Independent events do not depend on the actions and are just as likely to happen regardless of which action is chosen. For example, the output of the radiology department is not affected by an increase in volume in the lab but it is certainly reflected in overall volume and cash flow.

5. Create an outcome table: For each action in step 3 and event in step 4, determine a value describing the value that will occur with this combination of action and event. The resulting outcome table will appear as in TABLE 3.13.

    a. The value or metric used in the outcome table must be the same for each action and event combination related to the original objective.

    b. The measure can be any value but is most often a financial metric or a measure based on time or productivity.

    c. The figure often also includes the cost of each action in this figure rather than just the value of the return.

6. Draw the decision tree: Using the outcome table in TABLE 3.13, the decision tree in FIGURE 3.10 can be created. Note the use of the three types of shapes: a square for the decision, circles for each chance or opportunity (activity), and triangles for each outcome. The shapes are connected with arrows to show the flow of the decision process. Actions and events may either be written in full or as codes from the outcome table.

7. Use the decision tree to prioritize the choices: As in EXHIBIT 3.2, use the decision tree to determine the best actions by using a defined approach that takes into account the expected outcomes for each activity and subsequent events. It can be very difficult and costly to determine the exact financial outcome data, and so decisions may be made with less accurate data, making piloting the final selected decisions important to ensure that the best course(s) of action have been chosen. Thus in EXHIBIT 3.2

Table 3.13	Outcomes Table for Decision Tree		
		Events	
	Actions	E1 Increased Prices	E2 Decreased Prices
A1	Increased patient volume	3.4	1.4
A2	Increased lab volume	2.8	0.9
A3	Increased radiology volume	1.9	2.9

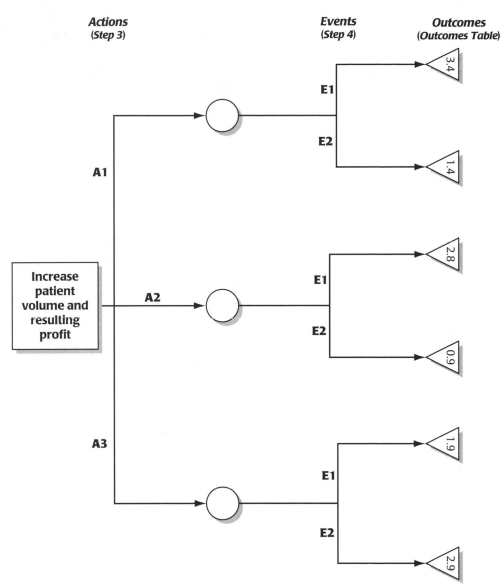

Actions (Step 3) **Events** (Step 4) **Outcomes** (Outcomes Table)

E1 3.4

E2 1.4

A1

Increase patient volume and resulting profit

A2

E1 2.8

E2 0.9

A3

E1 1.9

E2 2.9

FIGURE 3.10 Decision Tree

the organization will want to try each of the top three combinations with some specific patient populations before full-scale implementation.

Tips and Tricks

- Probability figures are usually shown as being a decimal value between 0 (no chance) and 1 (100% probability). Some diagrams, however, may use percentages that may be more familiar to the intended audience. The final probability values

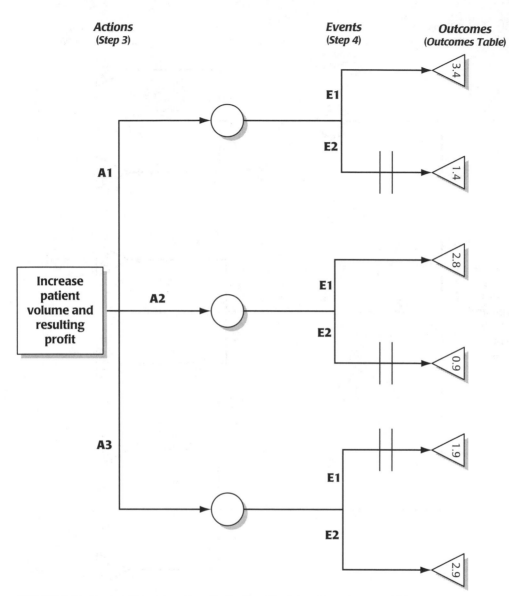

FIGURE 3.11 Revised Decision Tree Reflecting Decision Branches not Taken

may be placed on the decision tree diagram, usually in parentheses below the corresponding event lines.

- Once the decisions are finalized, the decision tree may be altered with double bars across the branches not selected, as shown in FIGURE 3.11. The revised figure may be redistributed to reinforce the decisions that were made while keeping all potential alternatives before decision makers. Note the double lines through the terminal branches that were not selected.

- Multilevel decision trees are extensions of the basic tree that often carry the scenario forward into the future. For example, in EXHIBIT 3.2 a multilevel tree could provide consideration of the consequences of the decisions that have been selected. These additional levels may extend over several pages, if needed. This approach is typically used when each level of decisions leads to further alternatives after the initial decisions have been implemented.

Cause and Effect Diagrams: Ishikawa Diagram

Although decision trees can also be used to relate effects to their underlying causes, other types of charts have been developed to accomplish this task. One of the most popular decision support diagrams was invented by Japanese chemical engineer Kaoru Ishikawa in the 1960s. The format for the Ishikawa diagram looks like a fish skeleton, so it is sometimes called the "fishbone diagram." Ishikawa popularized the graphic as a way of summarizing the various causes related to a specific effect. The causes are generally classified into one of six categories (the "6 M's"):

- Methods
- Machines (equipment)
- Manpower (people)
- Materials
- Measurement
- Milieu (environment)

Each one of the "ribs" in the fishbone diagram relates to one of these six categories, with branches on the rib representing a specific cause. The overall diagram thus provides the ability to identify which categories are major contributors to the effect.

When To Use

- When trying to define underlying causes for a problem
- When summarizing a number of causes for presentation to others, such as managers or senior leaders

Procedure

Although programs like Visio have sophisticated templates for creating fishbone diagrams, the initial phase is usually performed much like a brainstorming session. A group is assembled and ideas are generated using the "5 why's" of a root-cause analysis. That technique directs the brainstorming group to continue asking "why" as causes are being increasingly dissected into more specific issues and branches are added to the diagram. The process follows these steps:

1. Materials should include a flip chart and markers to create the diagram. If the group prefers an electronic session, then a computer running a program like Visio can be used with a projector.

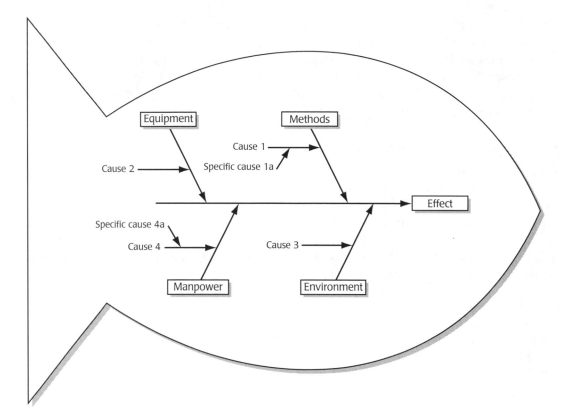

FIGURE 3.12 Ishikawa Diagram

2. Have the group agree on a problem statement, which is the effect, and put it at the center right of the flip chart or whiteboard inside the "effect box" (see FIGURE 3.12).

3. Get the group to brainstorm the major categories of problem causes and connect them via arrows to the main arrow. Because this step sometimes proves difficult, it is often helpful to use generic headings, such as those in FIGURE 3.12.

4. Have the group brainstorm all the possible causes of the problem in each category using the "5 why's." This technique starts by asking "Why does this happen?", and as each idea is given the facilitator writes it as a branch from the appropriate category. Causes can be written in more than one category if applicable.

5. Repeat the "Why does this happen?" question about each cause until all of the subcauses have been identified. In most cases the furthest that the "why" questions go is about five layers, which is the reason the technique is termed the "5 why's." As each subcause is identified, another branch arrow is added to the cause or subcause. The "layers" of branches help identify increasingly detailed issues in the causation of the effect.

6. When the group runs out of ideas, focus attention to places on the chart where ideas are few and ensure that the causation issues are sufficiently granular.
7. Finally, prioritize the categories, causes, and subcauses to begin to identify the sequence in which the issues are addressed.

Tips and Tricks

- As with any brainstorming process, ensure that the entire team understands and agrees on the problem statement before beginning.
- To get as much detail on the diagram as possible, it is necessary to be succinct in describing each cause and subcause.
- If some branches are relatively sparse, they may be "grafted" onto others to make the diagram more concise. Because some causes and subcauses may appear on more than one branch, pruning these sparse branches may allow the causes and subcauses to be addressed on another branch.
- Conversely, if some branches are overcrowded, they may represent more than one category. In those cases the overcrowded branches may be split into new categories. If the branches are overcrowded, then the effect that is being studied may also be too broad and may need to be broken into smaller pieces so that solutions can be manageable. In those cases a brainstorming session might help create a master list of issues that can be reduced to a prioritized few so that a better defined and more workable project can be initiated.

Special Diagrams

Workflow Diagram: Lean Spaghetti Diagram

Analysts have used the workflow diagram (see FIGURE 3.13) for many years to determine the pattern of movement within a process and to identify non–value added movement (a term from lean process management). Also called a spaghetti diagram or string diagram, this tool helps to establish the optimum layout for a work space based on observations of distances traveled by customers (patients), staff, or products like x-rays or lab specimens. Spaghetti diagrams uncover inefficiencies in flow, such as excessive travel between key steps, and provide a view of inadequate layouts so that improvements may be targeted to improving flow.

When To Use

- When designing a new process to set up optimum flow through the process
- When evaluating a process that involves movement of customers, staff, or products
- As a tool to determine non–value added time in a process due to transport or waiting

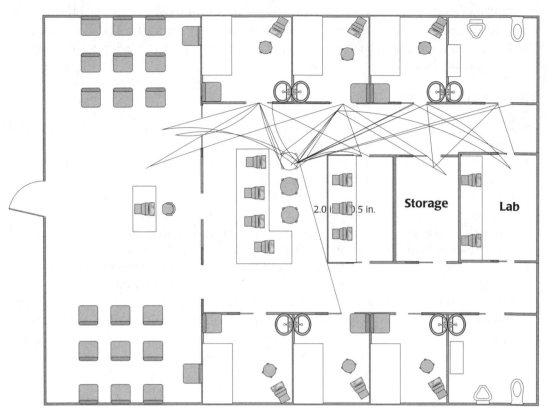

FIGURE 3.13 Workflow (spaghetti) Diagram

Procedure

1. Start with a floor plan of the work space to be used for the plot. Note the time, date, and process being evaluated but not the person being followed to track the process.
2. Explain the mapping process to the affected group and choose a volunteer who will allow observation of his or her workflow during the evaluation process.
3. Follow the individual through the process for several iterations to gain insight into the true process flow. During the observation, lines should be drawn between the various points on the floor plan that track the individual's steps.

   a. If a significant wait occurs, that waiting time should also be noted either in a table or directly on the diagram.

   b. Any unusual movement or nonconforming motions should be noted (e.g., reaching too high, twisting, lifting, etc.).

   c. Note any interruptions to flow, like need for donning a gown and mask or interruptions to attend to other urgent issues. If the trips or movements are not part of the flow, they should be recorded either on the chart or as notes to the chart.

4. Review the diagram with the affected group and determine areas for improving flow by removing redundant steps, rearranging the locations of stopping points in the flow, or automating steps in the process.

An example spaghetti diagram is shown in FIGURE 3.13 for a nurse working on one side of the emergency department's Low Acuity Clinic. The nurse moves frequently from the nursing station to the exam rooms, lab, and storage, with many steps retraced during the course of the observation period. This diagram can serve as a starting point for the team to determine the best approaches to reducing the unnecessary transport times for the nurse's work.

Tips and Tricks

- Creation of the spaghetti diagram occurs during a phase of review called "walking the process," meaning that the person creating the diagram actually walks through the process with one of the people involved in the process. Without this level of engagement, a spaghetti diagram is virtually impossible to create.
- A tablet computer with drawing capabilities is often very helpful in creating a work-flow diagram, because the resulting diagram can be stored in electronic format.
- The layout diagram and lines do not need to be drawn to scale at this stage, because process flow is of greatest importance. If rearrangement of the workplace becomes necessary, then scaled drawings may become important to ensure that everything fits in the new order.
- Remember that rearrangement of the workplace may entail moving equipment to new locations, so features like plumbing and electrical availability may become important when physical moves are considered.

■ Application of Improvement Tools

Root-Cause Analysis (RCA)

RCA is a "post hoc" approach to evaluating a process, that is, it is deployed in response to a problem or error that has occurred. For example, RCA may be used if a patient suffers harm because of a medication error to determine which steps in the medication administration process may have contributed to the error.

RCA assumes that problems are best solved by attempting to correct or eliminate root causes, as opposed to merely addressing the immediately obvious symptoms. By directing initiatives at these underlying issues, the improvement team strives to correct the system or process flow to solve the immediate issue and to prevent future problems. Although the goal of an RCA intervention is to repair all process steps that led to the process error, changes may create other glitches that lead to other errors, requiring more

RCA interventions. This continuous improvement approach works to ensure that the underlying system is reviewed and enhanced regularly to ensure top performance. RCA is based on a number of basic principles of problem analysis:

- Directing improvement efforts at the underlying causes of a process problem is more effective than simply trying to correct the erroneous process output.
- Effective RCA is methodical and reproducible. Following a set procedure for RCA produces the best results.
- Typically, defects and errors have more than one underlying cause (i.e., a defective process rarely has just one problematic process step). For the analysis and resulting interventions to be effective, the RCA must establish all root causes so that effective improvement initiatives may be generated.

Table 3.14	Elements of RCA
RCA Category	Examples
Materials	• Defective raw material • Wrong material for procedure • Lack of material
Machine/equipment	• Incorrect instruments or tools for procedure • Poor equipment maintenance • Poor equipment design • Defective equipment
Environment	• Organized workplace • Orderly workplace • Job design • Layout of workplace • Physical demands • Weather, other natural forces
Management	• Lack of management involvement • Inattention to work task • Hazards not foreseen and removed • Stress • Poor process oversight
Methods/procedures	• Lack of procedure definition • "Workarounds"—practice not following procedure • Poor communication
Work systems	• Lack of training • Lack of employee engagement • Misalignment of incentives • Little or no accountability

Procedure

Although the RCA procedure is designed to uncover the underlying problems that cause a process to malfunction, the overarching goal is to implement corrective action. A list of elements of RCA can be found in TABLE 3.14. The procedure is straightforward and follows many of the same procedures that have been outlined before:

1. Define the problem using the tools defined in the next section and by gathering and analyzing process data.
2. Identify causal relationships associated with the defined problem(s) using the "5 why's."
3. Brainstorm which causes can be removed to prevent recurrence.
4. Create solutions and associated measures to remedy the underlying causes. In some cases performing a pilot test with these solutions and using the measures to evaluate the effects may help determine the priority for implementing each solution. These initiatives can be initially screened using the SMART criteria:

   a. **S**imple: easy to design and put into service
   b. **M**easurable: capable of being measured relatively easily to determine effectiveness
   c. **A**ttainable: achievable by the team and resources available
   d. **R**elevant: directed at the specific problem identified by the team
   e. **T**imely: achievable within the allotted timeframe

5. Determine the sequence of implementation of the solutions, including the time for each improvement step to be applied. In many cases these process repairs can be staged so that cost is minimized and the effect of each solution can be well understood. However, if the process problem has been a sentinel event, such as significant patient harm, then the solutions may be implemented swiftly and simultaneously to reach the optimum solution quickly.
6. Measure the effects of the changes to ensure that the changes have produced the expected results.

RCA Tools

- *5 why's*: A question-asking method used to ascertain the cause-and-effect relationships underlying a particular problem. This technique is based on the assumption that asking "why" up to five times usually gets to the root cause of a problem. For example, for the problem "my refrigerator won't work" the sequence of questions might be:

  ○ *Why isn't the refrigerator working?* Does it have power? Yes
  ○ *Why isn't the refrigerator working, even though it has power?* Is the cooling system broken or leaking? No
  ○ *Why isn't the refrigerator working, even though it has power and the cooling system works?* Is the motor working? No

- ○ *Why isn't the motor working?* Is the inline fuse blown? Yes
- ○ *Replace the fuse: Does the refrigerator work?* HOORAY! It works!

- *Pareto analysis*: A statistical technique used in RCA and other applications to pare down an extensive list of possibilities to those that have the greatest effect on the desired variable based on the Pareto principle, the idea that 80% of an effect is often generated by 20% of the underlying causes. It consists of a formal technique in which each underlying cause is assigned an estimate of its effects on the final outcome, and then the estimates are graphed in sequence until 80% of the effect is determined (see EXAMPLE 2.1 for a simulated Pareto analysis). In most cases these causes comprise about 20% of the total number originally identified, making the list of potential targets more manageable.
- *Fault tree analysis:* A failure analysis in which a system error is analyzed using Boolean (if-then-else) logic to determine the probability of a safety hazard. Fault tree analysis diagrams are commonly used to illustrate events that might lead to a failure, so the failure can be prevented, and are commonly used in the analyze phase of six sigma processes. The analysis begins by defining the top event (or failure), then using event and gate shapes like those in FIGURE 3.14 to illustrate, top-down, the process that might lead to the failure. The diagram becomes a key

Symbol	Interpretation
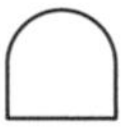	And gate
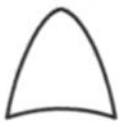	Or gate
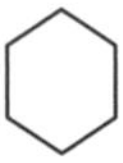	Inhibit gate
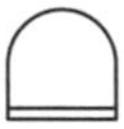	Priority and gate
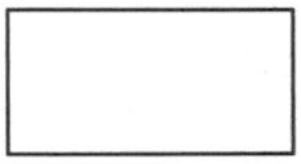	Event
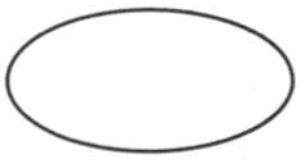	Conditional event

FIGURE 3.14 Fault Tree Analysis Chart Symbols

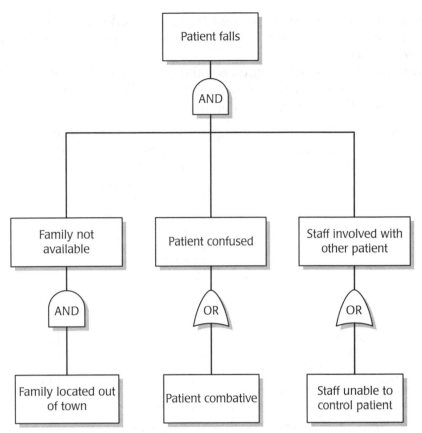

FIGURE 3.15 Fault Tree Analysis—Patient Falls

factor in tracing the fault and eliminating underlying causes, as shown in FIGURE 3.15 in the fault tree diagram for patient falls.

- *Ishikawa diagram*: The cause and effect, or fishbone, diagram discussed earlier and shown in FIGURE 3.12.
- *Barrier analysis*: A barrier in this paradigm is a control measure designed to prevent harm to vulnerable or valuable objects (e.g., patients, staff, organizational reputation, or the wider community); for RCA, the approach determines what barriers or controls should have been in place to prevent the incident or that could be installed to increase system safety. Barrier analysis offers a structured way to visualize the events that led to a process or system failure. Four types of barriers are usually considered as part of the analysis:
  - *Physical barriers:* examples include bar coding for medications, keypad controlled doors for computer security, automated drug dispensing units
  - *Natural barriers:* consisting of barriers of distance, time, or location, like spacing drug doses apart by several hours to prevent an adverse interaction, or surgical time out to ensure that all patient information is correct

- *Human action barriers:* exemplified by a nurse checking the temperature of the water used to bathe a newborn in the nursery, physician using a checklist to prevent a medical error
- *Administrative barriers:* protocols and procedures for hospital processes, supervision requirements for new nurses, the Joint Commission's Ongoing Professional Practice Evaluation program

- *Change Analysis*: This technique compares an error-free instance of a process with the situation in which the process created an error. For example, the RCA team

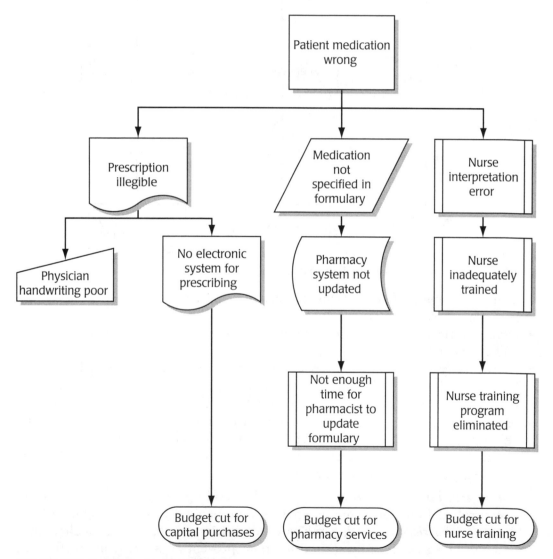

FIGURE 3.16 Causal Factor Tree Analysis

might compare the process used during a surgical procedure that created an error with the process used for the same procedure at a different time that did not produce the error. The differences in the two situations can help identify the changes in the process that led to the nonconforming outcome.

- *Causal factor tree analysis*: Use of a decision tree to track the root causes of an error. FIGURE 3.16 illustrates a causal factor tree developed for a medication error. The tree in the figure could be carried to produce further details using the 5 why's (e.g., "why was the budget reduced?").
- *TapRooT®*: A structured RCA system developed by Mark Paradies and coworkers in Knoxville, Tennessee, TapRooT provides an automated approach to RCA that has become widely used in a number of industries. The approach is based on human performance and equipment failure research and guides users through a computer algorithm to define root causes and develop solutions. More information can be found at http://www.taproot.com.

As should be evident, RCA is not a single, sharply defined strategy but rather a general concept of how to approach errors. RCA has become broadly, but inconsistently, used in health care to determine underlying root causes for medical errors. Unfortunately, the lack of consistent application of the RCA model to investigate underlying causes of errors misses many opportunities to improve the healthcare delivery system.

Failure Mode and Effects Analysis (FMEA)

Because RCA is a reactive approach, a preventive method was developed by safety engineers, called failure mode and effects analysis (FMEA). This technique is sometimes called failure mode effects and criticality analysis (FMECA) when error probabilities are calculated. The Veteran's Health Administration was one of the pioneers in applying FMECA in health care. Many quality professionals think of FMEA as RCA in reverse, that is, as a means of evaluating a process prospectively to prevent errors before they occur. Because healthcare organizations have been traditionally reactive rather than proactive, the Joint Commission began requiring use of FMEA as an accreditation standard (LD 3.20) in 2002. Because of the standard, FMEA has become a widely used tool in health care.

Procedure

As previously noted, RCA and FMEA are closely related, with the main difference being that FMEA is applied *before* a process results in an error. The FMEA procedure is as follows:

1. Choose a target process for FMEA: Typically, healthcare organizations will choose a process for FMEA that is associated with high risk of patient harm, identified by data using some of the decision tools that have been described previously or by brainstorming with process experts. Process selection can often

be accomplished by an executive team using operations and outcome data that can identify the risk level for the process. Tools such as the four-quadrant importance/performance matrix (see FIGURE 3.8), which relates risk (importance) to another parameter, like the number of patients affected (performance) or the expected cost of an error (performance), are useful in helping executives decide which project has highest priority.

2. Assemble the team: Multidisciplinary teams are often best suited to performing FMEAs, because failure modes in a process often cross functional areas. Subject matter experts are often helpful, as is a senior executive who can ensure that the FMEA procedure has necessary resources.

3. Flowchart the process: Using one of the flowchart methods described previously, a flowchart should be constructed that details process steps sufficiently to help the team identify potential failure modes (steps in the process where a failure may occur). The FMEA procedure numbers each step in the process so that a matrix can be created with a listing of the steps, failure modes, and the criticality analysis.

4. Perform a hazard analysis: Once the process steps are numbered, the numbers are transferred to a chart like that in TABLE 3.15.

   a. If the process has several potential failure modes, then each failure mode should be identified by a well-defined numbering system, such as 1a, 1b, 1c, for each failure mode in step 1. The numbering system may be carried to even more detailed levels, if needed (e.g., 1a1, 1a2, 1a3) for failure modes in

Table 3.15	Example of an FMEA Table							
Process Step	Failure Mode	Failure Cause	Failure Effect	Probability of Occurrence (1–10)	Probability of Detection (1–10)	Severity Level (1–10)	Risk Priority Number (RPN)	Corrective Action(s)
1								
2								
3								
4								
...								

Definitions:
Failure Mode: What can go wrong?
Failure Cause: What caused the failure?
Failure Effect: What happened as a result of the failure?
Probability of Occurrence: 1 represents low likelihood of occurrence, 10 represents high likelihood of occurrence
Probability of Detection: 1 represents a low likelihood of detecting the failure, 10 represents high likelihood of detection
Severity Level: 1 represents a low severity of the effect, 10 represents a high severity of the effect
Risk Priority Number: The value calculated from the three numeric parameters that is the combined priority of the failure mode
Corrective Action: The action initiated by the team to ameliorate the failure mode

Table 3.16	**FMEA Severity Ranking Examples**	
Example Score	Type of Event	Examples
10	Catastrophic	• Patient death or major permanent loss of function • Wrong surgery site • Infant abduction or discharge to the wrong family • Death of a visitor or a staff member • Damage to equipment or facility over $250,000
7	Major	• Permanent patient disability or disfiguration • Increased length of stay or level of care for three or more patients • Hospitalization of a visitor or staff member • Equipment of facility damage over $100,000
4	Moderate	• Increased length of stay or level of care for one or two patients • Need for treatment of one or two visitors or staff members • Equipment or facility damage less than $100,000
1	Minor	• No patient harm • Visitor evaluation but no treatment • Staff lost time • Minor equipment damage, not requiring repair

subprocess a of step 1. If the numbering system goes beyond three levels, then most likely the process being examined is too large for an effective analysis.

b. For each numbered step in the matrix, the team determines the cause and effect of the failure mode and enters this information into the matrix.

c. Each failure mode is then scored on three factors: the likelihood of the failure mode, the likelihood that the failure mode will be detected by the process owners, and the severity of the effect (see TABLE 3.16) of the failure mode. Each of these three parameters is scored on a 10-point scale, with 1 representing the lowest likelihood/severity and 10 representing the highest for both the likelihood of the failure mode and severity of the effect. The scale is *reversed* for likelihood of detection (i.e., a lower likelihood of detection is scored higher and vice versa). These relationships are detailed in TABLE 3.17.

d. A risk priority number (RPN) is then calculated from these three numbers according to the following equation:

$$\text{RPN} = P(\text{failure mode}) \times P(\text{detection}) \times L(\text{severity})$$

where $P(\text{failure mode})$ is the likelihood score for the failure mode to occur, $P(\text{detection})$ is the score for the likelihood that the failure mode will be detected, and $L(\text{severity})$ is the level of severity of the failure mode

Table 3.17	FMEA Factor Ranking Table			
	Score	Likelihood of Occurrence	Severity of Effect	Likelihood of Detection
	Low	1	1	10
		2	2	9
		3	3	8
		4	4	7
	Moderate	5	5	6
		6	6	5
		7	7	4
		8	8	3
		9	9	2
	High	10	10	1

e. The higher the RPN, the greater the risk. Obviously, the highest RPN is 1,000, and so the closer the RPN is to 1,000, the greater the risk. Although the RPN metric is of importance, even a relatively low RPN may be significant (e.g., if the severity score is 10, but the other two scores are each 2, the RPN will be only 400), but the high severity score may necessitate action.

f. Once all the RPNs are calculated, they are placed in rank order to determine those that have the highest priority for intervention.

5. Determine action steps and measures: Once the failure modes are prioritized using the RPN, the team can focus on corrective actions. Any improvement initiatives or process controls should be described in detail at this point, along with a business case analysis to demonstrate feasibility. For those initiatives that involve controls in the process, the team should determine process and outcome measures that can be used to test the new process.

Tips and Tricks

• Each failure mode may have multiple causes and effects. Failure modes include anything that could prevent the process step from being completed. For example, if nurse administration of a medication on time is the process step, possible failure modes are the nurse being diverted to other duties, the medication not being available, or the wrong medication being available (wrong dose, wrong form, wrong drug). Possible failure mode causes would include the lack of sufficient staff to manage all nursing duties, lack of nurse alerts for timely medication administration, medication shortage in the pharmacy, failure of the pharmacy to deliver the medication to the floor, incorrect prescription of the drug, incorrect interpretation of the medication order by the pharmacy, and so on.

- In general, as control interventions are developed for the process, they should be positioned as early in the process as possible. Multiple controls can be placed in the process to respond to a single hazard, and a single control can be used more than once in the process.
- Process owners are key members of any FMEA team, but in some cases the FMEA activity must be conducted without them. If process owners are not represented on the team, then their input should be sought as controls and process modifications are considered, because they will often know if a particular approach has been attempted in the past. Additionally, they have in-depth understanding of the process, the involved staff, and key indicators, which are all important as interventions are designed and involving the process owner in developing the solution ensures buy-in when implementation begins.
- Always consider a simulation or a pilot of a new intervention before deploying it system wide. This approach ensures that the projected performance is correct and can validate the business case for senior management.
- A very useful FMEA tool is available on the Institute for Healthcare Improvement's website (www.ihi.org). The tool leads users through the FMEA process using easily adapted forms, and the system provides a RPN as one of its outputs.

■ Summary

The first step in any improvement effort is to characterize and understand the underlying process. Process mapping tools provide a graphic representation of the process, which helps the team determine target areas for intervention. Using cause and effect analyses, Pareto analysis, and similar approaches, a quality improvement team can hone in on the root causes of process issues, and tools like matrices can help the team organize information for analysis. The next area for study will be the never-ending search for data in healthcare systems.

■ Discussion Questions

1. Describe the value proposition. What factors contribute to the value proposition for health care?
2. Quality improvement professionals frequently state that "all work consists of processes." Discuss what this means in health care. Does the physician–patient interaction lend itself to process analysis? Why or why not?
3. What is the value stream? Describe in your response the concepts of value added and non–value added work. Take a simple process from your work environment and describe the value stream.
4. Create a basic flowchart using a process from your experience.

Table 3.18	T-Matrix for Discussion Question 7			
Hospital A	8	9	8	8
Hospital B	12	8	7	8
	Service line offerings (number of lines)	Quality rankings (10-point index)	Cost index (10-point index)	Satisfaction rankings (10-point index)
MCO 1	34	8	7	8
MCO 2	56	8	8	10

5. When is it appropriate to use a program evaluation and review technique (PERT) chart? Create a PERT chart for a process from your experience using the cell template in FIGURE 3.4.

6. When is a deployment flowchart most useful? Draw a flowchart based on a workflow process from your experience.

7. How do matrices support decision making. Using the T-matrix from TABLE 3.18, justify the decision of XYZ Corporation's management to select Hospital B and MCO 2 for its employees.

8. What is the advantage of a decision matrix in helping a group come to a conclusion about alternatives? How are weights determined?

9. Create a four-quadrant matrix (such as the one in FIGURE 3.7) using an example from your experience, such as

   a. An importance (customer)/importance (staff) matrix for a visit to a fast food restaurant

   b. An importance (staff)/importance (leadership) matrix for a service line at your workplace

   c. An importance (customer)/performance (vendor) matrix for a service that your company purchases

   d. An importance (customer)/importance (lender) matrix for a loan application

10. Create a decision tree like that in FIGURE 3.10 for a decision with which you are familiar, for example, choice of food for dinner, determination of the best route to take to work based on traffic and construction, or from a business circumstance like choice of a new computer system, or a capital budget decision to expand or rebuild an office.

11. What is an Ishikawa diagram, and how is it used? Create an Ishikawa diagram for a clinical problem, such as low immunization rates, lack of health screening, failure to stop smoking, or physician failure to follow clinical guidelines.

12. How is a spaghetti diagram used in improving a process? How does a team use the spaghetti diagram to analyze workflow?

13. What is the difference between a root-cause analysis and a failure mode and effects criticality analysis? Explain how each would be used in a clinical situation or an administrative environment.
14. What does the acronym "SMART" mean? How is it relevant to performance improvement?

■ Additional Resources

Health care failure mode and effects analysis resources and forms. Retrieved October 2008 from http://www.va.gov/ncps/safetytopics.html

Kerzner H. *Project Management: A Systems Approach to Planning, Scheduling, and Controlling,* 8th ed. Hoboken, NJ: Wiley; 2003.

Klastorin T. *Project Management: Tools and Trade-offs,* 3rd ed. Hoboken, NJ: Wiley; 2003.

Milosevic DZ. *Project Management Toolbox: Tools and Techniques for the Practicing Project Manager.* Hoboken, NJ: Wiley; 2003.

MS Project 2007 tutorial: http://office.microsoft.com/training/training.aspx?AssetID= RC102106881033

Project Management Institute. *A Guide to the Project Management Body of Knowledge,* 3rd ed. Newtown Square, PA: Project Management Institute; 2003.

RFFlow software: http://www.rfflow.com; sample flowcharts at http://www.rff.com/flowchart_samples.htm

SmartDraw software: http://www.smartdraw.com

Tague N. *The Quality Toolbox,* 2nd ed. Milwaukee, WI: ASQ Quality Press; 2004.

TapRooT® system for root cause analysis. Retrieved October 2008 from http://www.taproot.com

Virine L, Trumper M. *Project Decisions: The Art and Science.* Management Concepts. West Sussex, UK: Kogan Paage Publishers; 2007.

Visio Tutorial: http://office.microsoft.com/en-us/visio/HP012077271033.aspx

Medical Informatics and Information Resources for Quality Improvement

CHAPTER

4

■ What Is Medical Informatics and Why Is It Important?

Medical informatics is a relatively new healthcare discipline that deals with the resources, devices, and methods required to optimize the acquisition, storage, retrieval, and use of data in health and biomedicine.[1] The medical informatics domain encompasses hardware and software but also includes processes and programs like clinical guidelines, formal medical terminology and computer syntax, and information management and reporting systems. The science of medical informatics has been evolving since the 1950s, when physicians and computer scientists at the Massachusetts General Hospital developed a computing language for medical applications called MUMPS (*M*assachusetts General Hospital *U*tility *M*ulti-*P*rogramming *S*ystem). Since that time countless physicians, computer scientists, nurses, and other health professionals have worked to automate clinical and administrative data collection, analysis, and reporting, leading to development of systems for streamlining and improving patient care. These professionals have moved the science and practice of medical informatics to new heights in the early 21st century.

One of the fundamental axioms of quality and performance improvement is stated as follows: *"You can't manage what you don't measure."* The effect of this statement has been seen across many industries in the past 50 years. After reviewing the approaches to process analysis in Chapter 3, the ability to make improvements in processes requires answering the following questions:

1. What is the gap between current process performance and the ideal expected performance?
2. What parts of the process can be targeted for improvement?
3. How does a team determine what parts of the process to improve?
4. How does a team determine when the process is improving as expected?

Using the fundamental axiom, it is clear that measurement of a process is key to answering these four questions. The science of medical informatics is the basis for creating measures, collecting data, and providing the information in a useable format for quality improvement professionals. Performance improvement work is impossible without the data that directs the team in determining solutions for the four questions.

109

Highly effective improvement teams include a medical informaticist as a core member who helps to find the appropriate data sources and craft *process* and *outcome* measures to characterize the process so that the team can prioritize opportunities for improvement. Once improvements are piloted, as described in Chapter 2, the medical informaticist can help design measures using existing data management systems so that the team can monitor initiatives as they are rolled out to the rest of the enterprise. This ongoing collaboration between quality improvement staff and medical informaticists can be crucial to ensuring the success of improvement efforts.

■ Types of Measurement Systems

As discussed earlier, measures are often distinguished by the point in the process at which the data are collected. Three major categories exist: *structural measures, process measures*, and *outcome measures*. Avedis Donabedian[2] was one of the first healthcare professionals to characterize the basics of medical quality as requiring three fundamental elements:

1. *Structure:* The necessary infrastructure needed to deliver medical care, which includes such elements as the medical equipment, staff, facilities, and information systems.
2. *Process:* The procedures and steps required to deliver healthcare services to customers.
3. *Outcome:* The net effect of the delivery of services to customers, including restoration of function, recovery from interventions, complications, and survival.

The relationship of these variables is shown in FIGURE 4.1. Structural variables must be in place so that processes can be completed to produce outcomes. Measurement systems must account for each of these domains and the parameters that exist within them.

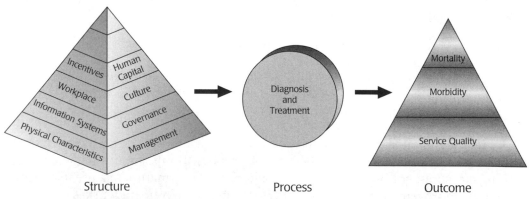

FIGURE 4.1 Donabedian Model for Healthcare Quality

Effective organizational capabilities, such as leadership, human capital, information management systems, culture, and incentive systems, are all critical as structural elements of a healthcare organization to ensure that processes may proceed effectively. Over the past two decades, as the healthcare industry has realized that further efficiencies are necessary for survival, each of these structural categories has become better characterized to allow more intense management scrutiny. Additionally, accreditation and certification organizations like The Joint Commission (TJC), the National Committee for Quality Assurance (NCQA), the Utilization Review Accreditation Commission (URAC), and the federal government through the Centers for Medicare and Medicaid Services (CMS) promote the assurance of an adequate infrastructure through their standards and certification requirements. Most of these accrediting organizations have developed standards and measures for all three of these domains.

Performance measures have three characteristics that must be incorporated into creation and deployment of any measurement system:

1. *Important:* Relevant to stakeholders, to the healthcare system being measured, and to any third parties that may use the measures for delivery or improvement of health care.
2. *Scientifically sound:* Based on current evidence of quality and efficacy, including cost effectiveness; numerator and denominator must be based on valid and reproducible data.
3. *Feasibility:* Data must be available for collection, analysis, and reporting; measures must be associated with processes that can be modified through reasonable methods and procedures.

Performance measures are used for quality improvement, accountability, and research. Some examples of situations in which metrics are used for accountability include:

- Pay for performance or pay for reporting programs
- Purchaser and/or consumer decision making
- Accreditation and external quality oversight

When used for accountability, measures must meet high validity and reliability standards, because the organization's reputation or financial performance may depend on the metrics. For example, in a pay for performance program, lower performance on a measure may cause a payer to lower reimbursement, and so the measure must be correct to ensure equity. This need for greater validity and reliability requires that each provider collect, analyze, and report data exactly the same using standardized and detailed specifications, called *operational definitions*, to ensure comparisons are fair. Typically, accountability data are used more by accrediting agencies, consumers, and payers than by the reporting healthcare entity, and the data are used to guide the selection of providers or to determine payments or financial incentives to providers for high performance. When results are used to compare provider groups to select providers based on performance, the financial survival of a healthcare organization may be at stake, necessitating the highest level of accuracy and validity to measurement systems.

Because of these risks, many practitioners argue that medical care is too complex to be measured. However, Donabedian's framework provides the rationale for developing metrics. If quality of care depends on the three domains in the Donabedian model, then quality improvement teams should be able to develop metrics for each. The next section describes some of these efforts in more detail.

Structure Measures

These metrics are sometimes described as "profile measures" because they can be descriptive of an organization's facilities, staff, and even culture. These types of indicators could include:

- Number of beds in a hospital
- Number of physicians or practitioners in a medical practice
- Presence of a positron emission tomograph (PET scanner) in an imaging center
- Gamma knife equipment in a surgical center
- Multidisciplinary teams for care
- Capability to perform patient education in self-care management
- Disease registries
- Electronic health records and decision support systems

These measures provide an indication of the available facilities for providing care without indicating if these facilities provide quality care. Unfortunately, some practitioners and consumers may equate the availability of advanced equipment or new facilities with quality care, but that logic is severely flawed. Even the newest and most advanced healthcare organizations may have quality issues if their processes are defective. For example, one of the most prestigious hospital systems in the world, Cedars Sinai of Los Angeles, overdosed actor Dennis Quaid's twins with heparin (see Chapter 1). Other renowned medical centers have had similar errors.[3-5] Unfortunately, just having the infrastructure in place is not a guarantee that quality care will follow, but lack of appropriate infrastructure can almost certainly create the possibility of significant errors from such mitigating factors as equipment failures or lack of proximity to the needed facilities in the event of an emergency.

Structure indicators can be classified using some of the cause and effect categories described in Chapter 3 during the discussion of the Ishikawa diagram:

- Manpower
- Materials
- Milieu (environment)

Manpower variables subsume a wide range in healthcare organizations. The first category that most people consider is the medical staff (i.e., physicians and other practitioners), but medical staff composition is only the tip of a very large iceberg. Although physicians drive a substantial amount of the volume in many healthcare enterprises, most of the daily work is carried out by other health professionals, such as nurses, therapists, pharmacists, nutritionists, and social workers, and support personnel, such as environmental services staff, food services, administrative staff, and customer service staff. Without all these professionals, the organization would not function. Thus because an organization's structure is characterized with measures, manpower metrics are of great importance. Thus structural variables in the area of manpower might include the following:

- Nurse staffing ratios: The number of nurses per patient, often measured as nursing hours per patient day.
- Nurse specialty certification: The number or percentage of nurses with appropriate specialty certification (e.g., as cardiac nurse specialists in a coronary care unit).
- Environmental service staffing ratios: The percentage of environmental staff per patient or some other measure of patient volume, like patient days.
- Availability of nutritionist services: Number of nutritionists per patient or measure of patient volume.
- Administrative staff ratios: Number or rate of administrative staff per patient or patient volume measure.
- Availability of certified therapy services: Therapists provide respiratory, speech, occupational, and physical therapy services, and each of these areas has certification requirements that should be met to ensure quality care.
- Pharmacist participation in patient care: Many hospitals and other types of organizations include a licensed pharmacist as an important member of the patient care team. This practice has been shown to reduce medication errors, and so including a pharmacist in the decision-making process (e.g., during patient rounds in the hospital) can be considered a structural variable relating to manpower.
- Availability of social services and/or care coordination: As health care has become increasingly complex, navigation of the system has become progressively more difficult. The ability for an organization to coordinate a customer's care adds significant value to the care and can promote higher quality care. Hospitals may employ social workers or nurses to perform the care coordination task, and many primary care practices are establishing themselves as "medical homes" to ensure that each individual's care is customized to her or his needs, as well as to ensure that needed care is delivered to each customer.

Materials measures include all elements of the supply chain, such as disposable medical supplies, surgical instruments, pharmaceuticals, and the myriad other resources needed to provide care. Most mid-sized to large healthcare organizations have developed supply chain management systems to ensure that needed supplies are immediately available at the point of care while optimizing efficiency by reducing costs of idle inventories, transportation, as well as item unit costs through group purchasing. Quality measures of materials management may vary from the availability of a specific resource to the speed with which these materials are made available to practitioners. The following are some examples of these types of measures:

- Turnaround time for surgical procedure trays in the surgical suite: The time it takes for the surgical staff to restock a surgical tray (instruments, sponges, etc.) after it has been used in a surgical procedure.
- Inventory turns: The number of times a particular item or group of items is renewed in the organization's inventory stores.
- Delivery time for an item or class of items: The time it takes to deliver an item or class of items from a central storage area or vendor to the point of care.
- Breakage rate for an item or class of items: Indirect measure of quality; the rate at which an item breaks during usage (e.g., suturing needle breakage).

Metrics developed for these purposes can serve to assess cost, as well as quality, and thus can be applied to the assessment of value according to the value proposition discussed in Chapter 3.

Finally, environmental ("milieu") variables are important to the structure metrics. The environment of care can involve any number of issues and types of measures but mostly gravitate toward the appearance and suitability of the locale in which care is delivered. The Joint Commission devotes an entire domain in its standards to the issue of the environment in which care is provided, with the following areas of importance:

- Safety
- Security
- Hazardous materials
- Emergency management
- Fire prevention
- Medical equipment
- Utilities management

An additional category was added to cover the appropriateness of the environment: the proper facilities for the level and type of care in the facility. Each of these categories has measures associated with the quality and performance of the area:

- Presence of policies and procedures, management plans, and vulnerability analyses (failure mode and effects analysis)
- Results of tests for toxins in the environment
- Test results for staff exposed to toxins

- Presence of safety and hazard management equipment
- Reports of disaster drills and actual events

These measures are all used for accountability to the accrediting body as well as for internal performance monitoring and improvement.

Other measures may also be used to evaluate the environment of care, based on customer evaluations and directed more at identifying opportunities for improvement. Many organizations include environmental questions in customer surveys directed at evaluating the "hospitality services" of the institution. Hospitals in particular use these metrics to determine if current food service and other hospitality services are attractive to patients and families. In most cases these metrics are included in the routine customer survey process, but in some cases targeted surveys may be conducted to focus on a specific service or patient population. For example, a hospital may include a "postcard survey" with food trays to ask patients if a new room arrangement in a particular care unit helps lead to calmness during hospitalization. These surveys are widely used and a highly valuable tool to gain important information about the milieu in which care is provided.

Process Measures

Process measures address the interaction between the patient and the provider (e.g., how are care and services provided) in the Donabedian model. Providers of care include everyone in the healthcare system, and because processes are the basis of all work performed, these measures are applied throughout the chain of care. Process measures are generally developed for specific steps in a target process to examine some characteristic of that step (e.g., cost, throughput, resource utilization, or customer satisfaction) with the performance of the step. The discussion of outcome measures in the next section demonstrates that these same types of measures can be used for the overall process as well.

Process measures usually fall into one of the following categories:

- Financial
- Utilization
- Compliance
- Disease specific
- Satisfaction with care

Each of these categories subsumes a specific aspect of the process or process step. As discussed in Chapter 3, the use of process management approaches for the evaluation and improvement of healthcare processes provides the ability to improve most healthcare services, but returning to our key principle for this chapter—you can't manage what you don't measure—the likelihood of achieving sustainable improvements without process metrics is quite small.

An important factor in health care is the cost of care, and so financial measures are of primary importance in determining if the cost of each step in the process is efficient. Financial measures might also include the revenue derived from a step as well, but in most cases cost is the primary target for these analyses. The following are some examples of financial measures:

- Cost of materials: The cost of any materials or supplies used in the step.
- Staff costs: The allocated cost of staff time and benefits for employees involved in the process step.
- Equipment amortization: The fractional cost of equipment used in a process step, based on the equipment's depreciation schedule.
- Building and utilities costs: The fractional cost incurred because of use of the building and utilities to provide the service.
- Administrative costs: Any costs for administrative services that might be related to the process step.

Although each of these metrics might be examined independently, often they are summed to a total cost for the process step. This approach to assigning actual costs to process steps is called activity-based costing and is widely applicable in healthcare industry accounting systems. Although many organizations find cost allocation to be a challenge, those who have achieved that goal can realize substantial benefits.

Measures of utilization of a particular process step can determine if the step is being used or if it is being avoided. Utilization measures help a quality improvement team recognize those steps in a process that are being bypassed by staff for reasons of practicality, lack of knowledge, failure to understand the process flow, and so forth. For example, during a "mandatory stop" preoperatively, a certain sequence of events is required to ensure that the correct patient is in the operating room, that the correct

Exhibit 4.1   Digression: Activity-Based Costing (ABC) in Health Care

Although a detailed discussion of ABC is beyond the scope of this book, numerous articles describe the potential benefits to healthcare organizations from adoption of ABC systems. As early as 1993, hospital systems noted that by combining ABC with existing standard costing systems, hospitals can better plan and control the cost of the services they provide. Pricing services has become an important factor in financial success, as well as marketplace competitiveness, and understanding costs is critical to cogent pricing practice. ABC provides the necessary information to better characterize the costs of services and has additional benefits, for example, the ability to identify target areas for cost reduction, to better manage customer demand, to optimize an organization's service/product line, and for use as a performance measurement tool. Many different types of healthcare organizations (e.g., hospitals, HMOs, and some medical practices) have developed ABC approaches to costing. See Additional Resources for more information.

site is marked for surgery, that the site has been prepared properly, that all preoperative laboratory and x-ray data have been collected and are on the chart, and that the operating room has all the necessary equipment and materials to perform the procedure. If the surgical team fails to check that the operating site is marked for the procedure, then utilization of that step in the process is inconsistent. In most cases utilization metrics are reported as rates (e.g., as the number of "defects" or nonconformities divided by the total number of cases). So for the situation just described, the utilization rate of the site marking check would be reported as:

$$Site\,marking\,check\,rate = \frac{Number\,of\,times\,site\,is\,checked}{Total\,number\,of\,surgical\,procedures\,performed}$$

Utilization measures such as these are frequently used to measure process quality. Nationally, the CMS has published a list of 134 measures, including some for process utilization measurement (the Physician Quality Reporting Initiative [PQRI]), which is used in the pay for performance and pay for reporting program, and some to measure and report the quality of care for physicians who accept Medicare payments. A partial list of these measures is shown in TABLE 4.1, and the complete list is shown in Appendix 1.1. Many of the measures assess process variables, but some target outcomes as well.

Table 4.1	Examples of CMS Process Measures From the Physicians Quality Reporting Initiative
Measure	Description
Screening for future fall risk	Percentage of patients aged 65 years and older who were screened for future fall risk (patients are considered at risk for future falls if they have had 2 or more falls in the past year or any fall with injury in the past year) at least once within 12 months.
Heart failure: angiotensin-converting enzyme (ACE) inhibitor or angiotensin receptor blocker (ARB) therapy for left ventricular systolic dysfunction (LVSD)	Percentage of patients aged 18 years and older with a diagnosis of heart failure and LVSD who were prescribed ACE inhibitor or ARB therapy.
Oral antiplatelet therapy prescribed for patients with coronary artery disease	Percentage of patients aged 18 years and older with a diagnosis of coronary artery disease who were prescribed oral antiplatelet therapy.
Diabetic retinopathy: documentation of presence or absence of macular edema and level of severity of retinopathy	Percentage of patients aged 18 years and older with a diagnosis of diabetic retinopathy who had a dilated macular or fundus exam performed that included documentation of the level of severity of retinopathy and the presence or absence of macular edema during one or more office visits within 12 months.

Another type of utilization measure relates to the efficiency of the process. Lean process management is based on improving the rate of throughput in a process by reducing non–value added work. Thus these measures are often for a process step or numbers of items passing through the step. Some measures in this category include:

- Number of blood draws per hour
- Rate of patients triaged in the emergency department per day
- Rate of patient room decontamination per hour
- Number of days from discharge to final bill

These types of utilization measures are directed at improving the efficiency and effectiveness of the underlying processes. For management purposes, these measures are indispensable for improving process throughput.

Another category of measures deals with compliance. The healthcare industry has numerous oversight bodies, from local and state health departments, to the Occupational Safety and Health Administration, to the CMS (see TABLE 4.2). State and federal laws address issues like disposal of medical waste, billing practices, and management of medical information. In some managers' minds adherence to Joint Commission standards entails a compliance activity as well. In any event, compliance measures are important to ensure that an organization has performed all the necessary process steps to comply with the multitude of regulations for healthcare organizations. Many times these measures are simple "binary" values (i.e., they have one of two values like "Meets"/"Does not meet" or "Compliant/Noncompliant"). Some measures may have multiple levels, such as an extra category like "Conditional Certification" to connote basic compliance with some exceptions that need to be improved for full compliance or certification.

Increasing effort is being directed at developing disease-specific measures for evaluation of performance in managing targeted diseases. Many such measures are listed in the compilation of PQRI indicators in Appendix 1.1. Disease-specific measures assess some element of performance in the care of a clinical condition (e.g., diabetes-specific metrics like performance of a retinal exam [Appendix 1.1, measures

Table 4.2	Compliance Measure Examples
Organization	Compliance Measure(s)
The Joint Commission	• Certified
	• Conditional Certification
	• Preliminary Certification Denial
Occupational Safety and Health Administration Voluntary Protection Program	• Star
	• Merit

14 and 15] or a foot exam [Appendix 1.1, measures 111 and 112]). Many of these metrics have been developed in recent years to begin to capture performance levels for various diseases, and the PQRI project is a good example of the breadth of these measurement efforts.

Finally, customer satisfaction measures are of increasing importance to many healthcare organizations. Most of these metrics are collected after a healthcare service is delivered (e.g., after being discharged from the hospital). Several national organizations perform patient satisfaction surveys, including Press Ganey (www.pressganey.com), Gallup (www.gallup.com), and HealthStream (www.healthstream.com). The major survey organizations have custom surveys and proprietary methods of analysis and comparison, but a relatively new approach has become available through the Agency for Healthcare Research and Quality (AHRQ, www.ahrq.gov) using the Consumer Assessment of Healthcare Performance Survey (CAHPS).

The CAHPS program divides healthcare quality into two major components: clinical aspects of care and consumers' experiences with healthcare services. To meet the challenges of capturing and reporting patient experiences, AHRQ led development of the CAHPS survey as a standardized, evidence-based survey for evaluating customers' experiences with the healthcare system. AHRQ launched the CAHPS program in the mid-1990s through the CAHPS Consortium, comprised of public and private research organizations that developed and refined the following principles that are the basis for all CAHPS products:[6]

1. *Emphasis on actual experience.* Although CAHPS surveys include both ratings and reports of experience, the emphasis is on respondents' reports of their experiences with health care, resulting in information that is more specific, actionable, understandable, and objective than general ratings alone.
2. *Standardization.* Survey tools and reporting measures are standardized, which allows for valid comparisons and benchmarking across healthcare settings.
3. *Use of the best science.* The development of CAHPS surveys and related tools incorporates the state-of-the-art in survey and report design. Thorough field testing ensures that survey administration guidelines and protocols are based on sound evidence of effectiveness and feasibility.
4. *Meaningful information.* To ensure that surveys generate information that has meaning for consumers and other audiences, report language and data displays are developed in conjunction with the survey instruments. The CAHPS Consortium also tests the language and formatting of survey instruments and sample reports with various audiences to maximize comprehension and usability.
5. *Input from all affected parties.* The survey development process includes frequent opportunities for major stakeholders, including clinicians, administrators, and accrediting bodies, to learn about the instrument and provide feedback.

6. *Public resource.* All CAHPS tools, resources, and services are in the public domain. Technical assistance, including general guidance as well as project-specific advice, is available to all users at no charge.

In the first few years of the CAHPS development project, the Consortium focused on creating and testing an integrated set of standardized questionnaires and reporting formats for consumers enrolled in health plans. AHRQ subsequently developed CAHPS II, which had an expanded agenda to:

- Create evidence-based and tested surveys that meet the needs of other components of the healthcare system, such as hospitals, nursing homes, and dialysis centers.
- Explore ways to improve the utility and suitability of CAHPS instruments for vulnerable healthcare populations.
- Study ways to use CAHPS results to evaluate and improve quality of care.

In June 2007 AHRQ launched CAHPS III, with a change in focus from the development of surveys to the creation of resources to support the implementation and use of CAHPS surveys for performance improvement and consumer choice.

CAHPS surveys have been developed for assessing the quality of care in both ambulatory and institutional settings. Each CAHPS bundle includes questionnaires, administration protocols, analysis programs, and guidance in reporting results. CAHPS was initially directed at commercial health plans, Medicaid and Medicare, and State Children's Health Insurance Plans, and it is now administered to over 120 million health plan beneficiaries. The National Committee for Quality Assurance includes CAHPS results in its health plan performance reports and as part of the accreditation process for health plans. CMS uses a version of the survey to poll Medicare beneficiaries in both traditional and managed care plans and reports the scores publicly (http://www.cms.hhs.gov/CAHPS/CAHPS/).

During the second phase of CAHPS development, the Consortium created standardized, evidence-based surveys customized for a number of other settings, including physician offices, managed behavioral healthcare organizations, dental plans, and tribal clinics. Ambulatory care survey products include several optional survey items that may be added to specific instruments. For example, surveys for physician services evaluation in a clinic include a number of core elements, including:

- Getting an appointment and health care when needed
- How well doctors communicate
- Courteous and helpful office staff

The Child Primary Care Questionnaire has two additional categories of measures:

- Doctor's Attention to Your Child's Growth and Development
- Doctor's Advice on Keeping Your Child Safe and Healthy

More information about the CAHPS Ambulatory Care Surveys can be found on the AHRQ website (https://www.cahps.ahrq.gov/content/products/PROD_Amb CareSurveys.asp).

CAHPS surveys have been adapted for specific subpopulations whose experiences may be different from those of the general populations. For example, a module for Children and Youth with Special Health Care Needs is available for the CAHPS health plan survey. Additionally, the CAHPS Consortium collaborated with the Choctaw Nation Health Service to develop a survey that addresses the needs and experiences of Native Americans.

The CAHPS Hospital Survey, often referred to as H-CAHPS or Hospital CAHPS, evaluates the inpatient experiences of adults. Hospitals using H-CAHPS can voluntarily report data to the CMS for consolidation and comparison reporting. Dialysis facilities and end-stage renal disease networks use the CAHPS In-Center Hemodialysis Survey to evaluate the experiences of patients receiving hemodialysis and developing improvement initiatives. The next phase of CAHPS will focus on nursing home surveys for both long-term and short-stay residents and their families.

A number of free services are available through AHRQ to support implementation of the surveys, interpretation of results, and use of the results for process improvement. The CAHPS User Network provides the following access:

- Phone and e-mail technical assistance
  - Toll-free number (800-492-9261)
  - E-mail (cahps1@ahrq.gov)
- Website (www.cahps.ahrq.gov)
  - CAHPS products and research findings
  - Information about managing survey projects and reporting survey results
  - Improvement projects to use results to improve the patient's experience
  - Product-specific CAHPS Survey and Reporting Kits: questionnaires, reporting composites, administration protocols, SAS analysis programs, and instructions for using the programs
  - Information about new CAHPS products, webcasts, and user meetings
  - Public reporting of survey results
  - Searchable bibliography and frequently asked questions
  - Networking information with brief profiles of CAHPS Health Plan Survey projects around the country, a link to AHRQ's Report Card Compendium, and links to related organizations, programs, and initiatives
- Updates on products and services
  - Announcements through *The CAHPS Connection* regarding product development, upcoming events, and changes to existing instruments

All the survey companies have amassed large databases for comparing each institution's performance to peer groups. Similarly, AHRQ has developed the National

CAHPS benchmarking database (CAHPS database), which currently contains 10 years of data from commercial and Medicaid plans. The CAHPS database has become the national repository for data from the CAHPS Health Plan Survey, and in 2005 H-CAHPS data were added to the database, submitted voluntarily by hospitals and vendors. The database will continue to grow as other CAHPS survey data are added in the future. Contributors to the database will have a number of privileges regarding access to the information:

- Access to reports that benchmark individual survey results to other organizations in the database
- Access to data from individual surveys
- Availability of customized analyses and reports on a fee-for-service basis
- Availability of raw data for specialized research related to consumer assessments of healthcare quality

More information about the CAHPS Database can be found at https://www.cahps. ahrq.gov/content/ncbd/ncbd_Intro.asp. Examples of the output from the database for health plans are provided in FIGURES 4.2 through 4.6. Similar results are anticipated for other healthcare entities as data are collected in the national database. An example of the pediatric primary care survey is included as Appendix 4.1. Complete kits for each of the CAHPS survey categories may be downloaded from the website above, including English and Spanish versions of the surveys. These kits not only contain the surveys, but they also have administration guidelines, data analysis guidelines and programs, and information about reporting results. Although specific surveys for subspecialty care are not yet available, many of the questions are equally germane for primary care physicians and specialists.

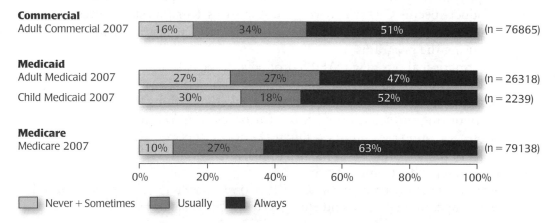

FIGURE 4.2 Responses to "Getting Needed Care" from National CAHPS Database 2007

Note: Response distributions may not sum to 100 percent due to rounding.

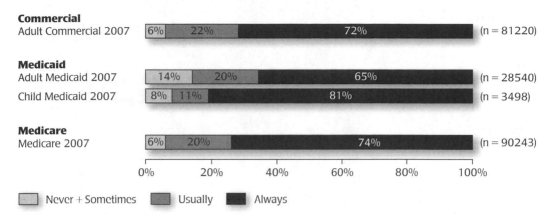

FIGURE 4.3 Responses to "How Often a Doctor Explained Things Understandably to Adults" from National CAHPS Database 2007

Note: Response distributions may not sum to 100 percent due to rounding.

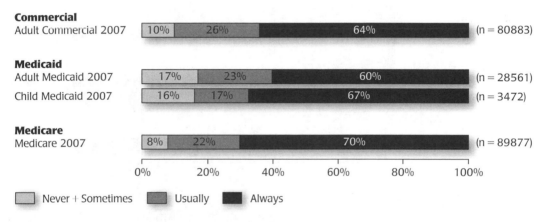

FIGURE 4.4 Responses to "How Often Did a Personal Doctor Spend Enough Time with Consumers" from National CAHPS Database 2007

Note: Response distributions may not sum to 100 percent due to rounding.

Outcome Measures

Whereas process measures are often directed at determining process efficiency, outcome measures usually assess process effectiveness. For many years the health-care industry concentrated on building the correct infrastructure and then on creating efficient processes. After the building phase, ensuring that the structure and processes lead to effective outcomes has become the foremost task. Two major categories of outcome measures exist in health care: business outcomes and clinical outcomes. Business outcome metrics are created to determine the business

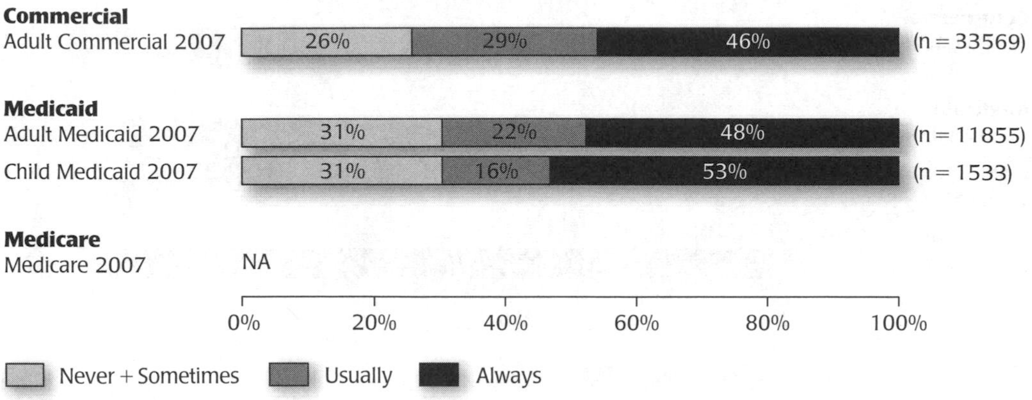

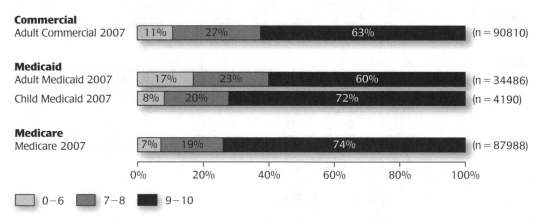

FIGURE 4.5 Responses to "How Often a Health Plan's Customer Service Provided Information or Help Needed by Customers" from National CAHPS Database 2007.

Note: Response distributions may not sum to 100 percent due to rounding.

FIGURE 4.6 Responses to "On a Scale of 1 to 10, How Would You Rate Your Personal Doctor or Nurse" from National CAHPS Database 2007

Note: Response distributions may not sum to 100 percent due to rounding.

effectiveness of a particular process. Some example business outcome metrics include:

- Collection rates for the accounts receivable collection process
- Return on investment to gauge management effectiveness
- Customer satisfaction for the ombudsman function at a hospital
- Insurance billing returns to measure the effectiveness of the billing system
- Room inspection passage rate for the environmental services processes
- Customer satisfaction with food service for the nutritional services department

Business measures are often generic and not specific for the healthcare industry, as shown in the list above. These metrics can and should be stratified, however, so they reflect any effects engendered by subpopulations of customers. For example, the accounts receivable collection rates may be different between customer groups, with some groups paying more rapidly and fully than others. By stratifying the data, managers can often find these differences and customize specific collection efforts for each customer segment. This segmentation approach improves management and process effectiveness and enhances results.

Clinical outcome measures are often very specific to the clinical condition being measured and must be appropriate to the usual healthcare needs and goals of the patient population in which they are used. Effective clinical outcome metrics take into account comorbidities (i.e., coexisting diseases and clinical problems that may affect the measure). Many clinical measures were originally developed in commercially insured populations and do not account for other comorbidities. One method of dealing with these comorbidities has been risk adjustment, which is a statistical method of trying to correct for the influence of a specific variable in the analysis. For example, if age may have an effect on an indicator, the analysis of the data will include a statistical adjustment for age, so that the information resulting from the analysis may be better understood in the context of a specific age grouping in the population. Although this approach can be rather statistically complex, it has been applied in a number of situations, for example, to adjust for comorbid conditions.

Another characteristic of clinical outcome measures is the need for validation of the metric. Every effective clinical outcome measure has been tested in real-world environments to ensure that it correctly measures what it is intended to measure. Validation of metrics requires a scientific approach that depends on the type of measure that is being deployed and is beyond the scope of this book. However, when choosing measures for a particular application, eight criteria must be considered:

1. Appropriateness of the measure: Does the measure provide information about the clinical entity that is being assessed?
2. Reliability: Is the measure reproducible and internally consistent?
3. Validity: Does the metric measure what it is supposed to measure?
4. Responsiveness: Is the measure sensitive to changes that are important to patients/customers?
5. Precision: Does the measure correctly differentiate between different levels of performance or responses?
6. Interpretability: Are the results of the measure easy to understand and use for determining improvement opportunities?
7. Acceptability: Are measurement efforts satisfactory to those being measured and those doing the measurement?
8. Feasibility: Are data for the measure easy to collect and analyze?

As clinical outcome measures are chosen for a performance improvement project, clinicians must play a key role in the planning process to ensure that the above criteria are met. Similarly, business process outcome measures should have adequate representation from subject matter experts in the area being considered for improvement initiatives. Some examples of clinical outcome measures include:

- Mortality from chronic renal disease
- Fracture rates in individuals treated for osteoporosis
- Rates of hearing loss in children after an episode of otitis media (ear infection)
- Suicide rates in patients hospitalized for behavioral health problems
- School performance in children treated for attention deficit disorder
- Pressure ulcer rates in bedridden patients
- Rate of school reintroduction in children with severe burns

As should be obvious, many such measures are possible. In fact, many outcomes measures have been created in the recent past, and a list of resources for these operational definitions and national performance levels is presented in Appendix 4.2.

■ Microsystem Data

For many analyses, data from microeconomic systems (i.e., individual firms or medical units) is collected and reported to payers or other accrediting bodies. For example, health plans report data from claims and chart audits to the National Committee on Quality Assurance to satisfy requirements for certification, hospitals report data to The Joint Commission to meet that organization's standards for accreditation, and even physicians are now being asked to report data as part of the CMS' Medicare PQRI (see Appendix 1.1). Data from all these sources are then aggregated in many of the available data sources (e.g., Health Effectiveness Data Information Set (HEDIS) reports are the result of aggregating data from certified health plans, culminating in the national data sources that are used for macroeconomic analysis).

The concept of "microsystems" in health care is slightly different from "microeconomic" systems. Based on the work of researchers at Dartmouth-Hitchcock Medical Center led by Paul Bataldan,[7] a microsystem in health care can be defined as a small group of people who work together on a regular basis to provide care to discrete subpopulations including the patients. A microsystem has both clinical and business goals, multiple linked processes, an environment in which information must be shared, and clinical outcomes for which the group is accountable. Clinical microsystems often evolve over time and frequently represent subgroups in larger healthcare organizations, like hospitals. Because these groups are accountable for clinical outcomes, they must ensure that the work of the microsystem is completed and simultaneously improve quality, meet the needs of the staff, and create an internal identity as a clinical unit. It is easy to recognize that clinical microsystems provide most of the frontline care in the healthcare delivery system. Successful clinical microsystems are focused on patients and customer service, and innovations in care are often discovered in these small groups. In theory, the overall quality of care produced by an institution is the sum of the levels of quality provided in each microsystem. Thus any organization is highly reliant on the frontline workers in microsystems to raise the overall level of performance by incremental operational excellence.

The clinical microsystem framework is useful for evaluating and improving quality of care in complex organizations. Often, the ability to measure quality in a large organization may seem daunting because of "all the moving parts," but using the concept of clinical microsystems, a quality improvement professional can divide the larger organization into smaller components, the clinical microsystems, which then can be analyzed using measures that have uniform operational definitions consistent across the enterprise and also with outside benchmarks.

■ Medical Record Systems

One increasingly important source of process and outcome data at the level of the individual patient encounter is the electronic medical record. Although medical insurance claims data provide the most widely used sources of information for analyzing utilization and quality of care, the most robust source of data is the medical record. To gain insight into patterns of care, the medical record, which is created by doctors and nurses as they provide care for patients, contains the most complete information about what services are provided as well as the sequence of findings and decisions leading to those services. The downside of using traditional medical record data, however, resides with the current paper records system that is commonly used in the United States: The only way of obtaining data for use in more complex quality improvement projects is to either create additional data collection forms to be completed in addition to the usual medical record entries or have an experienced clinician, such as a nurse, review the records one by one to extract the data from the written entries. Either approach is expensive and inefficient.

The ideal approach to collecting clinical data is to use information automatically recorded as patients are being treated. This information can serve as an accurate record of the services delivered as well as the process of delivering the care and the reasoning behind the selection of the clinical approach. A systematic approach to recording medical interactions has been developed in the nearly 300 electronic health record (EHR) systems available to physician practices.

Electronic Health Record Systems

Unfortunately, as of mid-2008, a survey of 2,758 physicians published in the *New England Journal of Medicine* indicated that only 4% have a fully functional EHR systems and 13% have a basic system.[8] Additionally, 16% of physicians said their practice had purchased an EHR system but had not used it yet. Another 26% said their practice was planning on purchasing a digital record-keeping system within the next 2 years. Thus the penetration of EHR systems into medical practice has been spotty at best. However, a number of incentives are being designed by payers to encourage EHR system adoption.[9] As these incentives are implemented, the business case for EHR adoption will become compelling, and medical practices are expected to embrace these more effective medical record systems. The value of EHR systems to implementing quality solutions, however, is clear and was outlined in a paper by The MITRE Corporation for the National Institutes of Health.[10] Several features of the EHR system provide the framework for improvement efforts:

- EHR systems must integrate systems that include laboratory, radiology (imaging), pharmacy, physician order entry, clinical documentation, and administrative modules.
- EHR systems must be subject to standards created by certification organizations for such features as:
  - Clinical vocabularies (i.e., descriptions of clinical conditions in a uniform way using the same group of words for a specific condition)
  - Interoperability, which allows one system to share data and messages with another
  - EHR ontologies, which consist of the content and structure of data entries in relationship to each other
- EHR user interfaces must be conducive to fitting with varying clinician workflow to facilitate data collection at the point of care.

These features improve the likelihood that data will be captured at the point of care in a form that is useful for conducting quality improvement analyses.

Clinical Data for Quality Analysis

The three major criteria above are important to ensure the validity of data used for performing quality improvement analyses. Integration of data sources, such as lab, radiology, and pharmacy, with clinical information is a fundamental requirement for performing quality improvement studies. Amalgamating these data sources in a clinical record for a medical office is usually part of the system's design but for larger enterprises, such as hospitals or regional health systems, usually requires more work. Many enterprise systems evolve using "best in class" software for each application, and the interoperability, or communication and ability to exchange information, becomes a major undertaking. Data-sharing standards have been established for some applications, like the HL-7 standard for data interchange in EHR systems.[11] HL-7 is one of the Standards Developing Organizations of the American National Standards Institute (www.ansi.org), and these Standards Developing Organizations (SDOs) have been instrumental in developing the specifications for the structure and function of the EHR system.

Many clinical applications, however, do not readily communicate with other programs. For that reason, another solution, the data warehouse, has become a viable approach to combining several disparate data sources into a single, central resource. Sometimes called a data repository, a data warehouse is a relational database that is designed for query and analysis rather than for processing transaction information. The fields in the database usually contain historical data derived from transaction files, but they can include data from other sources as well. For example, an insurance company data repository might contain claims data from providers, but it might also hold data from provider or patient satisfaction surveys, complaint database information, and results of quality reviews. The more information the data repository houses, the greater the ability of analysts to combine data sets to find relationships between variables. Using the insurance example, the analyst could use the combined data to identify high-volume procedures (transaction data) and match it to quality reviews for those high-volume procedures (quality review data) and relate costs of care (transaction data) to quality lapses (quality review data) and patient satisfaction (patient satisfaction data). These kinds of reviews are valuable for targeting opportunities for improvement or even areas of risk for the organization.

The data warehouse is particularly important for reducing the processing load for the transaction database. Transaction programs operate in real time and are used to record business transactions, like patient bills or clinical encounter entries, at the time that they occur. The computer is usually very busy with these activities, and adding queries to the list of tasks that the processor must perform can slow the system to a crawl. A data warehouse provides a way for queries to be performed on recent and historical data without interfering with transaction processing. A basic configuration of a data warehouse is represented in FIGURE 4.7. Notably, the data sources can come from not only databases within the organization, but also from other resources through direct connections or via the Internet.

In addition to the relational database holding data from a variety of sources, a data warehouse environment includes an extraction, transportation, transformation, and loading solution; an online analytical processing engine; client analysis tools; and other applications that manage the process of gathering data and delivering it to business users. These interface features provide end users, analysts, and decision makers with the needed access to accomplish their work more efficiently.

Availability of high-quality data is one of the keys to effective performance improvement, and tools like data warehouses and interoperability of data resources can facilitate the work of quality improvement professionals. Additionally, the combination of improved data collection, standardization of entries for most patient encounters, and availability of data in electronic formats that are more readily analyzed using advanced computer software packages makes the case for electronic medical records very compelling for quality professionals. Unfortunately, even EHR systems may store some data in the form

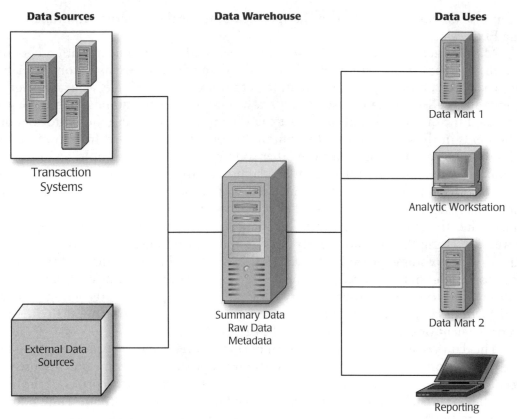

Data Sources

Transaction Systems

External Data Sources

Data Warehouse

Summary Data
Raw Data
Metadata

Data Uses

Data Mart 1

Analytic Workstation

Data Mart 2

Reporting

FIGURE 4.7 Data Warehouse Architecture

of freeform text rather than standardized fields with entries that are readily available for analysis. Many record systems use traditional physician dictation that is transcribed and then uploaded into the record as the method of recording clinical information. Some record systems, however, provide templates for data entry, allowing a practitioner to select from lists of potential entries to document an encounter. Templates can often be customized to accommodate a practitioner's workflow to facilitate a natural sequence for recording information from an encounter. A number of electronic medical record programs provide the ability to customize templates for this purpose, and creation of templates can be of tremendous benefit to making clinical data analysis doable.

■ Analysis Packages

A multitude of statistical analysis packages can be used for analyzing quality improvement data, but several features are important for these analyses:

- Capable of analyzing numeric or text data
- Ability to create specialized quality improvement graphics (e.g., control charts)

- Ability to perform the most common statistical analyses for quality improvement:
  - Analysis of Variance (ANOVA)
  - Regression analysis
  - Descriptive statistics
  - Power analysis
  - Design of experiments (DOE)
  - Capability analysis (Cp, Cpk, Ppk)
  - Time series
  - Chi-squared tests
  - *t*-Tests

Statistical packages can be freestanding or integrated with other programs, such as spreadsheet software. The primary shortcoming of spreadsheet programs arises when large data sets must be analyzed, but many add-ins have been written for programs like Microsoft Excel that perform well in a large number of medical applications. A list of programs commonly used in medical settings is provided in TABLE 4.3.

Statistical packages can help by applying techniques like *predictive modeling* and *data mining* to find patterns in large data sets. Predictive modeling is a statistical approach to identifying high-risk patients from historical utilization data (e.g., claims data from insurance companies or drug utilization data from pharmacy benefit management companies). The predictive modeling approach uses these electronic data sources to prognosticate the likelihood of future use of resources based on utilization trends from other patient experience. Perhaps the most common application of predictive modeling is identification of potentially high cost members of health plans for earlier preventive care interventions as a way of reducing future deterioration in health status that leads to higher costs and greater disability. Predictive modeling relies heavily on insurance and pharmacy data but soon could also rely on EHR data.

Another approach, data mining, is also showing promise for evaluating large data sets. Data mining identifies trends within data that may surpass traditional statistical analysis. Algorithms have been developed in software packages that help analysts identify key attributes within a data set that can be used to better understand processes and target opportunities for improvement. The algorithms are not perfect,

Table 4.3	Commonly Used Analytic Programs	
Program	Type	Link
SAS	Statistical programming system	www.sas.com
SPSS	Statistical programming system	www.spss.com
Minitab	Statistical programming system	www.minitab.com
QI Macros	Excel add-in	www.qimacros.com

however, and data mining analyses may yield false positives or no useful results at all. The approach is not new in the business world; for many years businesses have used powerful computers to sift through large volumes of data, such as grocery purchases, for market research. As more sophisticated computers have become ubiquitous, application of data mining to other data sets has become more feasible. Two techniques are typically used in data mining: knowledge discovery and prediction. Knowledge discovery provides explicit information in readable form that can be readily understood by users. Data mining can also be used to forecast future outcomes based on past data, much like predictive modeling. Both of these data mining techniques may use artificial intelligence procedures like rules engines, knowledge bases, or neural networks to perform the analysis. Moreover, some data-mining systems such as neural networks are inherently geared toward prediction and pattern recognition rather than knowledge discovery. More information regarding the use of data mining in health care can be found in the Additional Resources.

■ Summary

Nowhere in the healthcare system is data analysis more important than in quality management. One of the major challenges that quality improvement professionals face is gathering data for analysis, but the growing field of medical informatics is laying the foundation for better clinical data availability, and the ability to use the data effectively will create great opportunities for the healthcare system in the future. Statistical packages that perform predictive modeling and sophisticated data-mining programs can help find patterns of care that may create unsafe conditions for patient care, focusing improvement efforts more specifically and effectively. Using these advanced tools, the healthcare industry might finally be able to deliver on the promise of managing what is measured.

■ Discussion Questions

1. Explain the Donabedian model of performance improvement in health care. How does the model impact the work of the quality improvement professional?
2. Explain the difference between structure, process, and outcome measures. Give examples of these types of measures from your experience. How did you use these variables to improve your workplace?
3. Why is increased efficiency so important in health care? What business and societal factors have impacted the need for greater efficiency?

4. What three features must any quality metric possess? Explain each of these three features for a common measure used in healthcare systems: providing beta blocker therapy after a myocardial infarction (heart attack).
5. What is activity-based costing? How is it relevant to process analysis?
6. Under which domain do compliance measures fall? Why are compliance measures important to healthcare organizations?
7. Customer satisfaction measures have become much more important to healthcare organizations in recent years. Why are these measures important? How do organizations determine their performance relative to competitors?
8. What is CAHPS? Discuss the origins and advantages for using CAHPS.
9. Provide examples of clinical outcome measures. Why are these measures important for improving clinical care? What are the important features of effective outcome measures?
10. What is a clinical microsystem? Why is an understanding of clinical microsystems important as a basis for improving clinical care?
11. Define the concept of the EHR. How are EHR systems at the heart of a clinical improvement system?
12. How is a data warehouse used in a healthcare quality system? What features of a data warehouse make it valuable to a quality improvement practitioner?
13. Differentiate between predictive modeling and data mining. How are these approaches applied in a healthcare quality review system?

■ References

1. Health Informatics. Retrieved October 2008 from http://en.wikipedia.org/wiki/Medical_informatics
2. Donabedian A. The quality of medical care. *Science*. 1978;4344:856–864.
3. LaPointe N, Jollis J. Medication errors in hospitalized cardiovascular patients. *Archives of Internal Medicine*. 2003;163:1461–1466.
4. Two patients sue Stanford's Medical Center over objects left in after surgery. *San Jose Mercury News*, April 30, 2002. Retrieved October 2008 from http://www.highbeam.com/doc/1G1-120443059.html
5. Kaushal R, Bates D, Landrigan C, et al. Medication errors and adverse drug events in pediatric inpatients. *JAMA*. 2001;285:2114–2120.
6. CAHPS: Assessing healthcare quality from the patient's perspective. Retrieved October 2008 from https://www.cahps.ahrq.gov/content/cahpsOverview/CAHPS-ProgramBrief.htm
7. Clinical microsystems. Retrieved November 2008 from http://dms.dartmouth.edu/cms
8. DesRoches CM, Campbell EG, Rao SR, et al. Electronic health records in ambulatory care—A national survey of physicians. *New England Journal of Medicine*. 2008;339:50–60.
9. Certifying Commission on Health Information Technology (CCHIT). Incentive programs for EHR adoption growing—Certification Commission's research finds over $700 million in funding. Retrieved November 2008 from http://www.cchit.org/about/news/releases/2008/Incentive-programs-EHR-adoption-growing.asp

10. MITRE Center for Enterprise Modernization. Electronic health records overview. Retrieved November 2008 from http://www.ncrr.nih.gov/publications/informatics/EHR.pdf
11. Health Level 7. Retrieved November 2008 from http://www.hl7.org

■ Additional Resources

Medical Informatics Training Programs

National Library of Medicine training sites in United States:

- Harvard University
- New England Medical Center
- University of Pittsburgh
- Stanford University
- Yale University
- Duke University–University of North Carolina
- Oregon Health Sciences University
- Rice-Baylor University
- University of Missouri
- Columbia University
- University of Minnesota

Other U.S. programs:

- Vanderbilt University Medical School
- Johns Hopkins University
- University of Utah
- University of Alabama
- University of Washington
- University of Pennsylvania
- Philadelphia Veterans Administration Medical Center

Programs Outside the United States:

- Victoria (Canada)
- Geneva (Switzerland)
- Heidelberg/Heilbronn (Germany)
- Hildesheim (Germany)
- Luebeck (Germany)
- Manchester (United Kingdom)
- Campinas (Brazil)

Activity Based Costing Resources

Baker J. *Activity-based Costing and Activity-based Management for Health Care*. Gaithersburg, MD: Aspen Publishers; 1998.

McLean R. *Financial Management in Health Care Organizations*. Florence, KY: Delmar Cengage Learning; 2002.

AHRQ National Quality Measures Clearinghouse Measures

Agency for Healthcare Research and Quality. National Quality Measures Clearinghouse. About NQMC. Retrieved October 2008 from http://www.qualitymeasures.ahrq.gov/about/about. aspx

Agency for Healthcare Research and Quality. National Quality Measures Clearinghouse. About NQMC— Inclusion criteria. Retrieved October 2008 from http://www.qualitymeasures.ahrq.gov/about/inclusion.aspx

Agency for Healthcare Research and Quality. National Quality Measures Clearinghouse. Glossary. Retrieved October 2008 from http://www.qualitymeasures.org/resources/glossary.aspx

Agency for Healthcare Research and Quality. National Quality Measures Clearinghouse. Using the measures. Retrieved October 2008 from http://www.quality measures.ahrq.gov/resources/measure_use.aspx

American Medical Association Performance Improvement Resources

American Medical Association. Work groups. Retrieved October 2008 from http://www.ama-assn.org/ama/put/category/print/3106.html

American Medical Association. Physician Consortium for Performance Improvement. Retrieved October 2008 from http://www.ama-assn.org/ama/pub/category/print/2946.htm

National Quality Forum

The National Quality Forum's Consensus Development Process. Version 1.7. August 20, 2004. Retrieved October 2008 from http://www.qualityforum.org

Other Websites

AHRQ Innovations Exchange: http://www.innovations.ahrq.gov/

AHRQ National Clinical Guideline Clearinghouse: http://www.guideline.gov

Institute for Clinical Systems Improvement (ICSI): http://www.icsi.org

Institute for Healthcare Improvement (IHI): http://www.ihi.org

Intermountain Healthcare: http://www.intermountainhealthcare.org

Online Statistical Textbooks

StatSoft Electronic Textbook: http://www.statsoft.com/textbook/stathome.html

Hyperstat Online Statistical Textbook: http://davidmlane.com/hyperstat/

UCLA Probability and Statistics E-Text: http://wiki.stat.ucla.edu/socr/index.php/EBook

NIST Engineering Statistics: http://www.itl.nist.gov/div898/handbook/

Online Statistics: An Interactive Multimedia Course of Study: http://onlinestatbook.com/

Data Mining Resources

Chen H, Fuller S, eds. *Medical Informatics: Knowledge Management and Data Mining in Biomedicine.* New York: Springer-Verlag; 2005.

Lawrence K, Kudyba S, Klimberg R. *Data Mining Methods and Applications.* Pennsauken, NJ: Auerbach Publications; 2007.

Lenk Schilp J, Gilbreath R. *Health Data Quest: How to Find and Use Data for Performance Improvement.* San Francisco, CA: Jossey-Bass; 2000.

CAHPS® Clinician & Group Survey

Child Primary Care Questionnaire

[English Version]

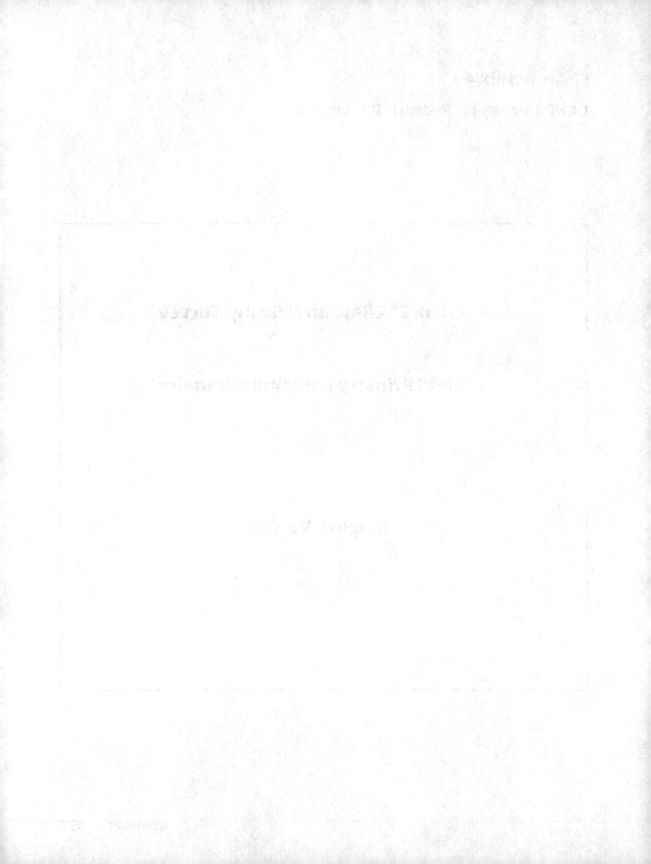

SURVEY INSTRUCTIONS

- ◆ Answer <u>all</u> the questions by checking the box to the left of your answer.
- ◆ You are sometimes told to skip over some questions in this survey. When this happens you will see an arrow with a note that tells you what question to answer next, like this:

☐ Yes → *If Yes, Go to Question 1 on Page 1*
☐ No

All information that would let someone identify you or your family will be kept private. {VENDOR NAME} will not share your personal information with anyone without your OK. You may choose to answer this survey or not. If you choose not to, this will not affect the health care you get.

*Your responses to this survey are completely **confidential**. Once you complete the survey, place it in the envelope that was provided, seal the envelope, and return the envelope to [INSERT VENDOR ADDRESS].*

*You may notice a number on the cover of this survey. This number is **only** used to let us know if you returned your survey so we don't have to send you reminders.*

If you want to know more about this study, please call XXX-XXX-XXXX.

About the Never/Always Response Scale

This survey employs a six-point response scale — "Never/Almost Never/Sometimes/Usually/ Almost Always/Always" — rather than the more common CAHPS four-point response scale of "Never/Sometimes/ Usually/Always." This expanded scale, which was tested by several early adopters of the survey, is recommended by the CAHPS Consortium.

Survey sponsors have the option of substituting the four-point scale. The Agency for Healthcare Research & Quality requests that users of the shorter scale notify the CAHPS User Network (cahps1@ahrq.gov) so that the Consortium can continue to examine the performance of the two response scales in the context of this survey.

Please answer the questions for the child listed on the envelope. Please do not answer for any other children.

YOUR CHILD'S DOCTOR

---

1. Our records show that your child got care from the doctor named below in the last 12 months.

   NAME OF DOCTOR LABEL GOES HERE

   Is that right?

   [1]☐ Yes → **If Yes, Go to Question 2**

   [2]☐ No → **If No, Go to Question 26**

   The questions in this survey booklet will refer to the doctor named in Question 1 as "this doctor." Please think of that doctor as you answer the survey.

2. Is this the doctor you usually see if your child needs a check-up or gets sick or hurt?

   [1]☐ Yes

   [2]☐ No

3. How long has your child been going to this doctor?

   [1]☐ Less than 6 months

   [2]☐ At least 6 months but less than 1 year

   [3]☐ At least 1 year but less than 3 years

   [4]☐ At least 3 years but less than 5 years

   [5]☐ 5 years or more

YOUR CHILD'S CARE FROM THIS DOCTOR IN THE LAST 12 MONTHS

These questions ask about <u>your child's</u> health care. Do <u>not</u> include care your child got when he or she stayed overnight in a hospital. Do <u>not</u> include the times your child went for dental care visits.

4. In the last 12 months, how many times did your child visit this doctor for care?

   $^1\square$ None → **If None, Go to Question 26**

   $^2\square$ 1 time

   $^3\square$ 2

   $^4\square$ 3

   $^5\square$ 4

   $^6\square$ 5 to 9

   $^7\square$ 10 or more times

5. In the last 12 months, did you phone this doctor's office to get an appointment for your child for an illness, injury or condition that <u>needed care right away</u>?

   $^1\square$ Yes

   $^2\square$ No → **If No, Go to Question 7**

6. In the last 12 months, when you phoned this doctor's office to get an appointment for <u>care your child needed right away</u> how often did you get an appointment as soon as you thought your child needed?

   $^1\square$ Never

   $^2\square$ Almost Never

   $^3\square$ Sometimes

   $^4\square$ Usually

   $^5\square$ Almost Always

   $^6\square$ Always

7. In the last 12 months, did you make any appointments for a <u>check-up or routine care</u> for your child with this doctor?

   $^1\square$ Yes

   $^2\square$ No → **If No, Go to Question 9**

8. In the last 12 months, when you made an appointment for a <u>check-up or routine care</u> for your child with this doctor, how often did you get an appointment as soon as you thought your child needed?

   $^1\square$ Never

   $^2\square$ Almost Never

   $^3\square$ Sometimes

   $^4\square$ Usually

^{5}☐ Almost Always

^{6}☐ Always

9. In the last 12 months, did you phone this doctor's office with a medical question about your child <u>during</u> regular office hours?

   ^{1}☐ Yes

   ^{2}☐ No → **If No, Go to Question 11**

10. In the last 12 months, when you phoned this doctor's office during regular office hours, how often did you get an answer to your medical question that same day?

    ^{1}☐ Never

    ^{2}☐ Almost Never

    ^{3}☐ Sometimes

    ^{4}☐ Usually

    ^{5}☐ Almost Always

    ^{6}☐ Always

11. In the last 12 months, did you phone this doctor's office with a medical question about your child <u>after</u> regular office hours?

    ^{1}☐ Yes

    ^{2}☐ No → **If No, Go to Question 13**

12. In the last 12 months, when you phoned this doctor's office after regular office hours, how often did you get an answer to your medical question as soon as you needed?

    ^{1}☐ Never

    ^{2}☐ Almost Never

    ^{3}☐ Sometimes

    ^{4}☐ Usually

    ^{5}☐ Almost Always

    ^{6}☐ Always

13. Wait time includes time spent in the waiting room and exam room. In the last 12 months, how often did your child see this doctor <u>within 15 minutes</u> of his or her appointment time?

    ^{1}☐ Never

    ^{2}☐ Almost Never

$^3\square$ Sometimes

$^4\square$ Usually

$^5\square$ Almost Always

$^6\square$ Always

14. **In the last 12 months, how often did this doctor explain things about your child's health in a way that was easy to understand?**

$^1\square$ Never

$^2\square$ Almost Never

$^3\square$ Sometimes

$^4\square$ Usually

$^5\square$ Almost Always

$^6\square$ Always

15. **In the last 12 months, how often did this doctor listen carefully to you?**

$^1\square$ Never

$^2\square$ Almost Never

$^3\square$ Sometimes

$^4\square$ Usually

$^5\square$ Almost Always

$^6\square$ Always

16. **In the last 12 months, did you talk with this doctor about any problems or concerns you had about your child's health?**

$^1\square$ Yes

$^2\square$ No → **If No, Go to Question 18**

17. **In the last 12 months, how often did this doctor give you easy to understand instructions about taking care of these health problems or concerns?**

$^1\square$ Never

$^2\square$ Almost Never

$^3\square$ Sometimes

$^4\square$ Usually

$^5\square$ Almost Always

$^6\square$ Always

18. **In the last 12 months, how often did this doctor seem to know the important information about your child's medical history?**

   ¹☐ Never

   ²☐ Almost Never

   ³☐ Sometimes

   ⁴☐ Usually

   ⁵☐ Almost Always

   ⁶☐ Always

19. **In the last 12 months, how often did this doctor show respect for what you had to say?**

   ¹☐ Never

   ²☐ Almost Never

   ³☐ Sometimes

   ⁴☐ Usually

   ⁵☐ Almost Always

   ⁶☐ Always

20. **In the last 12 months, how often did this doctor spend enough time with your child?**

   ¹☐ Never

   ²☐ Almost Never

   ³☐ Sometimes

   ⁴☐ Usually

   ⁵☐ Almost Always

   ⁶☐ Always

21. **In the last 12 months, did this doctor order a blood test, x-ray, or other test for your child?**

   ¹☐ Yes

   ²☐ No → **If No, Go to Question 23**

22. **In the last 12 months, when this doctor ordered a blood test, x-ray, or other test for your child, how often did someone from this doctor's office follow up to give you those results?**

   ¹☐ Never

   ²☐ Almost Never

3☐ Sometimes

4☐ Usually

5☐ Almost Always

6☐ Always

23. **Using any number from 0 to 10, where 0 is the worst doctor possible and 10 is the best doctor possible, what number would you use to rate this doctor?**

0 ☐ 0 Worst doctor possible

1 ☐ 1

2 ☐ 2

3 ☐ 3

4 ☐ 4

5 ☐ 5

6 ☐ 6

7 ☐ 7

8 ☐ 8

9 ☐ 9

10 ☐ 10 Best doctor possible

CLERKS AND RECEPTIONISTS AT THIS
DOCTOR'S OFFICE

---

24. **In the last 12 months, how often were clerks and receptionists at this doctor's office as helpful as you thought they should be?**

1☐ Never

2☐ Almost Never

3☐ Sometimes

4☐ Usually

5☐ Almost Always

6☐ Always

25. **In the last 12 months, how often did clerks and receptionists at this doctor's office treat you with courtesy and respect?**

1☐ Never

2☐ Almost Never

$^3\square$ Sometimes

$^4\square$ Usually

$^5\square$ Almost Always

$^6\square$ Always

ABOUT YOUR CHILD AND YOU

---

26. **In general, how would you rate your child's overall health?**
    $^1\square$ Excellent

    $^2\square$ Very Good

    $^3\square$ Good

    $^4\square$ Fair

    $^5\square$ Poor

27. **What is your child's age?**
    $^1\square$ Less than 1 year old

    _____ YEARS OLD *(write in)*

28. **Is your child male or female?**
    $^1\square$ Male

    $^2\square$ Female

29. **Is your child of Hispanic or Latino origin or descent?**
    $^1\square$ Yes, Hispanic or Latino

    $^2\square$ No, not Hispanic or Latino

30. **What is your child's race? Please mark one or more.**
    $^1\square$ White

    $^2\square$ Black or African-American

    $^3\square$ Asian

    $^4\square$ Native Hawaiian or other Pacific Islander

    $^5\square$ American Indian or Alaska Native

    $^6\square$ Other

31. **What is your age?**
    0☐ Under 18
    1☐ 18 to 24
    2☐ 25 to 34
    3☐ 35 to 44
    4☐ 45 to 54
    5☐ 55 to 64
    6☐ 65 to 74
    7☐ 75 or older

32. **Are you male or female?**
    1☐ Male
    2☐ Female

33. **What is the highest grade or level of school that you have completed?**
    1☐ 8th grade or less
    2☐ Some high school, but did not graduate
    3☐ High school graduate or GED
    4☐ Some college or 2-year degree
    5☐ 4-year college graduate
    6☐ More than 4-year college degree

34. **How are you related to the child?**
    1☐ Mother or father
    2☐ Grandparent
    3☐ Aunt or uncle
    4☐ Older brother or sister
    5☐ Other relative
    6☐ Legal guardian
    7☐ Someone else
    (Please print)

    _____

35. **Did someone help you complete this survey?**
    1☐ Yes
    2☐ **No → Thank you. Please return the completed survey in the postage-paid envelope.**

36. **How did that person help you? Mark all that apply.**

   $^1\square$ Read the questions to me

   $^2\square$ Wrote down the answers I gave

   $^3\square$ Answered the questions for me

   $^4\square$ Translated the questions into my language

   $^5\square$ Helped in some other way

   (Please print)

   _____

   _____

THANK YOU

Please return the completed survey in the postage-paid envelope

CAHPS Clinician & Group Survey – Child Primary Care Questionnaire
Supplemental Items

Doctor Communication With Child

Insert DC1-DC4 after core question 20.

DC1. Is your child able to talk with doctors about his or her health care?
- 1 ☐ Yes
- 2 ☐ No → If No, Go to Core Question 21

DC2. In the last 12 months, how often did this doctor explain things in a way that was easy for <u>your child</u> to understand?
- 1 ☐ Never
- 2 ☐ Almost Never
- 3 ☐ Sometimes
- 4 ☐ Usually
- 5 ☐ Almost Always
- 6 ☐ Always

DC3. In the last 12 months, how often did this doctor encourage your child to ask questions?
- 1 ☐ Never
- 2 ☐ Almost Never
- 3 ☐ Sometimes
- 4 ☐ Usually
- 5 ☐ Almost Always
- 6 ☐ Always

DC4. In the last 12 months, how often did this doctor listen carefully to <u>your child?</u>

1☐ Never
2☐ Almost Never
3☐ Sometimes
4☐ Usually
5☐ Almost Always
6☐ Always

Doctor Thoroughness

Insert DT1-DT2 before core question 21.

DT1. In the last 12 months, did this doctor ever examine your child?

1☐ Yes
2☐ No → If No, Go to Core Question 21

DT2. In the last 12 months, how often was this doctor as thorough as you thought your child needed?

1☐ Never
2☐ Almost Never
3☐ Sometimes
4☐ Usually
5☐ Almost Always
6☐ Always

Health Improvement

Insert HI1 after core question 17.

HI1. In the last 12 months, did you and this doctor talk about specific things you could do to prevent illness in your child?

1☐ Yes
2☐ No

Prescription Medicines

Insert PM1 after core question 20.

PM1. In the last 12 months, did this doctor talk with you about all of the prescription medicines your child was taking?

$^1\square$ Yes

$^2\square$ No

Provider Knowledge of Specialist Care

Insert PK1-PK2 after core question 20. Note: These items are recommended for use only if the sampled provider is not a specialist.

PK1. Specialists are doctors like surgeons, heart doctors, allergy doctors, skin doctors, and other doctors who specialize in one area of health care. In the last 12 months, did this doctor suggest your child see a specialist for a particular health problem?

$^1\square$ Yes

$^2\square$ No → **If No, Go to Core Question 21**

PK2. In the last 12 months, how often did the doctor named in Question 1 seem informed and up-to-date about the care your child got from specialists?

$^1\square$ Never

$^2\square$ Almost Never

$^3\square$ Sometimes

$^4\square$ Usually

$^5\square$ Almost Always

$^6\square$ Always

Scheduling Appointments and Contacting This Doctor

Insert SA1-SA2 after core question 12.

SA1. After hours care is health care when your child's usual doctor's office or clinic is closed. In the last 12 months, did you try to get any after hours care for your child at this doctor's office?

$^1\square$ Yes

$^2\square$ No → **If No, Go to Core Question 13**

SA2. In the last 12 months, did the after hours care available from this doctor's office meet your needs?

$^1\square$ Yes

$^2\square$ No

Shared Decision Making

Insert SD1-SD4 before core question 21.

SD1. Choices for your child's treatment or health care can include choices about medicine, surgery, or other treatment. In the last 12 months, did this doctor tell you there was more than one choice for your child's treatment or health care?

$^1\square$ Yes

$^2\square$ No → **If No, Go to Core Question 21**

SD2. In the last 12 months, did this doctor talk with you about the pros and cons of each choice for your child's treatment or health care?

$^1\square$ Yes

$^2\square$ No

SD3. In the last 12 months, did this doctor give you enough information about each choice?

$^1\square$ Yes

$^2\square$ No

SD4. In the last 12 months, when there was more than one choice for your child's treatment or health care, did this doctor ask which choice you thought was best for your child?

$^1\square$ Yes

$^2\square$ No

Child CAHPS Survey available at http://www.ahrq.gov/chtoolbx/measure2.htm

Table 4A.2.1 — HEDIS 2009 Measures

Measure	Application		
	Commercial	Medicaid	Medicare
Effectiveness of Care			
Guidelines for Effectiveness of Care Measures	☐	☐	☐
Adult BMI Assessment	☐	☐	☐
Weight Assessment and Counseling for Nutrition and Physical Activity for Children/Adolescents	☐	☐	
Childhood Immunization Status	☐	☐	
Lead Screening in Children		☐	
Breast Cancer Screening	☐	☐	☐
Cervical Cancer Screening	☐	☐	
Colorectal Cancer Screening	☐		☐
Chlamydia Screening in Women	☐	☐	
Glaucoma Screening in Older Adults			☐
Care for Older Adults			☐
Appropriate Testing for Children With Pharyngitis	☐	☐	
Appropriate Treatment for Children With Upper Respiratory Infection	☐	☐	
Avoidance of Antibiotic Treatment in Adults With Acute Bronchitis	☐	☐	
Use of Spirometry Testing in the Assessment and Diagnosis of COPD	☐	☐	☐
Pharmacotherapy of COPD Exacerbation	☐	☐	☐
Use of Appropriate Medications for People With Asthma	☐	☐	
Cholesterol Management for Patients With Cardiovascular Conditions	☐	☐	☐
Controlling High Blood Pressure	☐	☐	☐
Persistence of Beta-Blocker Treatment After a Heart Attack	☐	☐	☐
Comprehensive Diabetes Care	☐	☐	☐
Disease-Modifying Anti-Rheumatic Drug Therapy for Rheumatoid Arthritis	☐	☐	☐
Osteoporosis Management in Women Who Had a Fracture			☐
Use of Imaging Studies for Low Back Pain	☐	☐	
Antidepressant Medication Management	☐	☐	☐

Continues

Table 4A.2.1	HEDIS 2009 Measures (continued)		
	Application		
Measure	Commercial	Medicaid	Medicare
Follow-Up Care for Children Prescribed ADHD Medication	☐	☐	
Follow-Up After Hospitalization for Mental Illness	☐	☐	☐
Annual Monitoring for Patients on Persistent Medications	☐	☐	☐
Medication Reconciliation Post-Discharge			☐
Potentially Harmful Drug-Disease Interactions in the Elderly			☐
Use of High-Risk Medications in the Elderly			☐
Management of Urinary Incontinence in Older Adults			☐
Osteoporosis Testing in Older Women			☐
Physical Activity in Older Adults			☐
Flu Shots for Adults Ages 50–64	☐		
Flu Shots for Older Adults			☐
Medical Assistance With Smoking Cessation	☐	☐	☐
Pneumonia Vaccination Status for Older Adults			☐
Access/Availability of Care			
Adults' Access to Preventive/ Ambulatory Health Services	☐	☐	☐
Children's and Adolescents' Access to Primary Care Practitioners	☐	☐	
Annual Dental Visit		☐	
Initiation and Engagement of Alcohol and Other Drug Dependence Treatment	☐	☐	☐
Prenatal and Postpartum Care	☐	☐	
Call Abandonment	☐	☐	☐
Call Answer Timeliness	☐	☐	☐
Satisfaction With Experience of Care			
CAHPS Health Plan Survey 4.0H, Adult Version	☐	☐	
CAHPS Health Plan Survey 4.0H, Child Version	☐	☐	
Children With Chronic Conditions	☐	☐	
Use of Services			
Guidelines for Use of Services Measures	☐	☐	☐
Frequency of Ongoing Prenatal Care		☐	

Table 4A.2.1	HEDIS 2009 Measures (continued)		
		Application	
Measure	Commercial	Medicaid	Medicare
Well-Child Visits in the Third, Fourth, Fifth and Sixth Years of Life	☐	☐	
Adolescent Well Care Visits	☐	☐	
Frequency of Selected Procedures	☐	☐	☐
Ambulatory Care	☐	☐	☐
Inpatient Utilization-General Hospital/Acute Care	☐	☐	
Inpatient Utilization-Nonacute Care	☐	☐	☐
Identification of Alcohol and Other Drug Services	☐	☐	☐
Mental Health Utilization	☐	☐	☐
Antibiotic Utilization	☐	☐	☐
Outpatient Drug Utilization	☐	☐	☐
Cost of Care			
Guidelines for Cost of Care Measures	☐	☐	☐
Relative Resource Use for People With Diabetes	☐	☐	☐
Relative Resource Use for People With Asthma	☐	☐	
Relative Resource Use for People With Acute Low Back Pain	☐	☐	
Relative Resource Use for People With Cardiovascular Conditions	☐	☐	☐
Relative Resource Use for People With Uncomplicated Hypertension	☐	☐	☐
Relative Resource Use for People With COPD	☐	☐	☐
Health Plan Stability			
Board Certification	☐	☐	☐
Enrollment by Product Line	☐	☐	☐
Enrollment by State	☐	☐	☐
Language Diversity of Membership		☐	☐
Race/Ethnicity Diversity of Membership		☐	☐
Weeks of Pregnancy at Time of Enrollment		☐	☐
Health Plan Descriptive Information			
Years in Business/Total Membership	☐	☐	☐

Table 4A.2.2	Specialty Societies Involved in Measure Development and Reporting

- Professional Societies Measurement Development
- Alliance for Academic Internal Medicine
- American Academy of Family Physicians
- American Academy of Neurology
- American Academy of Ophthalmology
- American Academy of Orthopedic Surgeons
- American Academy of Otolaryngology
- American Academy of Pediatrics
- American Association for the Study of Liver Diseases
- American Association of Neurological Surgeons
- American College of Cardiology
- American College of Physicians
- American College of Rheumatology
- American College of Surgeons
- American Diabetes Association
- American Gastroenterological Association
- American Society for Bone and Mineral Research
- American Society for Gastrointestinal Endoscopy
- American Society of Clinical Oncology
- American Society of Echocardiography
- American Society of Nephrology
- American Thoracic Society
- Child Neurology Society
- Clinical Orthopaedic Society
- Congress of Neurological Surgeons
- Infectious Disease Society of America
- National Kidney Foundation
- Renal Physicians Association
- Society of Adolescent Medicine
- Society of Critical Care Medicine
- Society of Hospital Medicine
- Society of Thoracic Surgery

Source: Ferris TG, Vogeli C, Marder J, Sennett CS, Campbell Eb. Physician speciality societies and the development of physician performance measures. *Health Affairs.* 2007;26:1712–1719.

Economists generally divide economic activities into "macro-" and "micro-" economic systems. Macroeconomic systems encompass the broadest level of economic activity (e.g., the U.S. economy or the world economy). Microsystems deal with the economics of the firm (i.e., the business activities of individual businesses or business segments). The healthcare system can be viewed as a macroeconomic system, whereas the *individual entities* within its segments (i.e., insurers, providers, hospitals, pharmaceuticals, suppliers) are considered microeconomic systems. A great deal of effort has been expended in the past 30 to 40 years to create data resources for each of these components of the healthcare system, and because Medicare and Medicaid comprise the largest segments of payers, it is not surprising that the federal government publishes a number of data resources from its billing data:

■ Appendix 4.2

Sources for Benchmarking Data and Operational Definitions

Performance measures are developed by a variety of sources that consist of accrediting bodies, the federal government through the Centers for Medicare and Medicaid Services, medical societies, and other private entities. Some of these efforts are listed here:

- *AMA Physicians' Consortium for Performance Improvement* (http://www.ama-assn.org/ama/pub/category/4837.html): The consortium consists of subject matter experts, physicians, and experts in metric development convened by the American Medical Association (AMA) as a representative of national medical specialty and state medical societies, the Agency for Healthcare Research and Quality (AHRQ), and the Centers for Medicare and Medicaid Services (CMS). The consortium develops evidence-based clinical performance measures and clinical outcomes reporting tools from clinical guidelines for select conditions to support physicians in quality improvement efforts. CMS and other organizations work with the consortium to develop performance measures that are acceptable to physicians.

- *National Quality Forum* (NQF, www.qualityforum.org): A voluntary standards-setting organization that relies on consensus to create and recommend metrics. The organization endorses standards, including performance measures, quality indicators, preferred practices, and reporting guidelines using input from a variety of industry stakeholders. The NQF process starts with evidence-based metrics, and then the organization works to gain consensus from a multitude of stakeholders, but failure to gain complete consensus does not prevent adoption of valuable metrics. For example, some measures that do not have provider support have become NQF endorsed if they gain support of other member groups (health plans, consumers, and others). CMS generally adopts all measures developed by NQF, and so every effort is made to gain broad consensus.

- *National Quality Measures Clearinghouse* (NQMC, www.qualitymeasures.ahrq. gov): A website database, sponsored by AHRQ and the Department of Health and Human Services, that contains specific evidence-based healthcare quality measures and measure sets. The site is open to everyone and allows widespread access to quality measures by the healthcare community and other interested individuals. Any organization may contribute to the site, and any measures submitted are reviewed by AHRQ experts to ensure a level of rigor to ensure usability. NQMC's mission is to provide practitioners, healthcare providers, health plans, integrated delivery systems, purchasers, and others with access to detailed information on quality measures, and to further dissemination, implementation, and use to inform healthcare decisions.
- *The Joint Commission* (www.jcaho.org): The Joint Commission provides accreditation to healthcare organizations around the world, and as part of the accreditation process. The Joint Commission requires quality improvement activities and has developed sets of core measures, called ORYX measures, that must be reported. These measure sets for hospitals include:
  - Acute myocardial infarction (AMI)
  - Heart failure (HF)
  - Pneumonia (PN)
  - Pregnancy and related conditions (PR)
  - Hospital-based inpatient psychiatric services (HBIPS) (Starting with October 1, 2008 discharges)
  - Children's asthma care (CAC)
  - Surgical Care Improvement project (SCIP)
  - Hospital outpatient measures (HOP)

Hospitals must report four sets of measures to be accredited, and data for all applicable measures must be submitted through a performance measurement system evaluated and approved by The Joint Commission.

- *National Committee for Quality Assurance* (www.ncqa.org): This organization was an early adopter of performance metrics for healthcare payers through its Healthcare Effectiveness Data Information Set (HEDIS). These measures were initially used to evaluate Health Maintenance Organizations (HMOs) but have since been used in a variety of settings. A list of HEDIS measures for 2009 is included in TABLE 4A.2.1, and, as is evident, the metrics involve performance of network providers as well as health plans. For example, immunization rates may be considered a process outcome measure reflecting both the effectiveness of the provider and the health plan in promoting immunizations among target populations.
- *Medical Specialty Societies and Trade Organizations:* Some medical specialty societies and trade organizations have developed performance measures for their

respective areas of practice. Most of these organizations, however, are actively involved in other organizations (e.g., NQF and The Joint Commission) to help create specific measures. Some of these representative organizations are included in TABLE 4A.2.2.

- *Medicare data sources:*
  - Medicare utilization and quality data home page
    - Site: http://www.cms.hhs.gov/home/rsds.asp
    - Information resources: Portal to all Medicare utilization and quality data for research and statistical analysis

  - MEDPAR data set
    - Site: http://www.cms.hhs.gov/IdentifiableDataFiles/05_Medicare Provider Analysisand Review File.asp
    - Information resources:

      - Claims data for services provided to beneficiaries admitted to Medicare certified inpatient hospitals and skilled nursing facilities (SNF), including accumulation of claims from a beneficiary's date of admission to an inpatient hospital, where the beneficiary has been discharged, or to a SNF, where the beneficiary may still be a patient. Beginning in 1999, Managed Care Organization (MCO) bills were excluded.
      - Records include beneficiary demographic characteristics, diagnosis and surgery information, use of hospital or SNF resources (including detailed accommodation and departmental charge data, days of care, and entitlement data).
      - Death information is appended up to 3 years after date of discharge, which is useful for research into chronic disease outcomes in the elderly population.

  - Medicare Data Compendium
    - Site: http://www.cms.hhs.gov/DataCompendium/
    - Data resources:

      - Key historic, current, and projected statistics about CMS programs and healthcare spending. The tables are in Adobe or Excel files and provide expert analysis of the data CMS collects each year about its programs and the nation's healthcare system.
      - Data pertaining to budget, administrative and operating costs, individual income, financing, and healthcare providers and suppliers.
      - National data not specific to the Medicare or Medicaid programs may also be found throughout the publications.

- Medicare Current Beneficiary Survey
  - Site: http://www.cms.hhs.gov/MCBS/
  - Data resources:

    - Continuous, multipurpose survey of a nationally representative sample of aged, disabled, and institutionalized Medicare beneficiaries; it is the only comprehensive source of information on the health status, healthcare use and expenditures, health insurance coverage, and socioeconomic and demographic characteristics of the entire spectrum of Medicare beneficiaries.

- Medicare Cost Reports
  - Site: http://www.cms.hhs.gov/CostReports/
  - Data resources:

    - Data reported to the Healthcare Cost Report Information System (HCRIS) by Medicare Fiscal Intermediaries. Because the data come from fiscal intermediaries, CMS does not guarantee accuracy but does state that "authenticated information is only accurate as of the point in time of validation and verification."
    - Data files are available for hospitals, SNFs, renal facilities, hospice agencies, and home health agencies. Data are also available by fiscal year.

- Identifiable Data Files
  - Site: http://www.cms.hhs.gov/IdentifiableDataFiles/
  - Alternative site: http://www.resdac.umn.edu/Medicare/data_available.asp, the University of Minnesota Research Data Assistance Center (ResDAC), which processes requests for identifiable data files and extracts of Medicare data sets with individually identifiable data.
  - Data resources:

    - Beneficiary-specific and physician-specific information files which contain numerous claims and clinical data fields. Because the information in the files can identify individuals, access to the data requires a formal request to CMS, usually submitted through ResDAC.
    - Standard Analytical Files: Final claims data are available by type of claim. Each file can be ordered from CMS as a sample file by claim type, and more information can be found on the website.
    - Hospital Outpatient Prospective Payment System (OPPS): Records include diagnosis codes, bill type, outlier payments, and service revenue payments recorded by beneficiary that may permit identification of individual beneficiaries. At the time of this writing, the file includes more than 54 million claims for services paid under the OPPS, including multiple and single claims, and it is available twice a year.

- Hospital Outpatient Prospective Payment System (OPPS) Partial Hospitalization Program (PHP): Records contain data elements such as diagnosis codes, bill type, outlier payments, and service revenue payments and includes beneficiary identifiers. Derived from hospital outpatient prospective payment system claims, the file is presently created and available twice a year.
- Denominator File: This file contains data on all Medicare beneficiaries enrolled and/or entitled in a given year and has selected data fields from the Enrollment Data Base (EDB) only for beneficiaries who were entitled during the year of the report. The file is available annually in May of the current year for the prior year.
- Name and Address and Vital Status Files: Subset of the data elements in the Enrollment Database (EDB) created by CMS according to specific requests by either (1) numeric search using a list of Health Insurance Claim (HIC) numbers or social security numbers or (2) a demographic sampling. The data set contains personal identifiers and other private material which require CMS authorization for release to researchers. The *Names and Addresses File* contains name, address, state, sex, race, date of birth, date of death, and other demographic data. The *Vital Status File* contains the same demographic data with the exception of the beneficiary name and address.
- Renal Management Information System (REMIS): The primary resource to store and access information for the End Stage Renal Disease (ESRD) Program, REMIS tracks the ESRD patient population for both Medicare and non-Medicare patients. The database also includes operational interfaces to the Medicare Beneficiary Database and to the ESRD Network Organizations' Standard Information Management System. Because the data includes individual beneficiary information, permission for access must be granted by CMS.
- Long-term Care Minimum Data Set (MDS): A standardized, primary health status screening tool used to assess physical, psychological, and psychosocial factors for all residents in a Medicare and/or Medicaid-certified long-term care facility used to identify health problems in this patient population. This data set contains extensive health status information for this patient population.
- Health Outcomes Survey (HOS): Identifiable data files with the entire national sample for a 2-year cohort (including both respondents and non-respondents) and contain all of the HOS survey items with Medicare health plan identifiers, as well as several additional variables describing health plan characteristics. These files contain specific direct person identifiers (i.e., name and health insurance claim number), but these identifiers are eliminated from certain subsets that are created for specific purposes by request.

- *Resource-Based Relative Value System (RBRVS) data*
  - Site: http://www.cms.hhs.gov/PhysicianFeeSched/PFSRVF/list.asp#
  - Information resources: Relative value unit (RVU) conversions from CPT codes; many organizations now use work RVUs (wRVUs) as the denominator in calculating clinical productivity measures. A brief description of the RBRVS reimbursement system can be found in Appendix 4.3. The RVU data files provide the latest conversion units for the RBRVS reimbursement system.

- *Medicaid Statistical Information System (MSIS)*
  - Site: http://www.cms.hhs.gov/MedicaidDataSourcesGenInfo/
  - Information resources: These tables contain high-level aggregated statistics, as well as several subsets of the data:
    - Medicaid Managed Care Enrollment Report: Data elements include plan name, managed care entity, reimbursement arrangement, operating authority, geographic area served, and number of enrollees by plan
    - Description of State Programs: Includes information about each state Medicaid program, which managed care organizations serve the population, and what quality management programs are in place.
    - Medicaid Analytic Extract (MAX) Files: A data set of person-level data files on Medicaid eligibility, service utilization, and payments extracted from the Medicaid Statistical Information System (MSIS). The MAX development process combines MSIS initial claims, interim claims, voids, and adjustments for a given service organized into annual calendar year files.
    - Statistical Compendium: Medicaid Pharmacy Benefit Use and Reimbursement: Detailed state-by-state and national data on the use of and reimbursement for prescription drugs in Medicaid.

- *AHRQ data resources*
  - Site: http://www.ahrq.gov/data/
  - Medical Expenditure Panel Survey (MEPS) (http://www.meps.ahrq.gov/mepsweb/), which started in 1996, is a series of large-scale surveys of U.S. families and individuals, their medical providers (doctors, hospitals, pharmacies, etc.), and employers. Data collected include specific health services used, frequency of use, costs of the services, method of payment, and data on the cost, scope, and breadth of health insurance coverage. Major components include:
    - Household Component: Data from members of individual households, along with data from their medical providers. Data are collected from a sample of families and individuals in selected communities across the United States, drawn from a nationally representative subsample of households that participated in the prior year's National Health Interview Survey conducted by the National Center for Health Statistics. During the household interviews, the MEP Survey gathers detailed information for each person in the household on demographic characteristics, health conditions, health status, use of

medical services, charges and source of payments, access to care, satisfaction with care, health insurance coverage, income, and employment. The survey consists of several rounds of interviews over 2 full calendar years to provide a longitudinal view of health status, income, employment, eligibility for insurance coverage, health service utilization, and methods of payment for care. Using these data, household expenditures can be projected by specific demographic characteristics or by service and payment type. The household data are available on the MEPS website in downloadable form or as interactive charts and tables on the site.

- Insurance component: Also known as the Health Insurance Cost Study (HICS), the insurance component of MEPS consists of data from a sample of private and public sector employers about the characteristics of health insurance plans they offer employees, such as:

  - Number and types of private insurance plans offered
  - Premiums paid
  - Amounts contributed by employers and employees
  - Eligibility requirements
  - Benefits
  - Employer characteristics

  These data are available on the MEPS website in tables by national, regional, state, and metropolitan areas. Additionally, publications using the data and interactive data tools are available on the website.

- Medical provider component: Data covering hospitals, physicians, home healthcare providers, and pharmacies identified by the household component surveys. This information is included in the MEPS household component data either as supplements or replacements for the provider data received in the household component surveys.

○ Healthcare Cost and Utilization Project (HCUP, http://www.ahrq.gov/data/hcup/): A group of healthcare databases that includes a core set of clinical and nonclinical information found in a typical discharge abstract, such as diagnoses and procedures, discharge status, patient demographics, and charges in a uniform format to facilitate multistate and national/state comparisons and analyses. Some HCUP databases have associated charges for the electronic data, and more information is available on the website. HCUP databases include:

- State Inpatient Databases (SID): Inpatient discharge abstracts from healthcare organizations in more than 35 states that include more than 90% of all U.S. community hospital discharges and, in some cases, discharges from specialty facilities such as psychiatric hospitals.

- State Ambulatory Surgery Databases (SASD): Data from ambulatory care encounters in hospital-affiliated and freestanding ambulatory surgery sites in more than 20 states.
- State Emergency Department Databases (SEDD): Data from hospital-affiliated emergency department record abstracts for visits that do not result in a hospitalization. More than 15 states participate in the SEDD.
- Nationwide Inpatient Sample (NIS): NIS is the largest all-payer inpatient care database in the United States with data from approximately 8 million hospital stays from about 1,000 hospitals, representing a 20% stratified sample of U.S. community hospitals.
- Kids' Inpatient Database (KID): The only all-payer inpatient care database for children in the United States, although the number of states and discharges varies by year.

○ AHRQ software tools: AHRQ has also developed free software tools that can be used with the HCUP databases listed above as well as with other administrative databases. These downloadable software tools include:
- AHRQ quality indicators (QIs, http://qualityindicators.ahrq.gov): measures of healthcare quality that utilize readily available hospital inpatient administrative data, which consist of the following modules:

  • Prevention quality indicators: Indicators that identify hospital admissions that clinical evidence suggests may have been avoided, at least in part, through high-quality outpatient care.
  • Inpatient quality indicators: Measure quality of care inside hospitals, including inpatient mortality for medical conditions and surgical procedures.
  • Patient safety indicators: Measure quality of care inside hospitals but focus on potentially avoidable complications and iatrogenic events.
  • Pediatric Quality Indicators: Measure quality of care for children under age 18 and for newborns receiving care in hospitals and identify potentially avoidable hospitalizations among children.

- Clinical Classifications Software (CCS-ICD9, http://www.hcup-us.ahrq.gov/toolssoftware/ccs/ccs.jsp) for ICD-9-CM: Provides a method for classifying diagnoses or procedures from the *International Classification of Diseases, 9th Revision, Clinical Modification* into clinically meaningful categories. These categories can be used for various types of aggregate statistical reporting.
- Clinical Classifications Software (CCS-ICD10, http://www.hcup-us.ahrq.gov/toolssoftware/icd_10/ccs_icd_10.jsp) for ICD-10: Provides a method for classifying diagnoses from the *International Statistical Classification of Disease and Related Health Problems, 10th Revision,* into clinically meaningful categories. These categories can be used for various types of aggregate

statistical reporting. ICD-10 is expected to replace ICD-9-CM for most clinical and billing applications by 2012.

- Clinical Classifications Software (CCS-CPT, http://www.hcup-us.ahrq.gov/toolssoftware/ccs_svcsproc/ccssvcproc.jsp) for Services and Procedures: Provides a method for classifying current procedural terminology (CPT) codes and Healthcare Common Procedure Coding System (HCPCS) codes into clinically meaningful procedure categories.

- Mental Health and Substance Abuse Clinical Classification Software (CCS-MHSA, http://www.hcup-us.ahrq.gov/toolssoftware/mhsa/mhsa.jsp): Defines variables that identify general categories for mental health and substance abuse-related ICD-9-CM diagnoses in hospital discharge records for behavioral health data that is coded with ICD-9-CM diagnosis codes.

- Comorbidity Software (http://www.hcup-us.ahrq.gov/toolssoftware/comorbidity/comorbidity.jsp): Assigns variables that identify coexisting conditions on hospital discharge records that are coded using ICD-9-CM codes.

- Procedure Classes (http://www.hcup-us.ahrq.gov/toolssoftware/procedure/procedure.jsp): Allow categorization of ICD-9-CM procedure codes into one of four broad categories: minor diagnostic, minor therapeutic, major diagnostic, and major therapeutic.

- Chronic Condition Indicator (http://www.hcup-us.ahrq.gov/toolssoftware/chronic/chronic.jsp): Categorizes ICD-9-CM diagnosis codes into either chronic or not chronic or into 1 of 18 body system categories.

- Cost-to-Charge Ratio (CCR, http://www.hcup-us.ahrq.gov/db/state/costtocharge.jsp) Files: Hospital-level files designed to supplement the data elements in the HCUP NIS and SID databases and permit conversion of hospital total charge data to cost estimates.

- Utilization Flags (http://www.hcup-us.ahrq.gov/toolssoftware/util_flags/utilflag.jsp): Combines information from UB-92 revenue codes and ICD-9-CM procedure codes to create flags, or indicators, of utilization for specialized services such as intensive care unit, coronary care unit, and neonatal intensive care unit.

- Hospital Market Structure Files: Supplement the data elements in the NIS, KID, and SID databases and contain aggregate measures of hospital market competition that characterize the levels of competition that hospitals may face based on market area characteristics.

○ Clinical Practice Guidelines (http://www.ahrq.gov/clinic/cpgonline.htm): AHRQ maintains the principal clinical practice guideline repository in the United States. Between 1992 and 1996, the agency (then called the Agency for Health Care Policy and Research) sponsored the creation of a series of 19 clinical practice guidelines that set the standard for these evidence-based practice tools. Since that time, AHRQ has developed a repository of clinical guidelines from a number of sources, and all are available in the repository at the above website. The guidelines can be searched using the electronic full-text retrieval system called the Health Services Technology Assessment Text (HSTAT, http://www.ncbi.nlm.nih.gov/books/bv.fcgi?rid=hstat) at the National Library of Medicine website. Each guideline consists of several components: full clinical practice guideline, quick reference guides for clinicians, and consumer versions (English and Spanish).

- *National Center for Health Statistics* (http://www.cdc.gov/nchs/datawh.htm): The NCHS has a wealth of information about U.S. population health, a few of which include the following:
  - National Health and Nutrition Examination Survey (NHANES, http://www.cdc.gov/nchs/nhanes.htm): A national survey program that collects interview and physical examination data to assess the current health and nutrition status and examine trends over time in prevalence and risk factors for diseases. Data collected include:

    - Demographic data
    - Socioeconomic data
    - Dietary data
    - Health-related questions
    - Physical examinations with medical, dental, and physiological measurements
    - Laboratory tests

    Importantly, NHANES data are used to establish national standards for measurements like height, weight, and blood pressure as well as for epidemiologic studies and health services research.
  - National Ambulatory Medical Care Survey (NAMCS, http://www.cdc.gov/nchs/about/major/ahcd/ahcd1.htm): A national survey of a sample of visits to office-based physicians, not employed by the federal government, who are primarily engaged in direct patient care. Anesthesiologists, pathologists, and radiologists are excluded from the survey. Annual data from the survey are available from 1973 to 1981, 1985, and 1989 forward. Participating physicians are trained in how to complete the survey forms, and the data collected directly from providers are then used to create the database that also is used to augment data from other NCHS databases. Physicians are assigned randomly to a 1-week reporting period, during which a systematic random sample of visits are recorded on survey encounter forms that contain patients' symptoms, physicians' diagnoses, and medications ordered or provided, as well as demographic characteristics of patients and services provided.
  - National Hospital Ambulatory Medical Care Survey (NHAMCS, http://www.cdc.gov/nchs/about/major/ahcd/nhamcsds.htm): Similar to the NAMCS, this survey collects data on the utilization and provision of ambulatory care services in nongovernment hospitals, including both

emergency and outpatient departments. The survey samples visits to the emergency departments and outpatient departments of nongovernment general and short-stay hospitals and uses samples from hospital ambulatory programs in geographically defined areas from all 50 states and the District of Columbia. Hospital staff members are trained in use of the survey instrument and systematic random sampling methods that are used to select study participants. Data collected include:

- Demographic patient characteristics
- Expected source(s) of payment
- Patients' complaints
- Physicians' diagnoses
- Diagnostic/screening services
- Procedures
- Medication therapy
- Disposition
- Types of healthcare professionals seen
- Cause(s) of injury where applicable
- Characteristics of the hospital

The survey is being revised to include ambulatory surgical services in the future.

○ National Health Information Survey (NHIS, http://www.cdc.gov/nchs/nhis .htm): Perhaps the oldest systematic survey of health status in the United States, the NHIS has been collecting and reporting data since 1957. This information is collected from household interviews by the U.S. Census Bureau. Data from NHIS have been instrumental in helping shape national health policy. Interviewers visit 35,000 to 40,000 households to gather data about 75,000 to 100,000 people that includes demographic and health utilization information.

The NCHS has a number of other surveys that it maintains regarding the health of specific subpopulations, in addition to those described above.

- *The Commonwealth Fund* (www.commonwealthfund.org): The Commonwealth Fund is a private foundation that supports independent health services research through grants provided to researchers. The Fund's mission "is to promote a high performing healthcare system that achieves better access, improved quality, and greater efficiency, particularly for society's most vulnerable, including low-income people, the uninsured, minority Americans, young children, and elderly adults."[1] The Commonwealth Fund's website is a virtual treasure trove of data based on surveys that the organization's researchers perform in all areas of healthcare access, payment, and quality. The breadth of resources is beyond the scope of this book, and few raw data sets are available, but the Fund provides PowerPoint slides with many of the reports for use in presentations.

- *American Hospital Association* (www.aha.org): One of the best sources for U.S. hospital information, the AHA conducts a yearly survey of hospitals that serves as the basis for its State of America's Hospitals Report, which contains aggregate information on a number of hospital issues, like human resources, capacity levels for various departments, and disaster readiness. More extensive data are available to members and to the public for a fee. The organization also provides a chartbook with useful data on the U.S. healthcare marketplace and hospital economics in graphic format in PowerPoint and Adobe Acrobat files.
- *National Information Center on Health Services Research and Health Care Technology* (NICHSR, http://www.nlm.nih.gov/hsrinfo/datasites.html): This data resource, which is maintained by the National Library of Medicine, has a number of useful links to health services research data from the National Institutes of Health, foreign data sources, and links to university data resources. This website provides a good starting point for searching the Internet for data resources.

Reference

1. Commonwealth Fund Mission Statement. Retrieved November 2008 from http://www.commonwealthfund.org/about us_show.htm?doc_id=224805

■ Appendix 4.3

Resource-Based Relative Value System

In response to increasing costs of medical care and the inadequacy of the fee for service payment system for physicians, Medicare changed the payment system for physicians' services in 1992. At that time the federal government established a standardized physician payment schedule based on a resource-based relative value system (RBRVS), in which payments for services are determined by the resource costs needed to provide them. The cost for each service is divided into three components: physician work, expected practice expense, and professional liability insurance. Payments are calculated by multiplying the combined costs of a service by a conversion factor that is established annually by Congress, and each of the three components is adjusted by the Geographic Practice Cost Index (GPCI). The three GPCIs are computed every 3 years by CMS. GPCIs are constructed so they have national averages of 1.0. Geographic areas that have costs above the national average have index values above 1.0; areas with below-average costs have index values under 1.0.

The initial physician work relative values were based on the results of a study conducted by researchers at Harvard University and include factors like the time it takes to perform the service, the technical skill and physical effort, the required mental effort and judgment, and stress due to the potential patient risk. A work relative value unit (wRVU) is assigned to each current procedural technology (CPT) code, and these values are updated annually to reflect changes in the CPT codes and medical practice. The entire scale is reviewed and revised every 5 years. Approximately 52% of the entire RBRVS value is accounted for by the wRVU value.

Comprising about 44% of the entire RBRVS value, the practice expense component is based on a formula using average Medicare-approved charges from 1991, the year before RBRVS was implemented, and the proportion of revenues consumed by each specialty's practice expenses, depending on site of service. Starting in 2000, CMS added the resource-based professional liability insurance (PLI) relative value units.

Since 1991 annual updates to the physician work relative values are based on recommendations from the RVUS Update Committee, a committee composed of national medical specialty societies. This committee ensures that the RVU conversion table accounts for current CPT codes and medical practice changes.

Essentials of Statistical Thinking and Analysis

■ Art and Science of Statistical Thinking

All improvement requires change, but not all change results in improvement. The only way to determine if changes have been beneficial is through measurement, which consists of three steps: determining and defining key indicators, collecting an appropriate amount of data, and analyzing and interpreting these data. This approach was described by W. Edwards Deming[1] when he proposed the Theory of Profound Knowledge in his book, *The New Economics*, which serves as the basis for the concept of statistical thinking. Profound knowledge has four parts:

1. *Systems thinking*: Appreciation of the system as more than a sum of its constituents; comprehension of the interplay of the parts through coordination and collaboration to produce greater productivity and economy of operations. Systems consist of interconnected subsystems and processes that affect each other to produce an outcome that relies on the coordination and collaboration of work systems by managers.
2. *Process variation*: Recognition that all processes have variation that can either be inherent in the process or due to external influences. Variation is a major source of nonconforming output (nonconformities) that lead to reduced quality and higher cost. Identifying and reducing sources of variation is a major undertaking for performance improvement initiatives.
3. *Theory of knowledge*: Information must be tempered by experience and theory to become knowledge; that is, without theory and experience information cannot be translated into knowledge. Effective managers skillfully combine experience and theory to create knowledge for an organization.
4. *Psychology*: Understanding the variation in people is as important as understanding the variation in processes. Successful managers use the tenets of human psychology to effectively coordinate, collaborate, and motivate workers to optimize system outcomes.

These four elements of Deming's theory create expectations for managers to understand the system in which they work and to use data to create knowledge and share it with others throughout the enterprise to effect optimum system operations and high quality output. From these principles has evolved the concept of **statistical thinking**, which recognizes that managers are rarely high-level statisticians, but they must be able to grasp the meaning of statistical analyses to address both variation in processes as well as how statistical information can be transformed into knowledge. Statistical thinking also implies that application of the statistical data provides the best possibility of reducing variation and improving processes.

Ron Snee, a statistician who has published extensively on this topic, provided insight into statistical thinking in an article in 1986 that stated, "... statistical thinking is used to describe the thought processes that acknowledge the ubiquitous nature of variation and that its identification, characterization, quantification, control, and reduction provide a unique opportunity for improvement.... Every enterprise is made up of a collection of interconnected processes whose input, control variable, and output are subject to variation. This leads to the conclusion that statistical thinking must be used routinely at all levels of the organization."[2] In a later article, Snee refined his concept, saying, "I define statistical thinking as *thought processes*, which recognize that variation is all around us and present in everything we do, all work is a series of interconnected processes, and identifying, characterizing, quantifying, controlling, and reducing variation provide opportunities for improvement."[3] Thus from Deming's Theory of Profound Knowledge the concept of statistical thinking was born and serves as a guidepost for successful managers.

■ Statistical Process Control Puts Statistical Thinking Into Practice

Statistical process control (SPC) is a mature statistical tool for examining healthcare processes and identifying opportunities for improvement. Regardless of the improvement paradigm—six sigma, lean, plan-do-study-act, or their variants—measurement (data collection) is a key part of improving performance. Control charts are important at several stages of the improvement process. Traditionally, control charts are used after a quality improvement initiative has proven successful so that the gains made during the project can be sustained. However, in many cases SPC charts can be used to examine process measures before an intervention to determine what type of variation is present to provide direction to the improvement team.

The concept of control charts was invented by Walter A. Shewhart at Bell Labs in the 1920s to reduce the frequency of failures and expensive repairs of telephone equipment buried underground. Through carefully designed experiments based on mathematical statistical theories, Dr. Shewhart defined two types of variation: **common cause** and **special cause**. Common cause variation, originally called "chance cause" by Shewhart, is generally defined as variation that occurs within a process because of its design, and this type of variation has the following characteristics:

- Variation is based on the process materials and procedures.
- Variation is predictable using mathematics related to probability and chance.

- Variation is irregular (i.e., shows no particular pattern).
- High and low values within the measurements are statistically indistinguishable.

Special cause variation connotes performance outside the expected historical common cause variation and was termed "attributable cause" by Shewhart because it implied an external event or factor that created the variation in performance. Special cause variation is usually a surprise measurement on a control chart and can be distinguished from common cause variation as follows:

- Variation due to new, unanticipated, emergent, or previously unknown factors within the system
- Variation that is entirely unpredictable, even using statistical probability techniques
- Variation that is outside historical trends
- Variation that indicates an underlying change in the system or some previously unidentified factor

Shewhart defined the state of statistical control of a process as one in which all data points fell within ±3 sigma limits, which defines common cause variation, or variation that is 99.73% likely to be due to chance variation in the process. Processes that are in statistical control (i.e., have only common cause variation) have more predictable future outcomes and are generally more efficient. Quality improvement luminaries W. Edwards Deming and Joseph Juran capitalized on these principles to revolutionize manufacturing in Japan and other countries in the 1940s and 1950s. Managing process variation proved to be the catalyst to change a decimated industrial base in Japan into a world class, competitive business force that led the world in product and service quality for many years.

■ SPC Basics

Detecting change over time is not always easy. Measurement of the same clinical or administrative parameter, such as heart rate or errors on invoices, often yields slightly different results from one point in time to the next, but the question of whether this variation is significant is sometimes difficult to determine without more analysis. For example, a clinician may need to determine if a sudden change in a patient's heart rate from 70 to 100 requires treatment or is simply normal variation. Inherent variability is due to factors that are natural for the process, whether it is an individual's biological processes or the results of some slight change in an input to produce the patient's bill, or even a factor introduced by the measurement system itself. Statistical analysis of data sets, using techniques like SPC, can examine system performance to help identify both internal and external factors that lie behind variability within any process, not only providing insight into causes of system variation but also helping identify the effects and sustainability of improvement initiatives.

SPC is based on the same statistical principles used by other researchers, but these methods are used somewhat differently from traditional research. Formal research studies may require data collection at different points in time or place for comparison, using experimental models such as a randomized controlled trial, to evaluate the impact of a new medication via a null hypothesis to find whether there is a difference between an experimental group and a control group who did not receive the drug. On the other hand, the improvement practitioner may take a simpler approach to quality research design that does not involve the randomized controlled trial model, because the study may be directed at comparing the performance of a process at one site before and after a change has been introduced. In that case the randomized controlled trial model may be overkill, but the statistical rigor of measurement and analysis must still be ensured. The researcher and the quality improvement professional address the same question (i.e., the effects of an intervention on a system before and after the intervention event) to determine if the change was due to random variation or from the intervention itself.

One important advantage of SPC is the use of time series data. Many classical statistical methods use tests of large samples that ignore the time order (e.g., the mean medication error rate at intervention sites might be compared with that at nonintervention sites). These studies typically use statistical tests of significance to determine if one group is "significantly different" from the other. These methods have sufficient statistical power when based on large data sets. However, accumulation of ample amounts of data can limit the practical application of these methods in health care, and representation of

Exhibit 5.1 Quick Facts About Control Charts

Individual measurements from any process will demonstrate variation.

Variability of data within a stable (common cause) process is predictable within a defined range that can be computed from a statistical model such as the Gaussian, binomial, or Poisson distribution.

Measured values in a process with special causes will deviate unpredictably but in an observable way from the random distribution models that serve as the basis for control charts.

Data from stable (in control) processes are subject to establishment of statistical control limits that can be used to test for a change in performance after an intervention.

Knowing if a process has common or special causes can guide improvement teams in developing interventions based on the type of variation.

SPC and research approaches use similar statistical approaches but differ in the type of data collected and analyzed.

the data is often via simple bar charts, line graphs, or tables that may only be helpful in allowing a qualitative statement about whether or not an intervention worked.

SPC methods, however, retain the rigor of classical statistical methods but add the sensitivity of time series data that accumulate analyzable sample sizes in a shorter period of time. This integration of statistical significance tests with near–real-time analysis of graphs of summary data allows earlier detection of changes in trends due to process changes. Although many researchers may not be as familiar with the SPC approach, it has the same statistical validity and rigor of traditional experimental models. Another important feature of SPC is the way it supports statistical thinking among nonstatisticians through straightforward statistical theory and graphical displays.

The basic theory of SPC is based on the observations by Shewhart that a stable process has variation that is predictable and can be described by one of several statistical distributions. One commonly used model of random variation is the Gaussian (normal) distribution, which is familiar to most healthcare professionals. Although repeated measurements from many processes conform to the Gaussian distribution, there are many other processes that may not fit the normal curve, and other distributions, like the Poisson, binomial, or geometric distributions, may be more appropriate. In those cases the calculations of SPC chart parameters (upper control limit [UCL] and lower control limit [LCL]) are different from those used for charts based on the normal distribution. For example, the random variation in the number of postoperative surgical site infections coincides with a binomial distribution because there are only two possible outcomes: the infection either was or was not present after the surgical procedure. Common cause variation refers to the natural variation that is expected to occur according to the underlying statistical distribution if the mean and standard error remain constant over time. Thus the random variation between heart rates within a population of healthy people is a result of basic human physiology, but the random variation in monthly surgical site infection rates is a result of many factors like training, management of surgical supply sterilization, physician and nursing clinical practice, and application of universal precautions. As noted before, processes that exhibit only common cause variation are considered stable, predictable, and in statistical control. If the process remains in control, future measurements will consistently fit the same probability distribution as before. Thus if a stable process produces data that conforms to a Gaussian distribution and is not destabilized by one or more special causes, then about 99.73% of future data points will be ±3 standard deviations around the mean. In general, regardless of the underlying distribution, about 99.73% of all data will fall within ±3 standard deviations of the mean if the underlying process is stable.

Special (attributable) cause variation can be understood from a statistical point of view like the traditional hypothesis tests of data that exhibit statistically significant differences. A key distinction of SPC compared with traditional research is the use of time series data requiring smaller samples to test the null hypothesis that a single sample value is different from the other data points in the series. Special cause variation can be the result of either a deliberate intervention or an external event that is beyond the process owners' control. Attributable variation can be transient (e.g., a spike in office visits caused by a respiratory virus), or it can be longer term, such as when economic constraints require reduced staffing that prolongs waiting times in an emergency department. It is useful to think of interventions in research studies or quality improvement projects as "controlled" application of special causes of variation to a study group that require statistical tests to help determine the statistical significance of the pre- and postintervention differences.

The important difference between common cause and special cause variation is the approach taken to reduce or eliminate the source of variation. Because processes that exhibit special cause variation are unstable and unpredictable, the first target for intervention should be the cause of the out of control behavior of the process. Bringing the process into control by eliminating the special cause(s) often produces substantial cost savings and quality improvement, which often show the "quick gains" that reap the greatest benefits. On the other hand, processes that only demonstrate common cause variation continue to produce the same results, within statistical control limits, unless the process is fundamentally reengineered. Thus the approaches to identifying and improving special cause variation include root-cause analysis and rapid cycle interventions, whereas common cause variation generally requires more in-depth process analysis using techniques like Pareto analysis and value stream mapping. Control charts therefore define current process capability, and they can help define the approach that will be most likely to produce the greatest benefit based on whether variation stems from special or common causes.

■ Control Chart: Shewhart's Genius

Based on firm statistical theory and designed experiments, Shewhart developed a relatively uncomplicated process management tool, the control chart, to differentiate between common and special cause data points. SPC graphs generally consist of trend charts that have the basic form shown in FIGURE 5.1. The data are plotted on a trend chart with three other lines:

- **UCL**: Level three sigma values above the centerline
- **Centerline**: Mean or the median of the data, depending on the type of chart
- **LCL**: Line three sigma values below the centerline

Interpretation of a control chart consists of two related steps: identification of data points that fall outside control limits (special cause) and review of patterns of data within a time period. Either of these two steps may discover special cause data that directs the improvement team in looking for underlying attributable causes that are the first targets for intervention. Data values that fall randomly between the UCL and LCL, however, connote common cause variation.

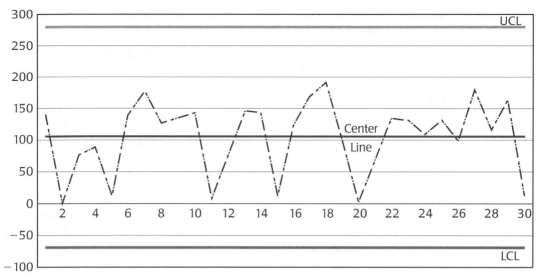

FIGURE 5.1 General Format of a Control Chart

Creation of the UCL and LCL is often left to a SPC programming package, but statistical thinking requires an understanding of the origin of these lines. Shewhart and other SPC experts recommend control limits set at ±3 standard deviations (sigma) for detecting meaningful changes in process performance while achieving a rational balance between two types of statistical errors:

- **Type I error (α error, false positive):** Mistakenly inferring that a statistical difference exists when no difference is present. In the case of SPC the mistake is to infer that a special cause is present when it is not. A type I error occurs when control limits are set too narrow.
- **Type II error (β error, false negative):** Failure to reject the null hypothesis when the alternative hypothesis is true; in the case of SPC the failure is to recognize a special cause when it is present. A type II error occurs when the control limits are set too wide.

For the normal distribution, as large quantities of data are plotted on the probability distribution, 99.73% of all data points fall within ±3 standard deviations of the mean, and 0.27% of all data points fall outside the 3 standard deviation limits. Thus a point outside the 3 sigma limits has only a 0.27% chance of being due to common causes (i.e., the type I error probability is 0.0027). The probability of a type I error is so small that it is reasonable to conclude that a point outside the 3 sigma limits is due to a special cause. These same thought processes are used in evaluating research studies involving acceptance and rejection of the null hypothesis for a designed experiment and apply to any control chart, regardless of the type of distribution. In fact, the 3 sigma limits have a higher threshold for type I error probability than the 2 standard deviations (α error of 0.05) typically used in most medical research studies, but unlike one-time hypothesis tests used in medical research studies, control charts usually consist of many (minimum of 20 – 25) points. Each point contributes independently to the probability of type I error, and so a control chart with 25 points using 3 sigma control limits has an overall false positive probability as follows:

$$\text{Type I error probability} = 1 - (0.9973) \times 25 = 0.0675 \text{ or } 6.75\%$$

The value of 6.75% for type I (α) error is considered by statisticians and performance improvement practitioners to be a reasonable risk of making a false-positive error and mislabeling a common cause to the category of special causes.

The use of control limits is one of two ways to identify special causes on a control chart. Statisticians developed criteria to apply to control charts that examine the chart data to determine if nonrandom patterns occur within the UCL and LCL. The three common rule sets listed in TABLE 5.1 are widely used to determine the existence of a special cause through assessment of the data pattern. Any of the three may be used to evaluate charts, and some control chart programs allow selection of the criteria set that best suits the end user. The Western Electric and Wheeler rules partition the control chart into zones, as shown in FIGURE 5.2.

Table 5.1	Rule Sets for Determining Special Cause Data Patterns
Rule Set	Rules
Western Electric	The control chart is divided into three zones on either side of the mean: Zone A is from 2 to 3 sigma from the mean, zone B is from 1 to 2 sigma from the mean, and zone C is from 0 to 1 sigma from the mean
	Mixture pattern rule: eight consecutive points on both sides of the c enterline with no points falling in zone C
	Stratification pattern rule: 15 consecutive points fall within zone A
	Instability pattern: points outside zone A
	Systematic negative autocorrelation: a long series of observations that alternate high-low-high-low
	Repetition pattern: the tendency for one chart to follow the same pattern as its predecessor
	Trend pattern: series of out-of-control points in the lower zones followed by a series of out-of-control points in the upper zones or vice versa or a series of points without a change in direction
Wheeler	The control chart is divided into three zones on either side of the mean: Zone A is from 2 to 3 sigma from the mean, zone B is from 1 to 2 sigma from the mean, and zone C is from 0 to 1 sigma from the mean
	Rule 1: any single data point falls outside zone A (>3 sigma from the mean)
	Rule 2: two of three consecutive points fall in zone A or beyond on the same side on the centerline
	Rule 3: four of five consecutive points fall in zone B or beyond on the same side of the centerline
	Rule 4: nine consecutive points fall on the same side of the centerline in zone C or beyond

Table 5.1	
Rule Set	Rules
Nelson	One point is more than 3 standard deviations from the mean
	Nine or more points in a row are on the same side of the mean
	Six or more points in a row are continually increasing or decreasing
	Fourteen or more points in a row alternate in direction, increasing and then decreasing
	Two or three out of three points in a row are more than 2 standard deviations from the mean in the same direction
	Four or five out of five points in a row are more than 1 standard deviation from the mean in the same direction
	Fifteen points in a row are all within 1 standard deviation of the mean on either side of the mean
	Eight points in a row exist with none within 1 standard deviation of the mean and the points are in both directions from the mean

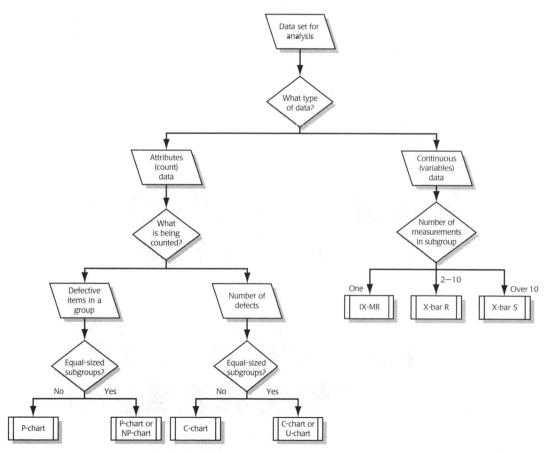

FIGURE 5.2   Control Chart Selection Algorithm

Calculation of the standard deviation (sigma) varies by type of chart because of the different statistical distributions and a few other parameters, such as the number of observations in each sample that is used to create a data point. For example, the formula for calculating the standard deviation for the Poisson distribution is different from that used for the binomial distribution. The formulas used to calculate these standard deviations are provided with each chart.

■ Types of Control Charts

FIGURE 5.3 provides a decision tree for selection of the most commonly used control charts, whereas TABLE 5.2 shows the basic types of control charts. As mentioned previously, **variables data** is defined as a measurement such as height, weight, time, or length. Generally, a measuring device such as a weight scale, stadiometer, or clock produces data in this format. Variables data are real numbers and so can have fractional or decimal values. **Attributes data** is defined as a count such as the number of employees, the number of surgical site infections, the number of medication errors, or the number of phone calls. Attributes data usually involves creating an operational definition of the event, and then when the defined event occurs, the event is counted. For example, when an infection occurs at the site of a surgical procedure within a week after the procedure, a surgical site infection is counted. The number of events meeting the operational definition is the total count. Attributes data never contains decimal places when it is collected; it is always whole numbers. However, when it is used to calculate a ratio, as in the p-chart, the attributes data may be converted to a fractional value.

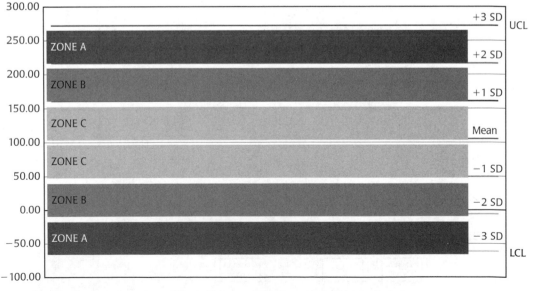

FIGURE 5.3 Control Chart Zones for Western Electric and Wheeler Rule Sets

Table 5.2	Basic Types of Control Charts
Attributes Charts	**Continuous Variable Charts**
p-chart	Individual X moving range
np-chart	X-bar moving range
c-chart	X-bar S
u-chart	

Sample or subgroup size is defined as the amount of data collected at one time as the process is sampled. Examples include the following:

- When assessing a patient's blood pressure using an automated sphygmomanometer, the pressure is checked once every 10 minutes, so the sample can be the average of six readings each hour, and the subgroup size is six.
- When measuring the height of a population of children in all the schools in a district, a sample of 10 children from each school is averaged to create a single measure for that school, providing a subgroup size of 10.
- When determining the number of phone calls that ring more than three times before being answered in each hour, the sample size is the total number of phone calls received per hour, which will likely vary for each hour. Thus the sample is the number of phone calls per hour meeting the criterion, whereas the subgroup size will vary, which is important when choosing a control chart (discussed further in the next section).
- When checking 20 patient invoices per day for errors, the sample size is 1 day and the subgroup size is 20.

The left branch of the decision tree helps determine the correct type of chart for the most frequently used attribute charts. The primary determinants for attribute SPC charts are what is being counted and whether the size of each sample subgroup is the same or different.

Steps in Choosing a Control Chart for Attribute Data

1. Is the count the number of nonconforming products or services (e.g., number of infections or number of medication errors)? If so, then use either the p- or np-chart. These charts can only be used when the number of nonconformities is less than or equal to the number of products or services.
   a. Is the sample size constant (e.g., the number of infections in a sample of 100 patients per week)? If so, then the np-chart is most appropriate.
   b. Is the sample size variable (e.g., the count of the number of infections in all the inpatients of the hospital per week)? If so, the p-chart should be chosen.

2. Is the count the number of nonconforming items within a product or service, such as number of infections per hospital unit, number of cleaning failures per room, or the number of surgical site infections per surgeon? If so, use either the c- or u-chart. These charts can be used even when the number of nonconformities exceeds the number of products or services.
   a. Is the sample size checked for the defect a constant number (e.g., the number of falls per day)? If so, then the c-chart is the best choice.
   b. Is the sample size checked for the defect a changing number (e.g., number of errors per insurance invoice, where the number of invoices per day varies)? If so, then the u-chart is most appropriate.

Some software programs have interactive wizards that follow this algorithm to help choose the appropriate attribute chart.

P-Charts

The p-chart is used when dealing with ratios, proportions, or percentages of conforming or nonconforming items in a given sample. A good example for a p-chart in health care is the proportion of Cesarean sections in total deliveries per month. The Caesarean section is considered to be a nonconforming event, and the ratio of Caesarean sections to total deliveries meets the criteria for a p-chart:

1. Data are counts of Caesarean sections divided by counts of total live deliveries.
2. The sample size varies within the selected time period (monthly).
3. The total number of nonconformities cannot exceed the total number in the sample.

The binomial distribution is used for p-charts, with p representing the nonconforming proportion and q (which is equal to $1 - p$) representing the proportion of conforming items or events. Because each delivery is an independent event, the measures are independent from one another.

Once the proportion of nonconformities is calculated (e.g., proportion of Caesarean sections per month), the centerline and control limits can be calculated as shown in TABLE 5.3.

For these formulas, p is the p value for each sample period and k is the total number of sample periods. Note that for this distribution the average of the nonconforming proportions defines the centerline and the control limits. Additionally, the parameters for the p-chart also have the sample size (n) as part of the calculation to accommodate the varying sample sizes.

NP-Charts

The np-chart relies on the binomial distribution, just like the p-chart; unlike the p-chart, however, sample size must be constant to use the np-chart. The np value represents

Table 5.3	Calculations for Centerline and Control Limits
Parameter	Formula
$\bar{p}$ (centerline)	$\bar{p} = \dfrac{\sum p}{k}$
UCL	$UCL = \bar{P} + 3\sqrt{\dfrac{\bar{P}(1-\bar{P})}{n}}$
LCL	$LCL = \bar{P} - 3\sqrt{\dfrac{\bar{P}(1-\bar{P})}{n}}$

Example 5.1 Using the P-Chart

The Medical Executive Committee of St. Cureall Hospital created a new scorecard to comply with The Joint Commission's Ongoing Professional Practice Evaluation standard, and one of the measures selected for analysis for family physicians and internists is mortality after myocardial infarction. The control chart in FIGURE 5.4 shows the performance of Dr. Heartfelt, a staff internist, over the past 20 months. The Chief of Internal Medicine, Dr. Patrick, noted that the majority of points were within control limits during the study period, but the mortality rate in the 15th month demonstrated special cause behavior. Dr. Patrick also noted that Dr. Heartfelt's chart indicated favorable special cause performance in periods 11, 14, and 20. The rest of Dr. Heartfelt's mortality rates fit within common cause limits and appeared to be in control. Dr. Patrick discussed the chart with Dr. Heartfelt and performed chart reviews for the 10 patients and six deaths in period 15, which indicated that the patients admitted in that period were older and had long histories of cardiac disease, with several who had longstanding congestive heart failure. Dr. Patrick also reviewed a selected number of charts from periods 11, 14, and 20, which indicated that Dr. Heartfelt had begun using a new therapy that he had learned at a cardiology conference that was showing promise in a subset of patients. Dr. Patrick asked Dr. Heartfelt to present the new technique and his experience at Medicine Grand Rounds.

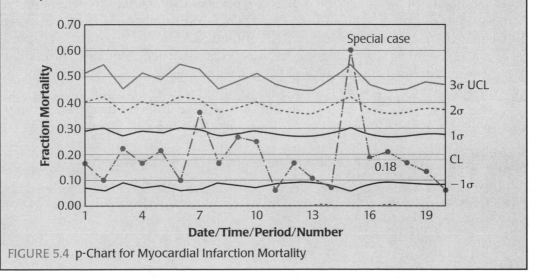

FIGURE 5.4 p-Chart for Myocardial Infarction Mortality

the actual number of nonconformities, rather than the proportion, and the formulas for calculating the parameters for this chart are as shown in TABLE 5.4.

Although constant sample sizes are fairly unusual in health care, in some cases *n* values may be the same, as shown in EXAMPLE 5.2.

Use of control charts for both diagnosis and follow-up control is the most common application of this quantitative approach. Without the data, determination of the causative factor is much harder and in some cases could be nearly impossible. Having data to indicate the success of an intervention helps confirm the causative factor and verify the efficacy of the intervention.

The difference in control limits between p- and np-charts deserves comment, because the p-chart has "wavy" control limits, but the np-chart limits are flat. This difference is due to the different sample sizes in the p-chart data, leading to different common cause control limits on the p-chart. Because the np-chart has constant sample size, the control limits are flat.

U- and C-Charts

The u-chart monitors process variation due to fluctuations in defects per item or group of items and is useful to determine not just how many items are not conforming, as in p- and np-charts, but also how many defects there are per item or service. The unit being evaluated (e.g., a service, a patient, a work unit) is often termed an "area of opportunity," which is the frame or area in which a nonconformity may occur. A commonly used explanation for the difference between the number of defective items and the number of defects uses an automotive example. Suppose a piece of metal is being fabricated for an automobile and to be used it must be scratch free. As the metal pieces proceed down the assembly line, defective parts are removed from the line and counted. That count is the number of defective items, analyzed using a p- or np-chart. In addition, though, each defective piece is also assessed to determine the number of scratches on each surface. That count is the number of defects, analyzed by a u- or c-chart. Nonconformance must be distinguished from defective items because there can be several nonconformances on a single defective item. Similarly, the number of patients registering complaints can be counted and analyzed (p- or np-chart) or the number of patient complaints may be assessed and evaluated (c- or u-chart). c- and u-charts are based on the Poisson distribution and have different properties from p- and np-charts. If the sample size does not change and the defects on the items are

Table 5.4	Formulas for Calculating the Parameters for the NP-Chart
Parameter	Formula
np (centerline)	np
UCL	$UCL = n\bar{p} + 3\sqrt{n\bar{p}(1-\bar{p})}$
LCL	$LCL = n\bar{p} - 3\sqrt{n\bar{p}(1-\bar{p})}$

Example 5.2 Using the NP-Chart

Mary Davis, the supervisor of medical records, was shocked when she was confronted by Dr. Goodwriter, the clinic director, with the results of an audit by Medicaid that indicated a high level of nonconforming charts that lacked sufficient documentation to justify billing charges. Mary reviewed the records of a group of 22 "frequent fliers" (patients who make frequent visits to the clinic) to determine the documentation deficiency levels for the prior 21 months and plotted the data on the np-chart shown in FIGURE 5.5. The graph clearly indicated that the special cause event (the Medicaid audit finding of incomplete charts) had been preceded by a rise in variation in the 7 prior months. Mary reviewed the charts that created the special cause point in month 20 and found that most of the charts that were deficient were completed by pediatric residents who were training in the clinic during that time. She observed that variation in the deficiency rate began to rise around month 15 and recalled that the clinic began participating in the pediatric training program during month 14. Mary immediately created an in-service educational program for the residents that she repeated for each new group of residents at the beginning of their month-long rotations in the clinic starting in month 21, with a resultant return of the documentation deficiency measure to prior levels of performance and variation.

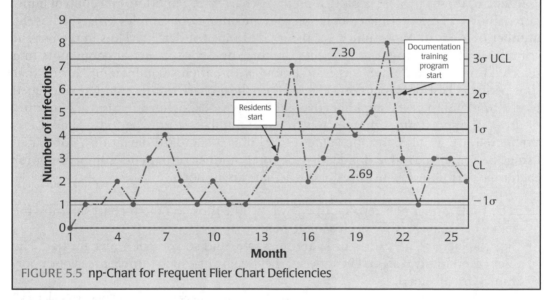

FIGURE 5.5 np-Chart for Frequent Flier Chart Deficiencies

fairly easy to count, the c-chart becomes an effective tool to monitor the quality of a process. As is evident from the decision tree in FIGURE 5.3, the c-chart requires equal sized subgroups, whereas the u-chart may have unequal sized subgroups. Thus the c-chart is actually a special case of u-chart in which sample size is fixed rather than variable. The u-chart parameters are calculated as shown in TABLE 5.5.

Data values (u_j) are defined by the number of defects per sample of size n_j as follows:

$$u_j = \frac{(count)_j}{n_j}$$

Table 5.5	Calculation of U-Chart Parameters
Parameter	Formula
$\bar{u}$ (centerline)	$$\bar{u} = \frac{\sum\limits_{j=1}^{m}(count)_j}{m}$$
UCL	$$UCL = \bar{u} + 3\sqrt{\frac{\bar{u}}{n_j}}$$
LCL	$$LCL = MAX\left[0, u - 3\sqrt{\frac{\bar{u}}{n_j}}\right]$$

Each of these u_j values is plotted on the u-chart with centerline and control limits noted above. The centerline calculation uses the number of samples (m), which is the **number of areas of opportunity** *not* the total number of defects. Thus in the patient complaint sample, $(count)_j$ represents the total number (count) of complaints in a selected time period, and n_j is the total number of patients complaining during that time period. These data points are entered onto the u-chart with a centerline calculated by the total number of complaints over all time periods, divided by the total number of areas of opportunity (m), which is the total number of time periods. The UCL is calculated using the centerline value (u-bar) plus 3 standard deviations, computed using the centerline value divided by the total number of patients complaining for each time period. A few features of the u-chart are of note:

- The UCL (and a non-zero LCL) is "wavy" like those on the p-chart, because the value of n_j can vary for each sample point.
- For the c-chart, all values of n_j are the same, and so control limits are flat. The c-chart is simply a special instance of the u-chart in which sample areas of opportunity are all equal.
- Note that the LCL cannot be less than zero, because there can be no "negative defect" counts, and so the LCL will be no less than zero as noted in the formula that equates the LCL to the greater of zero or 3 standard deviations below the centerline.

EXAMPLE 5.3 demonstrates the application of a u-chart.

The increasing use of u-charts in patient safety applications, as in the catheter-related bloodstream infections described in EXAMPLE 5.3, has made them indispensable in a number of different situations. Not only can they be useful in identifying special causes, but they are also helpful in monitoring trends in appropriate safety metrics.

Example 5.3 Using the U-Chart

Dr. Marv Ellis heads the infection control surveillance group at St. Cureall Hospital. He tracks catheter-related bloodstream infections (bloodstream infections probably caused by insertion and maintenance of a central vascular catheter line) as part of the hospital's infection surveillance program using a u-chart (FIGURE 5.6). He noted a spike in the infection rate during month 8 of the analysis and a special cause "out of control" point in month 9. Thereafter, the rate returned to its usual levels and remained in control. Since the out of control point indicated a special cause, Dr. Ellis reviewed the patient charts to determine if some characteristic of these ICU patients contributed to the high rates. Although the ICU cares for burn patients, there did not seem to be any changes in case mix or APACHE scores for those months, and so he dug deeper into the problem. Checking with the nursing staff, Dr. Ellis discovered that the catheters used during that period had come from the manufacturer with inadequate quality control, and the seals on the wrappers were found to be defective, leading to unsterile conditions. The head nurse in the ICU, Caitlin Sharp, had become alarmed when she noted a higher rate of catheter-related bloodstream infections during the month and subsequently had launched her own root-cause analysis that identified and remedied the problem. To improve surveillance, Dr. Ellis decided to share the infection control charts with all nursing and medical staff members so they could better determine if rates were exceeding control limits.

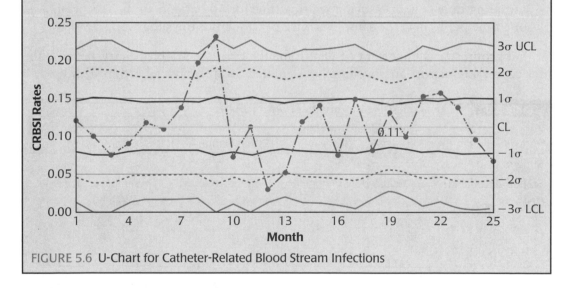

FIGURE 5.6 U-Chart for Catheter-Related Blood Stream Infections

■ Choosing and Using Continuous Variable Charts

The three most commonly used control charts for continuous variables (real numbers) are

1. Individual X moving range chart
2. X-bar range chart
3. X-bar S chart

The three charts differ primarily in the number of measurements in each subgroup, which determines the method by which the standard deviation is calculated. The primary differences between the three charts are listed in TABLE 5.6. The calculations in TABLE 5.6 use multipliers to correct for the small sample size for the variables data, and the values for these "bias correction factors" are shown in TABLE 5.7. Because variables control chart theory stems from the statistics of the normal (Gaussian) probability distribution, the population from which the measurements are taken should be approximately normally distributed.

Fortunately, the only major criterion considered for choosing the type of variables chart is the number of items in the subgroup for each sample. The concept of a subgroup is straightforward but often is confusing at first. To determine the size of a subgroup, consider the following:

- What is being sampled? A sample is the act of taking one or more pieces of information from a process in a particular period of time (e.g., measuring waiting time for patients in the reception area one time per hour).
- The subgroup size is the number of pieces of information that are taken at each sampling time (e.g., measuring waiting time for 10 patients in the reception area one time per hour). The sample is once per hour, but the subgroup size is 10.

Subgroup size is important to determine the correct variables chart, because the bias correction factors are specifically calculated for differing subgroup sizes.

Table 5.6	Characteristics of Variables Control Charts		
Parameter	Individual X Moving Range	X-bar Range	X-bar S
Subgroup size	1	2–9	>9
Standard deviation measure	Adjusted moving range	Adjusted average range	Sample standard deviation
X-chart centerline	$\overline{IX} = \dfrac{\sum IX}{k}$	$\overline{\overline{X}} = \dfrac{\sum \overline{X}}{k}$	$\overline{\overline{X}} = \dfrac{\sum \overline{X}}{k}$
X-chart UCL	$UCL_{IX} = \overline{IX} + (\overline{MR} \bullet A_2)$	$UCL_{\overline{X}} = \overline{\overline{X}} + (\overline{R} \bullet A_2)$	$UCL_{\overline{X}} = \overline{\overline{X}} + (\overline{S} \bullet A_3)$
X-chart LCL	$LCL_{IX} = \overline{IX} - (\overline{MR} \bullet A_2)$	$LCL_{\overline{X}} = \overline{\overline{X}} - (\overline{R} \bullet A_2)$	$LCL_{\overline{X}} = \overline{\overline{X}} - (\overline{S} \bullet A_3)$
Standard deviation centerline	$\overline{MR} = \dfrac{\sum MR}{k-1}$	$\overline{R} = \dfrac{\sum R}{k}$	$\overline{S} = \dfrac{\sum S}{k}$
Standard deviation UCL	$UCL_{MR} = \overline{MR} \bullet D_4$	$UCL_R = \overline{R} \bullet D_4$	$UCL_S = \overline{S} \bullet B_4$
Standard deviation LCL	$LCL_{MR} = \overline{MR} \bullet D_4$	$LCL_R = \overline{R} \bullet D_4$	$LCL_S = \overline{S} \bullet B_4$
Definitions	k = number of subgroups	k = number of subgroups	k = number of subgroups

	X-bar Chart					
Table 5.7	**Bias Correction Tables for Variables Control Charts**					
Subgroup Size	Range	S		S Chart	MR or R Chart	
	A2	A3	B3	B4	D3	D4
2	1.886	2.659	0	3.267	0	3.268
3	1.023	1.954	0	2.568	0	2.574
4	0.729	1.628	0	2.266	0	2.282
5	0.577	1.427	0	2.089	0	2.114
6	0.483	1.287	0.03	1.97	0	2.004
7	0.419	1.182	0.118	1.882	0.076	1.924
8	0.373	1.099	0.185	1.815	0.136	1.864
9	0.337	1.032	0.239	1.761	0.184	1.816
10	0.308	0.975	0.284	1.716	0.223	1.777
11	0.285	0.927	0.322	1.678	0.256	1.744
12	0.266	0.886	0.354	1.646	0.283	1.717
13	0.249	0.85	0.382	1.619	0.307	1.693
14	0.235	0.817	0.407	1.593	0.328	1.672
15	0.223	0.789	0.428	1.572	0.347	1.653
20	0.18	0.68	0.51	1.49	0.414	1.586
25	0.153	0.606	0.565	1.435	0.459	1.541

Adapted from Stephenson RW. Control chart construction. Retrieved November 2008 from http://www.public.iastate. edu/~wrstephe/stat495/shewhartcc.pdf

Among other differences, a major distinction between attribute charts and variables charts is the inclusion of a second control chart for the variability measure for continuous variable charts. This second control chart performs the same kind of SPC analysis for the variability measure used for the X indicator to determine the degree of variation *within* each subgroup. For example, the X-bar R SPC chart may have as many as nine measurements within one subgroup. These measures should be fairly close to a Gaussian distribution, but if the subgroups are consistently skewed toward the left or right, the samples taken may not be randomly selected or the population from which the samples were taken may not be close to a normal distribution. In those cases the analysis of the X-bar chart may not be valid, and it may be impossible to determine the presence or absence of special causes in the X-bar data. Thus for variables charts the variation measure chart (MR, R, or s) should be reviewed and found to be within control limits before analyzing the IX or X-bar chart. If the variation measure chart is not in control, then the assumptions of a normal distribution and random sampling approach that are the basis for the use of variables charts need to be reexamined.

An example of just such a situation is demonstrated in the data set in TABLE 5.8. The control chart used in this example is the IX-MR shown in FIGURE 5.7. Note the two charts, one for the IX metric and the other for the range. The range chart has two signs of an out of control indicator: point 18 is above the UCL and a run of 12 points below the centerline from point 6 to point 17. The out of control MR chart indicates that one of the assumptions, either a non-Gaussian data distribution in the population or a nonrandom sampling strategy, led to the anomalous results. Another way of examining the data in the control chart sample is through the use of a histogram, which shows the distribution of the metrics. FIGURE 5.8 displays the histogram for this data set, and the lack of normal distribution of the measures is intuitively apparent from

Table 5.8	Data Set for IX-MR Chart Demonstrating Out of Control Range Chart
Time	Value
1	12
2	18
3	2
4	16
5	2
6	3
7	4
8	2
9	3
10	4
11	1
12	1
13	3
14	1
15	2
16	4
17	5
18	29
19	18
20	1
21	12
22	19

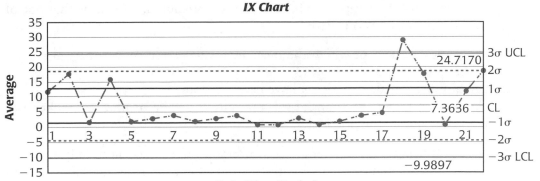

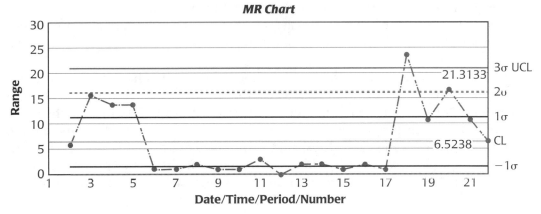

FIGURE 5.7   IX-MR Chart Demonstrating Out of Control MR Chart

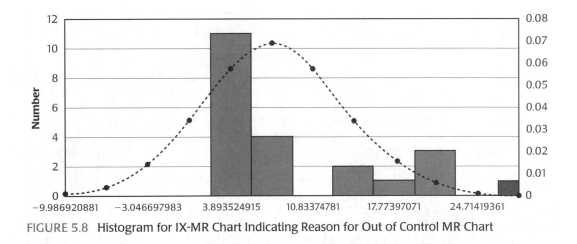

FIGURE 5.8   Histogram for IX-MR Chart Indicating Reason for Out of Control MR Chart

the graph. In fact, the data appear to be binomially distributed, indicating that one of three possibilities must be considered:

1. The population from which the measures were taken may not be normally distributed.
2. The sampling method may not have been random.
3. The process may have changed substantially (i.e., one or more special causes may have altered the process).

If the sampling process were set up to ensure random extraction of indicators for analysis, then the first and third possibilities are most likely. Further investigation can help disclose the root cause for the pattern in the data and help to revise the analysis or seek other ways of evaluating the process.

The continuous variable control chart is a powerful tool for determining if a process is in control and for monitoring a process during and after an improvement intervention. EXAMPLE 5.4 will help demonstrate how this statistical approach can be of help.

EXAMPLE 5.4 demonstrates the power of control charts in changing opinion into data and helping improvement teams establish performance targets. The lab turnaround time team not only reduced the variation and special causes in the mean time for phlebotomists to draw blood for immediate complete blood counts, but the mean time was reduced nearly 40% from 20 minutes to about 12 minutes. In both cases the range chart remained within control, indicating that the appropriate analysis was done and that the data collection process met the criteria for randomness.

Example 5.4 Continuous Variable Control Chart for Laboratory Turnaround Time

Dr. Lawrence Livermore at the International Laboratories Reference lab was concerned by the number of complaints by clinicians about the speed with which lab results were reported. The most common test was the complete blood count (CBC), and physicians from the emergency department (ED) and the intensive care unit (ICU) both said they thought the rapidity of getting results back had become a problem. Being a good scientist, Dr. Livermore decided to collect data on the CBC process to determine the source of the problem. He first called together everyone involved in the process, from ordering clerks in the ED and ICUs, and the group constructed the process flowchart in FIGURE 5.9. The group supervised collection of times at each point in the process and determined that the greatest variation and time delay was in the phlebotomist step, because the phlebotomist had to access the EHR to find the order and the patient's location. The team's collection technique involved random sampling five times per day for 3 weeks, with the results for the phlebotomist time listed in TABLE 5.9. They then graphed the results on the control

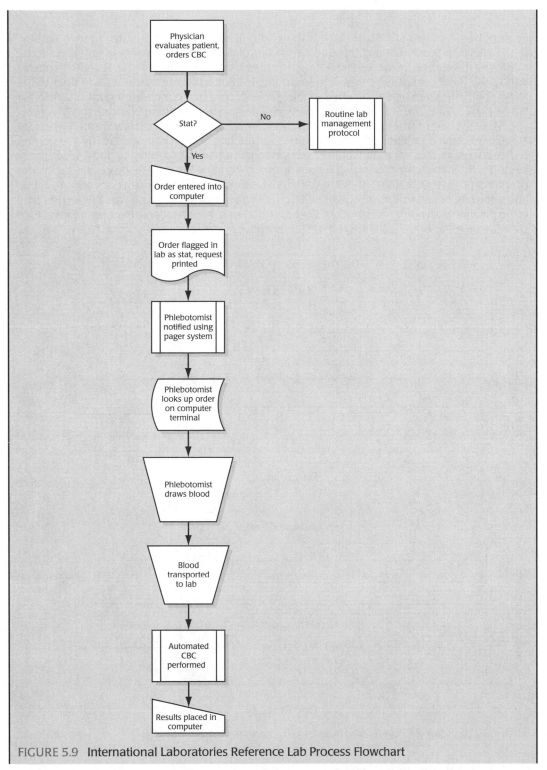

FIGURE 5.9 International Laboratories Reference Lab Process Flowchart

chart (X-bar R) shown in FIGURE 5.10. Starting with the R-chart, the team determined that the data collection procedure appeared to be in control, and the data collected appeared to be randomly distributed. However, the team also noted that the variation in the R-chart increased during the latter part of the study, but not to the level of a special cause. Turning then to the X-bar chart, the team was astonished at the special causes in the time from notification to the time of collection. The first run of six points was below the centerline, indicating a favorable special cause with turnaround times, and the team surmised that the Hawthorne effect had actually improved phlebotomist performance for the first week. However, during the second and third weeks, three of control points emerged on a Sunday, a Friday night, and a Wednesday night. The team performed a root-cause analysis to determine the underlying causes for the out of control performance and found three different reasons for the performance, involving volume and criticality of patients in the ED and ICU, but the true underlying cause was the wasted time in the phlebotomist notification process. The team made recommendations that were implemented over the next 2 months, with the resulting improvement in the process shown in FIGURE 5.11.

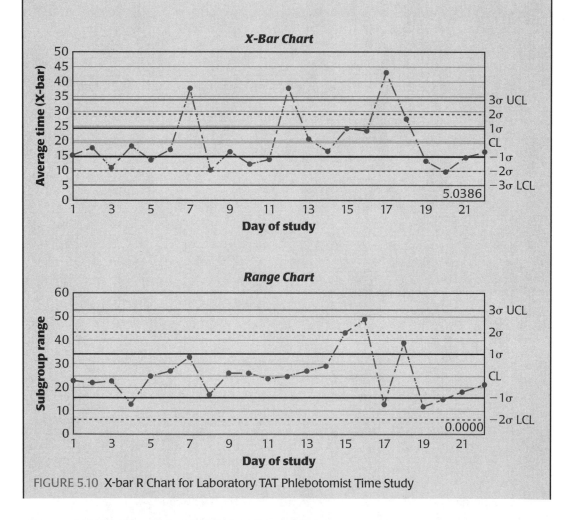

FIGURE 5.10 X-bar R Chart for Laboratory TAT Phlebotomist Time Study

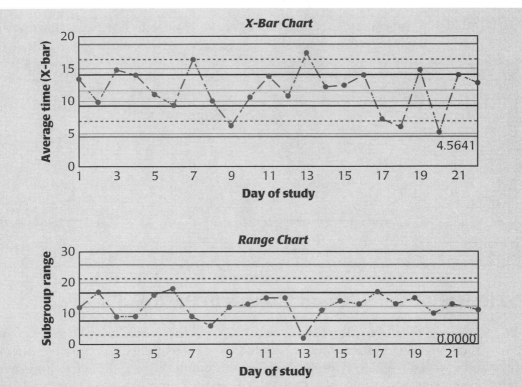

FIGURE 5.11 Post-Intervention Control Charts for Laboratory TAT Phlebotomist Time Study

Table 5.9	Laboratory Turnaround Time Data for Phlebotomist Steps (in minutes)				
Day	Obs 1	Obs 2	Obs 3	Obs 4	Obs 5
1	12	10	27	16	24
2	18	27	6	18	19
3	2	29	19	14	25
4	16	29	8	12	18
5	2	23	5	23	3
6	3	3	22	8	4
7	38	51	42	18	39
8	2	29	24	21	26
9	3	28	23	23	26
10	4	18	18	3	25
11	1	12	13	29	30
12	29	53	37	42	28
13	3	22	18	18	22

Table 5.9	Laboratory Turnaround Time Data for Phlebotomist Steps (in minutes) (continued)				
Day	Obs 1	Obs 2	Obs 3	Obs 4	Obs 5
14	1	19	3	18	14
15	2	42	18	45	28
16	4	22	25	53	15
17	38	45	51	39	42
18	29	48	27	27	25
19	18	9	23	2	13
20	1	27	27	30	10
21	12	24	14	11	4
22	19	9	2	4	30

■ Limitations of SPC and "Bumps in the Road"

SPC is a powerful tool for improving healthcare performance, but like any "great thing" there are always some limitations. SPC has been applied in a number of circumstances with outstanding results, but even this quantitative approach to improvement must be used judiciously. Perhaps the most common error that leads to inappropriate use of SPC is the selection of the wrong chart. Although the algorithm in TABLE 5.3 can help eliminate these types of errors, unfortunately the wrong analysis is sometimes performed, leading to misidentification of a process as out of control. Thus whenever a process is deemed to have one or more special causes, the first question to be asked is, "Have I used the right chart?" A review of the chart decision using the algorithm often discovers that error.

Another limitation of the approach is the concept that Deming called "tampering," which is simply ascribing special cause characteristics to common cause variation. Veteran quality professionals have experienced this problem several times in a career. For example, a managed care chief financial officer might look at two or three points on a chart tracking medical loss ratio and infer a special cause, even though the data do not indicate an out of control process. Intervening in this type of erroneous decision process is important to prevent misspent time trying to track down and correct a special cause when none is present. As discussed previously, the approaches to common cause and special cause variation are substantially different, and tampering (i.e., using special cause investigation techniques to evaluate a common cause) only leads to frustration, added expense, and wasted time. SPC can be applied in many areas in health care but should be applied with the knowledge base to ensure appropriate analysis and intervention.

Another limitation to anticipate is the assumption that once a special cause point is found, a quick review of the situation by subject matter experts will reveal the underlying problem and suggest a quick solution. EXAMPLE 5.4 is evidence of just such a limitation. Although the team identified a wave of critically ill patients as obvious causes for delays in phlebotomist response, in fact, the underlying problem was the communication system for getting information from the site of an order for a stat CBC to the phlebotomist. Because the team could not predict when critically ill patients would appear in the emergency department or deteriorate in the ICU, the next solution turned out to be the best (i.e., expedite delivery of the stat request to the phlebotomist). The danger of having a quick, but poorly informed, response is that time and money can be wasted on an inadequate solution, simply because the SPC chart suggested a solution. In the example, the team was led by an experienced improvement professional that helped delve into the issue deeply enough to avoid the obvious, but erroneous, conclusion.

SPC must be practiced by professionals but used by statistical thinkers. Although front-line workers can be taught how to use the data in an SPC chart to make better decisions, they often may not be able to effectively track down the cause of an out of control point when it occurs. Most healthcare processes are intimately intertwined with other related processes, leading to a web of interactions that can make root-cause determination complex. When an SPC signal appears, front-line staff need to know when to make rapid adjustments and when to alert others that more thought and analysis is needed regarding the underlying cause, which could be in a process completely different from the one that is showing the signal. Experience helps this situation, but a lack of response protocols can lead to poor reactions to out of control signals and decrements in performance.

In most cases it is virtually impossible to measure all indicators for a process under study. Selection of the best indicators often relies on the judgment of subject matter experts, but if a poorly functioning process is measured and no abnormal metrics surface, then the team must assume that the wrong indicators were chosen and adjust the measures accordingly. Again, an experienced performance improvement (PI) professional can provide insight in these situations.

Although most measurement systems perform reliably, the limitations of the measurement system may become a factor. For example, if a machine is used to make a measurement (e.g., a clock to measure time), an inherent error is present that may affect the indicator and lead to an error in the interpretation of the SPC output. An entire science of gage repeatability and reliability has been developed to address this issue in the manufacturing industry, but similar approaches have not been applied to healthcare measurement systems to the same extent. In any measurement situation the reliability of the tool or individual doing the measurement must be taken into consideration if aberrant results are reported. In some cases interrater reliability studies that do repetitive testing of different individuals involved in collecting data may be helpful in reducing the error related to measurement reliability and repeatability.

Keeping all these possible problems in mind should help preclude many of the common problems related to SPC and enhance the value of the approach in most healthcare systems. Fortunately, many analysis systems have been developed to help reduce the likelihood of these limitations causing problems with most assessments.

■ Analysis Packages for SPC

A number of statistical analysis software are available to perform SPC, and a complete exposition of all these software programs is beyond the scope of this book. However, the control charts constructed for the examples in this chapter were created using a Microsoft Excel add-in called QI Macros. A number of other packages for this purpose and their websites are listed in TABLE 5.10.

■ Approaches to Refining SPC Analyses

In some cases data may be too aggregated to yield significant differences when these differences exist. For example, a group of physicians may have substantially different costs of care and wide variation from case to case for a particular clinical episode of care, but an aggregate measure of the cost of care for all physicians treating the condition may not show any out of control points or substantial variation. Larger samples often "hide" underlying variation because of the statistical smoothing that occurs with large samples of data. In these situations two strategies may be of value: stratification and analysis of means (ANOM).

Stratifying data is essentially the separation of data into categories by characteristics that are shared or not shared. For example, the large group of physicians may be stratified by specialty to determine if the cost of care is higher within one specialty compared with another. Stratification is often done iteratively, that is, after one level of stratification other more specific levels are found, but each stratum should make sense from a decision-making standpoint. At some point stratification can be overdone:

Table 5.10	SPC Analysis and Charting Software
Software Package	Website
QI Macros	www.qimacros.com
StatIt	www.statit.com
SQCPack	www.pqsystems.com
JMP Software (SAS)	www.sas.com
SPC for Excel	www.spcforexcel.com
Minitab	www.minitab.com
QI Analyst	www.spss.com

Samples can be made so small that insignificant differences can appear statistically significant (a type I error) simply because the sample size is too small. However, stratification can be a useful tool to uncover important targets for intervention.

By sorting data into multiple levels of logical groupings with shared characteristics, it is sometimes easier to pinpoint the root cause of a problem. For example, stratification of physicians and specialties by region of the country was one of the seminal insights of the small area analysis that is the basis for the Dartmouth Atlas (www.dartmouthatlas.org) findings of substantial differences in the cost and quality of care in different areas of the United States. Using Medicare data John Wennburg and analysts at Dartmouth College stratified the cost and quality of care by zip code and aggregated the information into comparative assessments of medical care. Using an analogous approach on the cost of care example described above, the cohort of physicians may first be stratified by specialty, then by location (zip code), and then perhaps by patient insurance source. Applying control charts to these strata then may find trends and variations that could lead to improvement initiatives. Some other tools that are often applied to stratify a population include Pareto charts, bar charts, pie charts, and histograms, all of which display counts of objects in different categories. Additionally, a decision tree could be used to build a branching algorithm that can help with the stratification decision process.

ANOM is another method of teasing out otherwise hidden differences. This approach helps to determine if sample means are equal; if they are not equal, the visual analysis can reveal the level of significance of the differences by providing upper and lower decision limits (UDL and LDL). These limits account for individual variation among strata, based on one or more of the specific characteristics that created the strata. For example, the physician cost differences in treatment of a specific condition described above could be analyzed by evaluating each provider using ANOM, with output similar to that in FIGURE 5.12 that provides individual mean and 3 sigma limits (the UDL and LDL). The visual representation of these differences and variation outside decision limits is much easier to interpret than many other types of analysis. Although the ANOM is not an SPC chart, the LDL and UDL make interpretation of the results similar (i.e., the data that falls outside the decision limits is significantly different from that within the LDL and UDL).

The first task of ANOM is to determine the UDL and LDL, and the formulae for making those calculations can be found in statistics textbooks and other locations.[4] The UDL and LDL depend on several factors:

- Samples' means
- Grand mean (the mean of all the samples' means)
- Standard deviation
- Desired alpha (type I error) level (usually 0.05, but at 3 sigma levels $\alpha = 0.003$)
- Number of samples
- Sample sizes

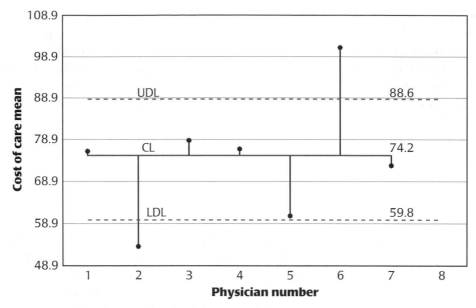

FIGURE 5.12 Analysis of Means for Physician Cost of Care

ANOM compares the natural variability of every sample mean with the mean of all sample means. When running an ANOM, the user is usually prompted for the alpha level, and the level of 0.0027 provides 3 sigma limits for the LDL and UDL. FIGURE 5.12 provides a sample graph of an ANOM chart. Note that two physicians fall outside the decision limits for the analysis. Physician 6 is above the UDL, whereas physician 2 is below the LDL. The remaining providers are within the decision limits. Interpretation of this information is important, not only because the physician with the high cost requires attention, but the physician who is below the LDL also should be evaluated, either for best practices that can be emulated by others or for potential problems with quality of care because of less utilization of appropriate services.

■ Barriers to Implementation of SPC

Although SPC and other analyses are of great importance in helping understand data and make better decisions, there are still barriers to implementing these methods. The three broad divisions of barriers—people, data and chart construction, and information technology—indicate what areas need to be addressed when introducing SPC in a health-care organization. As an increasing emphasis is put on data and comparisons of performance, many clinicians feel threatened (statistically, half will be below the median for any performance measure and will feel particularly threatened), and so the focus of the use of data in the organization must be on improvement, not punishment. Educational programs on the use and analysis of the data defuse some of the resistance, but consistent use of the data for performance improvement with the use of punitive measures reserved only for the most recalcitrant of practitioners ensures broader acceptance of the evidence-based management approach that so prominently features SPC. Making quality the center of the effort will gain the support of clinicians, staff members, patients, and members of the governance body, because the entire system will provide safer, more cost-effective care.

■ Advanced Statistical Tools

SPC is a useful tool for quality improvement programs, and the use of control charts is generally easily implemented in most organizations. Moving from a trial and error culture to one that bases decisions on data is one achievement that can move any organization to higher levels of performance. When a performance improvement team begins to use techniques that may require comparisons of two or more interventions, or perhaps designed experiments that may try several interventions in a system to achieve the best results, then other statistical approaches may be necessary. For example, a process that is not in control must be examined to determine the underlying cause, requiring approaches to establish relationships. When the team determines that more than one solution might be possible to improve a process, a trial and error approach to improvement would take time and cost substantially in human and financial resources. In that circumstance an approach similar to that used in clinical research is applied, called design of experiments (DOE). The next three sections address the methods used for each of these situations.

Establishing Relationships

Typically, after a special cause is identified the quality improvement team expends effort to identify the underlying reason(s) for the out of control performance. In most cases more data are necessary to find the cause, and additional analysis may be helpful in determining which of the potential causes are of greatest importance. Although many statistical methods are available to determine the nature and statistical strength of a relationship between one or more causes and an effect or outcome, one method that is used frequently is regression analysis. Researchers from a wide range of disciplines routinely use regression analysis to try to quantify the direction, strength, and magnitude of relationships between variables as well as to test hypotheses and subsequently predict future behavior of the dependent variable based on changes in one or more independent variables. Regression extends the capability provided by other statistical procedures by quantifying the level or amount of change expected in an outcome (termed the "dependent variable") based on a measured level of change in a predictor (termed the "independent variable"). Regression analysis has been

Exhibit 5.2 Fundamentals of Regression for Statistical Thinkers

Regression is a mathematical technique that helps determine relationships between dependent (y) and independent (x) variables

The relationship between the variables has a certain level of statistical significance that is provided in the form of the r-value.

The sign of the coefficient (β) for the independent variable tells the direction (up or down, plus or minus) of the x-variable's effect on the y-value.

The value of β provides the magnitude of the effect of the independent variable on the dependent variable.

Regression analysis can be done on a single y-x combination (simple linear regression) or on a single y-value with multiple x-variables (multivariate regression).

Although regression is designed to analyze numeric values, even non-numeric data can be transformed into numbers using dummy variables.

Mathematical transformations are possible to ensure that the data being analyzed meet the requirements effectively.

applied to a number of areas in health care, from managed care to clinical research, and has helped decision makers understand cause and effect relationships for predictive purposes in numerous performance improvement initiatives.

Applied to performance improvement, these techniques are useful in defining relationships and also in helping to find potentially confounding factors such as comorbidities (coexisting clinical conditions), prior healthcare treatment, staffing patterns, utilization, and demographic characteristics. Researchers are afforded the ability to understand and describe the association of various predictor variables with phenomena such as changes in clinical outcomes for a given therapeutic intervention or process change in the delivery system. Correlation is a major tenet of basic regression and is used to establish relationships that are used to target specific interventions to improve quality.

Regression has many forms, and a variety of methods is available that refine the regression approach to specific circumstances. The focus of this discussion, however, is on its use to find relationships to target improvement initiatives.

Correlation connotes the strength of a linear association between two variables, and although there are several measures of correlation, the most commonly used is the **Pearson product–moment correlation coefficient** (usually abbreviated with a lowercase r). The Pearson correlation is an expression of the association between two continuous variables (real numbers), which are the most commonly used for defining quality relationships. As with SPC charts, other correlations are used when other types of variables, like ranked variables, are used. Correlation coefficients measure two facets of a relationship: the magnitude (with absolute coefficient values ranging from zero to one) and the direction (either positive or negative). For the Pearson correlation the larger the absolute value of the correlation coefficient, the stronger the linear association (e.g., a correlation of −1.0 indicates a perfectly negative linear association, whereas 0.0 indicates no linear association and 1.0 indicates a perfectly positive linear association). Thus if the r-value for the relationship between two variables is −1.0, then the dependent variable can be expected to always decrease as the independent variable increases. For example, a positive correlation may exist between a patient's overall healthcare costs and the number of physician visits or hospital stays, indicating that expenditures increase as a function of use of medical services. Similarly, a negative correlation may exist between the number of medical errors occurring in a hospital setting and the magnitude of the quality assurance program in place in the hospital, which would confirm that the quality improvement program was having the expected effect. It should be emphasized that the Pearson correlation measures a *linear* association between two variables, and so if a nonlinear relationship exists, the Pearson r-value might not be a reliable indicator. If, for example, the r-value from analysis of a data set is zero, then there may be either no relationship or a nonlinear relationship defining the association between the variables. Although statistical software packages routinely report correlations and related tests of statistical significance, graphical analyses of scatter plots similar to that shown in FIGURE 5.13 can indicate if other types of relationships exist that may not conform to the linear model reflected by the Pearson r.

Although correlation and regression are linked conceptually, differences between correlation and regression are important. Correlation expresses the strength of a linear association between variables, whereas regression involves the estimation of a mathematical equation based on selecting an appropriate mathematical model that includes all relevant variables. As such, correlation does not depend on the scales of

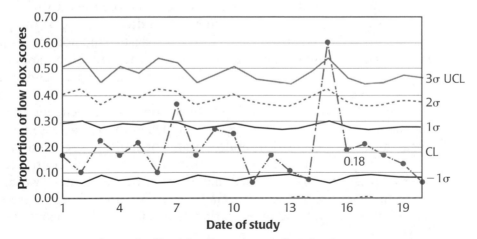

FIGURE 5.13 Low Box Scores for Physician Promptness – Exercise 3

measurement of the comparison variables, whereas changing measurement units in regression can change the interpretation of the results dramatically. In regression analysis, correlation statistics are used to assess the levels of relationships between variables. The **coefficient of determination** (r^2) is particularly important because it connotes the degree to which a dependent variable is explained by an independent (predictor) variable. The coefficient of determination is the square of the Pearson correlation coefficient and so is always between zero and +1.0. When multiple independent variables are involved in the relationship, which is often the situation in a quality improvement study, r-squared value is replaced by the **coefficient of multiple determination**, or **R-squared** (R^2). The **adjusted R-squared coefficient** may also be reported and corrects for the number of independent variables that are specified in a multiple regression equation when more than one predictor variable is involved. The R^2 coefficient provides useful information in evaluating the overall goodness of fit of a given regression equation, with a higher value signifying a better fit. Although these statistics establish a relationship, the quality improvement team should evaluate the nature of the association (i.e., if the relationship is causative). In addition to these important statistics, the F-statistic for the regression analysis also provides insight into the statistical significance of the relationships defined in the regression equation. However, even a high degree of statistical significance can only specify an association, not a causative relationship.

As mentioned previously, the quality improvement team begins by assessing possible underlying causes of an out of control process, and using measures associated with these potential causes, relationships are hypothesized for analysis through regression analysis. Each variable selected is thus part of the hypothesis of causation (i.e., becomes an independent predictor of the outcome variable). Each variable could be analyzed separately, but most often multiple indicators are analyzed simultaneously (multiple regression). Frequently, the team will conduct a literature review to determine if others have encountered a similar problem and then select variables to analyze from these sources. Regression itself embodies a diverse range of analytical techniques, such as multivariate, proportional hazards, logistic, and nonlinear methods. Despite the existence of more advanced methods, linear regression remains the most useful. Linear regression describes the relationship between a dependent and an independent variable as a straight-line function. **Simple linear regression** refers to the specific case with a linear relationship between only one dependent variable and one independent variable. When more than one independent variable is involved, the simple linear model is extended to **multivariate (or multiple) regression**. For example, a relationship between a medication error rate that exceeds control limits and the number of prescriptions processed may be modified with other variables, such as nurse staffing factors, physician specialty, etc. The simple linear regression model may be enhanced by adding other variables to explain the reasons for the special cause event.

Regression models attempt to estimate a "line of best fit" through a set of data points that then can serve to describe the relationship of the population from which the sample is taken. A linear equation estimate takes the following form:

$$y = \alpha + \beta X + \varepsilon$$

where y is the dependent variable of interest; α is the intercept, or constant, of the equation; β is the slope coefficient, often referred to simply as "beta"; x is the independent variable of interest; and ε is the *residual*, disturbance, or error term.

In simple linear regression the line of best fit represents a line drawn on a typical *xy*-graph as shown in FIGURE 5.14. As variables are added to the analysis, the graph becomes increasingly complex and after two or three variables becomes multidimensional. In a multivariate regression analysis the line of best fit is a two-dimensional plane when there are two independent variables, but the graph becomes an *n*-dimensional object when there are *n* independent variables. In the multivariate model the β terms represent estimates of the effects of each independent variable on the dependent variable with all other independent variables held constant. Because a sample of data is typically used to estimate the population parameters α and β, the estimates are denoted with the letter "a" for the alpha term and the letter "b" for β; the estimated value of the dependent variable is often expressed with a caret as Y and called "Y-hat." The most common method of estimating the regression coefficients is ordinary least squares, which is designed to minimize the sum of the squared error term. More details of the ordinary least squares approach can be found in free online statistical texts listed in the Additional Reading section at the end of the chapter.

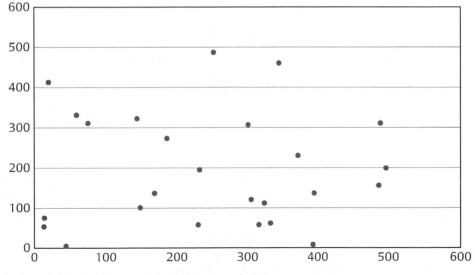

FIGURE 5.14 Scatter Plot Demonstrating no Correlation

The equation defines the relationship between the dependent variable (y) and the independent variables (x). The alpha (α) term represents the point on the y-axis where the line intersects the axis or the value of y when x is zero. In many cases the x value may never be zero, and so the α term may not be of interest. The slope, or β coefficient, indicates the change in the dependent (y) variable for each unit change in the independent (x) variable. The mathematical sign of slope indicates the direction of the correlation: A positive β corresponds to a positive correlation, and a negative β corresponds to a negative correlation. Most of the time, the β coefficient is interpreted as defining the change in y for every unit of x, but when a nonlinear relationship exists, more sophisticated data transformations may be necessary to establish linearity between the dependent and independent variables, leading to a somewhat different interpretation of β. A more extensive discussion of data transformations follows.

Like SPC, regression models are based on some basic assumptions of the nature of the underlying data:[5]

1. The parameter coefficients of the model describe a linear relationship between the dependent and independent variables, described as follows:

$$Y_i = \alpha + \beta X_i + \varepsilon_i$$

2. The predictors (X_i) of the model are nonrandom (called *nonstochastic*).
3. The **expected value** of the residual ε_i for any given value of the independent variable is equal to zero, as follows:

$$E(\varepsilon_i | X_i) = 0$$

4. The residual term has a constant variance (var) across observations, represented mathematically as follows:

$$\text{var}(\varepsilon_i | X_i) = \sigma^2$$

5. The residual terms of any two independent observations, X_i and X_j, are independent and unrelated, indicating a random distribution, or lack of *autocorrelation* (i.e., correlation between data values in the observations). The lack of correlation in the residuals of two independent observations is represented as a covariance (cov) as follows:

$$\text{cov}(\varepsilon_i, \varepsilon_j | X_i, X_j) = 0$$

6. The residual term is unrelated to all independent variables. That is, the conditional covariance with respect to an independent variable and the residual is equal to zero:

$$\text{cov}(\varepsilon_i, X_i) = 0$$

7. The residual term, ε_i, is normally distributed.
8. No perfect linear correlation exists between any of the independent variables (i.e., no *multicollinearity* is present).

To derive parameter estimates, the number of observations must exceed the number of parameters estimated, that is, the number of data points collected must exceed the number of beta coefficients. The number of observations per independent variable required for reasonable precision of the estimates is a function of the magnitude of the beta value, but social scientists suggest 15 observations per independent variable as a general guideline. Additionally, if some level of multicollinearity exists between some of the independent variables, then larger numbers of observations may be necessary to achieve a useable model.

Parametric statistical methods (those that start with the assumption that data are distributed according to a specific probability function, e.g., the normal distribution) are often used in conjunction with regression techniques, and so additional factors should be considered for a regression analysis:

- Data are randomly sampled.
- Data in the sample are independent of each other.
- Sample means are normally distributed.
- Data come from an interval scale (equal distance between two numbers on the scale).

The condition of normally distributed sample means is typically achieved through the **law of large numbers,** which states that a mean value from a randomly drawn sample from a population is highly probable to equal the population mean if the sample size is large.

The need for regression variables to be real numbers can be circumvented by creating **binary**, or **dummy**, **variables,** binary values of 0 or 1 that represent categorical values like male–female, treated–nontreated, etc. This approach allows inclusion of qualitative variables in multivariate regressions and treats categorical variables like continuous variables.

Multicollinearity is a significant issue in multivariate models, particularly as the number of independent variables increases. When independent variables are highly or perfectly correlated with each other, the individual effects of the predictors cannot be precisely estimated. If multicollinearity is present, then both the precision and accuracy of coefficients are reduced. Multicollinearity may arise from the following:

- Failure to collect sufficient amount of data.
- Non-Gaussian distribution in the sample population.
- Wrong regression model (i.e., use of a linear model for a nonlinear data set).

Multicollinearity generally is not significant at low levels of correlation between independent variables, but when predictors are highly correlated or if multiple variables are moderately correlated with one another, then the standard errors of the regression coefficients may be unusually large, leading to a weak model. Several signs of multi-collinearity can be found in the regression statistics:

- Large R^2 value with relatively few statistically significant t ratios.
- High pairwise correlations between independent variables.
- High values for the condition index or the variance inflation factor (e.g., values of the condition index ≥ 15 or variance inflation factor ≥ 10); these two statistics are reported by most regression software and reflect the presence of multicollinearity.

If multicollinearity is not addressed, the resulting model will likely have large variances for parameter estimates, resulting in statistically insignificant parameter coefficients with relatively wide confidence intervals. Several approaches are used to reduce the problem, such as dropping one or more variables, combining correlated variables, applying transformations to the model (e.g., logarithmic transformations discussed later), or increasing the number of observations in the study.

One of the important parts of the output from a regression software program is analysis of residuals (the error [ε] terms in the regression equation), which can provide a determination of the validity of assumptions of homoscedasticity (equal variance for the dependent variable across all the data), independence of predictors, model linearity, and distribution normality. Because residuals represent the difference between the actual value of the dependent variable and the value of the dependent variable that is estimated from the line of best fit, if the assumptions of linear regression are violated or if the regression equation is incorrect for the data set, the error term demonstrates inconsistencies. These inconsistencies may require reformulation of the model and use of transformation methods to ensure that the data set fits a linear model. The error term values should be distributed randomly around an average value of zero, and often a scatter plot of the residuals against the predicted value of the dependent variable can provide a visual indication of random distribution of the terms. When a linear regression equation is proposed for a nonlinear data set, the resulting graph of residuals is curved or follows a regular pattern. In short, any nonrandom distribution of the residuals indicates multicollinearity and should prompt further evaluation of the model and its fit to the data set. A histogram of the error terms is often reported to test for normally distributed residuals.

Serial correlation or **autocorrelation** connotes a lack of independence of the error terms and is another indicator of a poorly fitting regression model. The Durbin-Watson d test reported in the regression output is used to determine the level of autocorrelation, although other tests are also available. If the residuals demonstrate autocorrelation, the model requires revision that may involve more sophisticated statistical techniques that are beyond the scope of this text but are found in the statistical texts listed in the Additional Reading section at the end of the chapter.

Logarithmic Transformation of Data

Data sets that do not conform to the normal distribution may be transformed mathematically into a distribution that meets the criteria for regression. Healthcare utilization or cost data are typically not normally distributed and often demonstrate heteroscedasticity, with distributions that are positively skewed. In these cases, transforming the data set may achieve the goal of creating a distribution that is close enough to linear to allow use of regression analysis. For example, the original distribution shown in FIGURE 5.15 could define a relationship between a dependent and independent variable, and the use of linear regression to analyze the data set would yield the line shown on the graph with the relationship:

$$y = 541410x - 4 \times 10^{-6}$$

and an R^2 value of 0.21, indicating that only about 20% of the variation in y is explained by the independent variable. Additionally, the data set has a significant outlier at the upper end of the distribution. On the other hand, if the distribution is changed so that the y values (dependent variables) are transformed to the natural logarithm of y ($\ln y$), then the graph in FIGURE 5.16 results, with the relationship:

$$\ln(y) = 0.5\,x + 4.25,$$

and an R^2 value of 0.93, which indicates that about 93% of the variation in y is explained by x (i.e., a much better fitting model). Further, analysis of the residuals in each situation would reveal that the model calculated from the original data set had residuals that were not randomly distributed; however, in the transformed data set

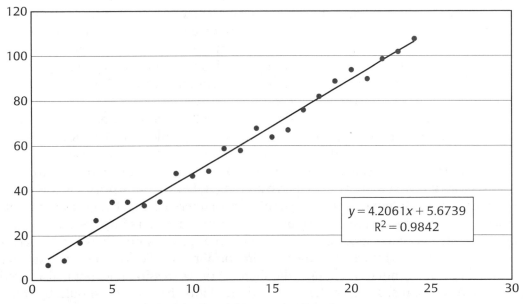

FIGURE 5.15 Graph of a Simple Linear Model Regression Equation

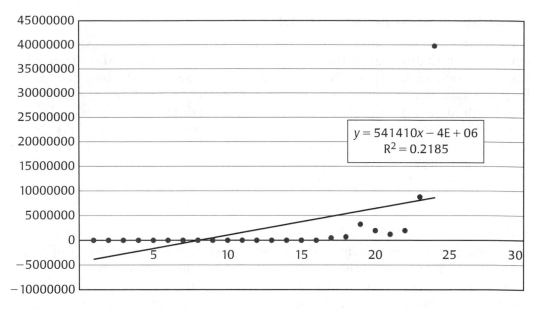

$$y = 541410x - 4E + 06$$
$$R^2 = 0.2185$$

FIGURE 5.16 Original Non-Linear Data set Graph with Linear Regression Model Overlay

model, the residuals were much more randomly distributed. The transformed distribution thus provides a much more robust regression model. A key point to remember, however, is that the interpretation of the relationship between the dependent and independent variables is not the same as before. The independent variable predicts the behavior of the **natural logarithm** of the dependent variable, *not* the measured or expected values of the dependent variable. Thus, when interpreting the equation, the relationship between the independent and dependent variables must be adjusted to this new understanding. For decision makers, this alteration may have significant implications, because the changes in the dependent variable will be substantially accentuated as the independent variable increases.

Transformation of the y-value using the natural logarithm is only one of many possible transformations. Any of the variables, independent or dependent, can be transformed, and other types of mathematical transformations may be applied, such as log base 10 ($\log_{10}$), log base 2 ($\log_2$), square root, or other mathematical treatments. In most cases it is best to transform the y-values first, because transforming the x variable does little to change distribution of the data in reference to the regression line but rather is like cutting the joint distribution of the x,y data pairs into vertical sections and changing the spacing of the sections. This change does not change the vertical spacing of the data, which is often the more important issue. Performing a transformation on the y-values not only changes the shape of the regression line, but it also alters the relative vertical spacing of the observations. Thus the y-values should be transformed first to determine if other alterations will be needed. In most cases, if data

Example 5.5 Use of Regression Analysis to Predict Risk of Hospitalization

Quality Over Cost (QOC) managed care company is trying to determine its medical loss ratio for a specific clinical condition, disease D. The analysts at QOC, led by Dr. Matt H. Chang, have the claims and pharmaceutical utilization data sets and, using that information, they would like to determine if certain patterns of care are of greater value to reducing hospitalization rates (i.e., increased morbidity and complication rates) in the population of health plan members with disease X. The dependent variable of interest is thus hospitalization versus no hospitalization, which is represented by a binary variable (0 for no hospitalization, 1 for hospitalization). The predictors they surmise will be of value include member age; gender; presence or absence of three potential comorbidities (A, B, and/or C) represented by binary variables; average monthly dosage of drugs M, N, and/or O over the 12 months before the evaluation; and whether the member has undergone surgery for disease D in the past 2 years, represented by a binary variable (0 for no surgery, 1 for surgery). They note that with nine independent variables they need at least 10 observations, but, fortunately, they have over 1,000 members in the two databases that would qualify for the analysis. Using a SAS program, the analyst team created a data set that combined the drug and utilization data and ran a multivariate analysis to obtain the β coefficients in TABLE 5.11 with their associated p values for presentation to senior managers. Dr. Chang reviewed the residuals and determined that no anomalies were present, indicating the model was reasonable. He also noted that the R^2 value is 0.58, indicating that about 58% of the risk of hospitalizations could be explained by the chosen variables. Senior managers noted that although all the variables showed significant p values (except for gender and disease C, with p values around 0.1), the highest beta values were found with comorbid disease B and drug N, indicating that these two factors contributed the most to hospitalization rates for members with disease D. This initial analysis of the data prompted the analyst team to begin to develop a strategy to study the influence of disease B and drug N on the hospitalization rates for disease D, including further analysis of members with these two predictors to see if they are different from the remaining members of the health plan's beneficiaries with disease D.

Table 5.11	Statistics for Managed Care Example 5.5	
Independent Variable	Beta	p Value
Age	0.001	0.001
Gender	0.0001	0.1
Disease A	0.3	0.05
Disease B	1.2	0.019
Disease C	0.04	0.12
Drug M	0.21	0.011
Drug N	0.43	0.001
Drug O	0.003	0.0021
Surgery	0.005	0.003

transformations are required to achieve linearity, the involvement of a statistician familiar with these approaches is desirable.

Examples of the use of log transformed data for regression analysis abound in the healthcare literature. Armstrong and Malone[6] conducted an assessment of asthma-related costs associated with fluticasone versus three different leukotriene modifiers. The dependent variable was log-transformed post-asthma cost with predictors that included age, sex, log-transformed pre-asthma cost, presence of chronic obstructive pulmonary disease, treatment group (i.e., fluticasone or leukotriene modifier), and the use of certain medications before the study period, like number of short-acting beta-agonist inhalers used and binary variables representing the use of long-acting beta agonists, theophylline or mast cell stabilizers, or oral corticosteroids. In 347 patients from a database of 350,000 managed care organization members, they reported that patients taking a leukotriene modifier obtained more short-acting beta-agonists than patients receiving fluticasone (6.49 ± 4.05 vs. 4.30 ± 3.41, $p < 0.0001$). Survival analysis of time to receive any additional controller therapy revealed that patients receiving fluticasone were significantly less likely to receive another controller than were those receiving a leukotriene modifier ($p = 0.0014$). These results were helpful to the managed care organization in determining how to include each of the four medications in its formulary.

Regression is a powerful and widely used statistical technique that allows quality improvement professionals to make statistically valid associations between dependent and independent variables for the purposes of better understanding processes and outcomes. Correlation is a key ingredient in a regression analysis, making it particularly useful in such tasks as root-cause analysis and other investigative studies in all segments of the industry. Statistical thinkers may not need to be adept in performing the calculations and transformations of data sets, but knowing the application of the technique and some of the caveats can help managers use this powerful tool to maximum advantage. The flexibility of regression makes it particularly useful in a number of settings, from relatively straightforward simple linear regression to highly complex multivariate models. The increased availability of administrative databases containing medical and pharmacy claims data may provide more opportunities for performing regression studies in a number of different settings, but as clinical data become more standardized and computerized, the use of these techniques will prove a powerful method for optimizing clinical care.

Design of Experiments

Sir Ronald Fisher, a scientist at a small agricultural research station in England in 1926, developed a strategy for planning research known as *design of experiments* (DOE) to conduct valid experiments in the presence of naturally fluctuating conditions such as temperature, soil condition, and rainfall. These principles have been successfully adapted to industrial and military applications since the 1940s, and in the past

Exhibit 5.3 DOE for Statistical Thinkers

DOE is a method for validating processes and identifying important factors and levels that drive process output.

Experiments consist of multiple runs using factors that influence an outcome variable, with each factor at different levels in each run.

Experiments are designed using statistically valid methods that examine main effects of individual factors and the effects of interactions of these factors. Most experiments use two levels for each factor and are denoted as 2^n experiments (i.e., two levels of n factors).

Using approaches like blocking and randomization, the experiment can be optimized to provide the most significant relationships between factors and outcomes.

30 years the application of DOE has gained acceptance throughout the world as an essential tool for improving the quality of goods and services. Newly applied in the healthcare industry, DOE is becoming an essential part of a quality improvement programs in many different types of healthcare organizations.[7] The work of Japanese quality expert Genichi Taguchi promoted the use of DOE in designing robust products in the telephone and other industries, leading to products that were developed and tested using statistical experimental design. These methods were applied at Ford Motor Company with great success, leading to wider adoption of DOE in American industry in the 1960s and 1970s. As computing power became more ubiquitous, many user-friendly software packages provided the capability to perform the statistical analyses to support more sophisticated DOE procedures.

Interestingly, DOE techniques have been applied by medical researchers for decades but have not been readily adopted for quality improvement interventions and new product/service design. Medical device manufacturers, however, are being directed by the U.S. Food and Drug Administration to apply this engineering approach to improve reliability of devices under a plethora of conditions but to do so economically. For that reason DOE has become a major factor in that sector. Properly designed and executed experiments generate more precise data while using substantially fewer experimental runs than alternative approaches. Results can be interpreted with relatively simple statistical techniques, with the same power as randomized controlled trials that have become standard in medical research.

The concept of **process validation** involves collecting and storing data that demonstrate with a high degree of statistical confidence that a particular process will continue to deliver services or produce products that meet standards that are either established by the industry, regulators, accrediting bodies, and other oversight organizations. Because this capability is the basis for patient safety and process reliability, these approaches are receiving much attention from healthcare administrators and clinicians alike. Such techniques as failure mode and effects criticality analysis (see Chapter 3) can use DOE to design systems and processes to alleviate safety and quality issues by judiciously experimenting with the process variables before implementation. In DOE this approach is sometimes called **process characterization**, in which key elements of the process are methodically varied during the design phase to optimize operating combinations and identify variation that lead to reduced quality outcomes.

Not only will this approach help with the optimization effort, but the results from the DOE can provide information that allows anticipation of outputs should process inputs change or deteriorate. These combinations of variables can be carefully recorded and used to troubleshoot processes when output does not meet expectations. In particular, simple two-level factorial and fractional factorial designs are useful techniques for worst case scenario studies.

Traditional experimentation in health care evaluates only one variable (or factor) at a time, with all other variables held constant during the experiment. Although this experimental model demonstrates the effect of the selected variable under controlled conditions, when other variables change the experiment must be repeated to understand how those changes modify the output. For example, an experiment might be designed to determine fixed expiratory volume at 1 second (FEV_1) results at one of two specific concentrations of an inhaled β-agonist in a sample population of people with asthma, some of whom were using a steroid inhaler and some not, with two levels of steroid dosage; however, to measure the effect of varying concentrations of the drug, the experiment would need to be repeated with all other variables held constant. Fisher proposed varying all factors at once using a factorial design, in which experiments are run for all combinations of levels for all factors. With such a study design, testing reveals what the effect of one variable would be when the other factors are changing. Using a factorial design for the asthma drug example, running a test with both variables at their high level might yield a FEV_1 average of 90% of predicted, but to evaluate the synergistic effect of the two drugs, combinations of the two must be tested, which is the goal of the factorial experimental approach.

Three aspects of a process are analyzed in an experimental design:

1. **Factors,** or inputs to the process. Factors can be classified as either controllable or uncontrollable variables. People are generally considered a noise factor (i.e., an uncontrollable factor that causes variability under normal conditions but which can be controlled during the experiment using techniques like blocking and randomization). Potential factors can be categorized using the Ishikawa chart (cause and effect diagram) discussed in Chapter 3.
2. **Levels,** or settings of each factor. The levels of factors in an experimental design are generally within controllable ranges.
3. **Response,** or output of the experiment. Experimenters often desire to avoid optimizing the process for one response at the expense of another. For this reason important outcomes are measured and analyzed to determine

the factors and their settings that will provide the best overall outcome for the critical-to-quality characteristics—both measurable variables and assessable attributes.

Consider the process of baking a cake. In this case, the controllable factors are the ingredients for the cake and the oven in which the cake is baked. The baker can be considered a "noise factor" because he may sleep on the job or leave the building before the process is completed. There could be other types of factors, such as the mixing method or tools, the sequence of mixing, or even other people involved. Levels in this example include the various oven temperature settings and the amounts of sugar, flour, and eggs. Response variables in the case of cake baking include the taste, consistency, and appearance of the cake, which are measurable outcomes potentially influenced by the factors and their respective levels.

The purpose of designed experiments is to optimize the output, given various levels of the factors that serve as inputs into the process. Thus for cake baking, the goal is to provide the best cake possible (taste, consistency, appearance) by finding the best levels of the major inputs: oven temperature settings, sugar amount, flour amount, and number of eggs. The goals then become as follows:

- Comparison of alternative combinations of factors.
- Identifying significant inputs (i.e., which factors are of greatest significance and are there any other factors of significance).
- Achievement of optimal response (process output).
- Reduction of variation in the output as well as input factors.
- Targeting a response (output) by minimizing or maximizing response levels (i.e., balancing critical to quality factors to achieve true optimization).
- Improving process robustness or fitness for use regardless of conditions. Taguchi mastered this issue by finding ways of designing experiments to produce outputs regardless of variation in inputs.

The design of an experiment addresses the issues listed above by specifying factors to be tested, levels of the factors, and the conditions for the experiment. As discussed in the SPC section previously, experimental results rely on a capable measurement system and a stable process. If either of these assumptions is violated, then the likelihood of success of the experimental design is small. In some cases using SPC to monitor the measurement system or process capability can help ensure that the experimental results are valid. Additionally, four potential fallacies may create invalid results in experimental runs:

1. Other sources for error and unexplained variation (i.e., any factor that has not been previously recognized that affects the experiment's inputs or outputs). Properly designed experiments are capable of identifying these extraneous sources of error.

2. Noise factors are those inputs that induce variation into the process but are not controlled by the experimenter. For example, the baker in the cake-baking example can be a source of noise, as could environmental variables like different ovens, different brands of flour, etc.

3. Confusing correlation with causation. As discussed in the section on regression modeling, although two variables move in tandem, they may only be correlated. One may not be exerting a causative effect on the other to create the movement, but rather the correlated changes may indicate that each may simply be changing without any relationship. Often, subject matter experts may need to establish the appropriate relationship.

4. The **combined effects or interactions between factors** require careful consideration before conducting the experiment. For example, consider an experiment to grow plants with two inputs: water and fertilizer. Interactive effects may be as important as main effects in producing a specific output. For example, the eggs and flour may interact in a heated environment (oven) to produce an unanticipated effect that changes the response variables. Factor interactions may generate nonlinear effects that are not additive, but these interactions can only be studied with more complex experiments. Two levels for each factor is defined as linear, that is, two points define a line, whereas three levels are defined as quadratic (three points define a curve), and four levels define a cube, and so on.

The experiment design process consists of the steps illustrated in the flowchart in FIGURE 5.17. The process involves group work throughout the process, because the team

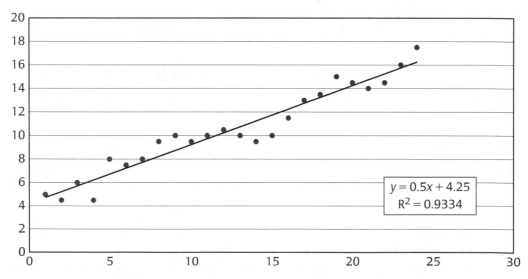

FIGURE 5.17 Natural Log Transformation of Data set with Linear Regression Model Applied

needs to design the experiment by determining the factors, responses, and levels, and once the experiments have been run, the group then comes together to determine if the experimental hypothesis was confirmed.

One of the most common types of experiments is the comparison of two process methods, or two methods of treatment. There are several ways to analyze such an experiment depending on the information available from the population as well as the sample. One of the most straightforward methods to evaluate a revised process method is to plot the results on an SPC chart that includes historical data from the baseline process using the control limits established by the prior process. Another method of comparing two process methods is to perform an analysis of variance (ANOVA), which reports the results of the **Fisher F-test** (F-ratio) as the method of comparing the means of alternate treatments. The F-test was designed by Fisher to test the hypothesis that two different variances are equal (the null hypothesis for the F-test). The F-test for ANOVA is stated as follows:

$$F = \frac{Between\ group\ variability}{Within\ group\ variability}$$

ANOVA is used to test hypotheses about differences between two or more means. Thus, in a DOE application, ANOVA tests which group means are significantly different from others. ANOVA can be used to test differences among several means for significance without increasing the type I error rate. The goal of ANOVA is to determine if the variance levels of group means divided by the variance within each group exceeds a certain value, termed Fcrit (critical F); if so, then the difference is significant and the null hypothesis that states there is no difference is rejected. Fcrit varies with the risk of type I error, which is usually set at 0.05, or a 5% risk of accepting an incorrect null hypothesis (false positive). Lookup tables of F values related to each risk level are available, but nearly all statistical packages, and even some spreadsheet programs like Excel, provide the F-value and p value as part of the output from an ANOVA run. EXAMPLE 5.6 demonstrates the use of ANOVA, and the ANOVA output in TABLE 5.13 provides the common parameters output for this analysis. Any experimental design must include randomization of the variables in the process. For instance, in EXAMPLE 5.6 each run was selected randomly using a random number generator. Randomization of the experimental design ensures that the ANOVA statistical requirement for independence of measurement is satisfied.

A column in the ANOVA output reports the degrees of freedom (df) for the numerator (between groups) and denominator (within groups). In this case there are two degrees of freedom in the numerator because three numbers were used to calculate the variance of the means, minus one degree of freedom for the error term. The denominator of the F-ratio, called the pooled variance within each treatment, has 27 degrees of freedom (30 individual data points less 3 degrees of freedom for

Example 5.6 Design of Experiments for Days' Accounts Receivables

Like many durable medical equipment vendors, Dr. Ivy Slopé (pronounced slo-pay) had problems with cash flow. One major issue that she faced was the slowness with which insurers were returning payments for the invoices that her office staff submitted. She had taken a course on improving performance using DOE and decided to review the billing process with her staff, using days in accounts receivable (AR days) as the metric for determining process effectiveness and efficiency. The staff discovered three possible methods of improving the billing system, but none of the three was clearly superior using AR days. The data in TABLE 5.12 shows the effect of each of the three procedures with 10 runs of each. The team used a randomization procedure that ensured effective use of ANOVA, using each of the process modifications randomly over a 60-day period. The AR days data in TABLE 5.12 were analyzed using single-factor ANOVA, with results reported in TABLE 5.13. The summary section in TABLE 5.13 provides the average AR days and variance for each of the three process improvements. Process A demonstrates the lowest average and variance, which would indicate that procedure as the best choice if the F-test confirms a significant difference between the groups. In the ANOVA table, the Fcrit value is noted to be 3.35, and the between-groups F-test is 9.995, which is significant at $p < 0.0005$. Thus the observed difference between process A and the other two processes is statistically significant. Dr. Slopé and her staff changed the process for accounts receivable to the revised procedure A.

Table 5.12	Data for Days' Accounts Receivable (Example 5.6)		
	Accounts Receivable Days		
	A	B	C
Run 1	24	25	35
Run 2	25	31	29
Run 3	25	27	28
Run 4	25	29	30
Run 5	24	25	27
Run 6	26	24	45
Run 7	24	29	31
Run 8	24	32	32
Run 9	22	30	28
Run 10	23	33	29

Table 5.13	ANOVA Output Days' Accounts Receivable (Example 5.6)			
Single-factor ANOVA				
Summary				
Groups	Count	Sum	Average	Variance
A	10	242	24.2	1.288889
B	10	285	28.5	9.833333
C	10	314	31.4	28.26667

Table 5.13						
ANOVA						
Source of Variation	SS	df	MS	F	p Value	Fcrit
Between groups	262.4667	2	131.2333	9.995205	0.000564	3.354131
Within groups	354.5	27	13.12963			
Total	616.9667	29				

calculating the sample averages). In total, the degrees of freedom add up to the total number of data points in the analysis (2 numerator + 1 error + 27 denominator = 30). The higher the degrees of freedom, the more powerful the analysis and most statistical analysis software will calculate the degrees of freedom automatically.

This example represents a simple experimental design where one factor is evaluated at several levels, but more complex experimental designs are possible using DOE. Multifactor experiments are designed to evaluate multiple factors set at multiple levels. One approach is called a **full factorial** experiment, in which each factor is tested at each level in every possible combination with the other factors and their levels. Full factorial experiments that study all paired interactions can be economic and practical if there are few factors and only two or three levels per factor, but the number of runs goes up exponentially as additional factors are added. For example, an experiment with two levels and three factors must have 2^3, or eight, runs to evaluate all possible combinations. Similarly a two-level, four-factor experiment would need 2^4, or 16, runs to evaluate all the possibilities. Full factorial experiments are denoted using the following notation:

$$N^k$$

where N is the number of levels and k is the number of factors. It should be evident that as the number of factors and levels grows, the number of runs needed becomes exponentially larger and prohibitively expensive, mandating another approach.

To deal with these situations, the concept of **fractional factorial experimental design** was developed. Fractional designs are cost effective because they apply statistically valid methods to reduce the number of combinations tested. Although a thorough examination of setting up fractional factorial experiments is beyond the scope of this text, statistical thinkers need to understand the basic principles behind the approach. Understanding the approach requires comprehension of the concept of **main effects** and **interactions**. The main effect of a factor is the direct effect of the factor alone on an outcome or dependent variable. Interactions connote the combined effect of two or more factors on an outcome or dependent variable. For example, an increased dosage of an antihypertensive drug may have an effect on reducing blood pressure (main effect), but the drug may have a greater effect in smokers than in nonsmokers (interaction). These effects are generally represented mathematically as follows:

$$y = aX_1 + bX_2 + c(X_1 \times X_2) + \varepsilon$$

where X_1 is factor 1, X_2 is factor 2, a is the main effect for factor 1, b is the main effect for factor 2, c is the interaction effect for the combination of factor 1 and factor 2, and ε is the "error term," representing all the sources of errors encountered when estimating this model to represent the actual relationship between the dependent variable and predictors X_1 and X_2.

If only main effects were significant (e.g., if the antihypertensive drug affected all individuals in exactly the same way), then the interaction effect would be zero, a situation rarely seen in health care. Proper design of the experiment can determine each of the main and interaction effects. The goal of a fractional factorial designed experiment is to create experimental runs that identify the main and interaction effects but, through intelligent organization of the experiments, keep the number of runs to a reasonable level. Fractional factorial designs are denoted as follows:

$$N^{k-p}$$

where N is the number of levels, k is the number of factors, and p is the numeric factor representing the fraction of the full factorial experiment used in the fractional experiment.

For example, in a two-level, five-factor experiment, the full factorial notation would be 2^5 with a total of 32 runs to complete the experimental model. If only eight experimental runs are possible (i.e., one-fourth the number for a full factorial experiment), the fractional factorial design of eight runs would be denoted by 2^{5-2}. Design of the fractional factorial experiment requires a process called **blocking**, which helps control the influence of **nuisance factors**, which affect the outcome of the experiment but are not of interest as part of the relationship. For example, in the antihypertensive drug experiment a number of factors like gender, age, and ethnicity might have very minor effects that are not anticipated to be significant as main effects. However, these factors may be involved in interactions that can affect the outcome measure (systolic blood pressure) and so they must be accounted for in the experimental design. Blocking is the approach used to deal with these other factors without making the experiment too large and expensive.

One of the great enemies of any experimental design is intended or unintended bias. Bias of any kind can alter the results of an experiment, leading to incorrect conclusions from either type I or type II errors. In planning an experiment it is necessary to limit any bias that may be introduced by the experimental units, conditions, or time factors. Randomization and blocking can be used to minimize these effects by identifying and isolating or eliminating nuisance or noise factors. Randomization is familiar to most professionals in health care as a method based on chance alone by which study interventions are assigned to a group. Randomization minimizes the differences among study groups by equally distributing interventions using a process that is based on chance alone. Using this approach, a table of random numbers is used to assign the order of each intervention in the experiment. The interventions are then applied according to the random order, often in a sequence that is not known to those conducting the experiment to eliminate bias. In EXAMPLE 5.6 the three interventions were randomly assigned to 60-day time blocks over the time of the study, ensuring at least two payment cycles for testing the insurers' responses to the interventions.

Blocking is the process of grouping similar experimental units (e.g., insurers with similar durable medical equipment coverage patterns in EXAMPLE 5.6). Blocking reduces known but irrelevant sources of variation between experimental units, allowing the experiment to focus on a specific source of variation. For example, insurers can be grouped in a block based on coverage and copayment percentages in EXAMPLE 5.6 to determine if the level of coverage (i.e., the amount that the insurer is required to pay) is related to speed of payment. Blocking can also be used to prevent experimental results being influenced by variations from batch to batch, machine to machine, day to day, or shift to shift. A more detailed discussion of blocking and randomization in experimental design can be found online in the *Engineering Statistics Handbook* published by the National Institute of Standards and Technology.[8]

When selecting the factor levels for an experiment, it is important to have a broad enough range to adequately capture the natural variation of the process. Most experiments are designed with two levels, usually denoted as a high level (+) and a low level (−). In some cases a third level between the high and low level may be added to create a three-level experiment, where the middle level is denoted by a zero (0). Levels close to the process mean may hide the significance of a factor over its range of values, and for factors that are measured on a variable scale, selected levels may be as much as three standard deviations on either side of the mean. These levels are likely to provide sufficient differences to demonstrate the main effects and interactions.

Carefully planned, statistically designed experiments offer clear advantages over traditional single-factor approaches. Full and fractional factorial experiments provide useful tools for process validation, where the effects of various factors acting simultaneously on the process must be discerned. DOE is easily understood by medical industry professionals, and factorial experimental designs are relatively easy to construct, efficient, and, more importantly, able to examine interactions as well as main effects. Results are statistically valid and can lead to robust conclusions regarding the importance of specific factors at defined levels and with defined interactions. Effective experimental designs block out extraneous factors, and randomization can be applied to eliminate bias. Computer software is essential for developing and running factorial experiments, and a number of packages listed in TABLE 5.14 are available to assist with the more complicated designs.

■ Discussion Questions

1. What is systems thinking? Why is the concept important in quality improvement?
2. Describe Deming's Theory of Profound Knowledge. How do the four elements of his theory relate to improving performance?
3. Describe the theory of control charts. How is the use of a control chart like performing a hypothesis test? What is the null hypothesis for a control chart?
4. What are the two major categories of control charts? Name and briefly describe the most common charts in each of these two major categories.
5. Define special cause and common cause variation. How do they differ? What approaches are taken to eliminate these causes of variation?
6. What is the difference between statistical process control and a randomized control trial? How are the two approaches similar?
7. Surgical site infections are of continuing concern for many hospital systems. Discuss the use of control charts to evaluate the following problem and report recommendations.

   The Infection Control Surveillance Committee (ICSC) at St. Very Clean Hospital, a 300-bed hospital with an active surgical service, noticed an increase in the infection rate for thoracic surgical patients. A nurse on the committee suggested that a possible contributor to this increase could be

Table 5.14	Software Packages for DOE
Program	Website
ReliaSoft	http://doe.reliasoft.com
Stat-Ease	http://www.statease.com
JMP	http://www.sas.com
Statistica	http://www.statistica.com
Statgraphics	http://www.statsoft.com
QI Macros	http://www.qimacros.com

the increasing use of flash sterilization more routinely in the operating rooms, rather than as an emergency method of sterilizing an instrument that had been dropped during a procedure. However, two physicians on the committee posited that one of the older cardiothoracic surgeons might be the underlying problem (i.e., a special cause). The discussion became somewhat heated at times, and Dr. Dugan, the chair of the ICSC, decided to task the administrative staff to collect data to determine the underlying cause.

The committee recommended review of the use of flash sterilization to determine if its rate of use had increased over time and if it had become a problem. Rather than debating opinions, the committee decided to take a closer look at this hypothesis by analyzing data on the rate of flash sterilization per 100 surgical procedures to see how it has varied over time.

Question: What chart should be used, and how should the data be analyzed?

8. Dr. Ignatius M. Goode, a family physician, is working hard on improving appointment wait times and is tracking several performance measures monthly for his five physician and three advanced practitioner office. The staff created a short six-question survey using a five-point Likert scale to assess patient satisfaction for several aspects of appointment efficiency (front desk delays, ease of sign in, nurse intake, use of time during wait, physician promptness, and ability to see the provider of choice, etc.). The proportion of patients who respond "poor" or "very poor" to the question of physician promptness is plotted on a p-chart shown in FIGURE 5.18. What can you infer from the p-chart? What are the next steps for Dr. Goode and his staff? How can the staff determine if any changes they make will be helpful?

9. What are the major limitations of statistical process control? How can a quality improvement professional circumvent or avoid these problems?

10. Describe stratification of data sets. What benefits might be realized by stratifying data? What criteria are used to define strata?

11. Why is analysis of means useful in further developing hypotheses for differences in strata?

12. Discuss the barriers to implementing SPC and evidence-based management. How can a quality improvement professional deal with these challenges?

13. What are the major elements of regression techniques that are important for statistical thinkers? How can linear regression be applied in health care?

14. Create a matrix for a 2^3 full factorial experiment using ± notation. (Hint: Use Excel and the pattern in TABLE 5.15.)

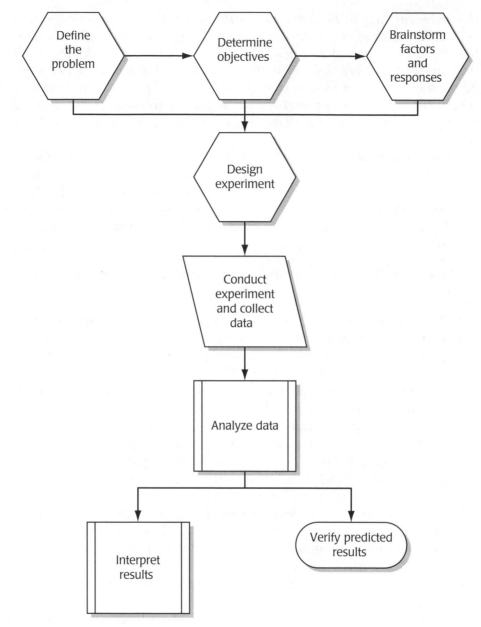

FIGURE 5.18 DOE Process

Table 5.15	Design of Experiments Matrix for a Two-Level, Four-Factor (2^4) Design			
	Factor 1	Factor 2	Factor 3	Factor 4
Run 1	+	+	+	+
Run 2	−	+	+	+
Run 3	+	−	+	+
Run 4	−	−	+	+
Run 5	+	+	−	+
Run 6	−	+	−	+
Run 7	+	−	−	+
Run 8	−	−	−	+
Run 9	+	+	+	−
Run 10	−	+	+	−
Run 11	+	−	+	−
Run 12	−	−	+	−
Run 13	+	+	−	−
Run 14	−	−	−	−
Run 15	+	−	−	−
Run 16	−	−	−	−

■ References

1. Deming WE. *The New Economics*. 2nd ed. Cambridge, MA: MIT Press; 2000.

2. Snee RD. In pursuit of total quality. *Quality Progress*, 1986;20:25–31.

3. Snee RD. Statistical thinking and its contribution to total quality. *American Statistician*, 1990;44: 116–121.

4. Bass I. Analysis of means—ANOM. Retrieved November 2008 from http://www.sixsigmafirst.com/ANOM.htm

5. Gujarati DN. *Basic Econometrics*. 3rd ed. New York: McGraw-Hill; 1995.

6. Armstrong EP, Malone DC. Fluticasone is associated with lower asthma related costs than leukotriene modifiers in a real-world analysis. *Pharmacotherapy*, 2002;22:1117–1123.

7. Neuhauser D. Why design of experiments just may transform health care. *Quality Management in Health Care*, 2005;14:217–218.

8. National Institute of Standards and Technology. How do you select an experimental design? Engineering Statistics Handbook. Retrieved December 2008 from http://www.itl.nist.gov/div898/handbook/pri/section3/pri33.htm

■ Additional Reading

Statistical Process Control

Berwick DM. A primer on leading the improvement of systems. *British Medical Journal* 1996;312:619–622.

Berwick DM. Controlling variation in health care: a consultation from Walter Shewhart. *Medical Care* 1991;29:1212–1225.

Berwick DM, James B, Coye MJ. Connections between quality measurement and improvement. *Medical Care* 2003;41(1 Suppl):I30–I38.

Blumenthal D. Applying industrial quality management science to physicians' clinical decisions. In Blumenthal D, Scheck A, eds. *Improving Clinical Practice: Total Quality Management and the Physician*. San Francisco: Jossey-Bass; 1995:25–49.

Carey RG. *Improving Healthcare with Control Charts: Basic and Advanced SPC Methods and Case Studies*. Milwaukee, WI: ASQ Quality Press; 2003.

Control Chart Wizard online, an online query system to determine the best control chart for an application. Retrieved April, 2009, from http://www.isixsigma.com/control_charts/

Curran ET, Benneyan JC, Hood J. Controlling methicillin-resistant *Staphylococcus aureus*: A feedback approach using annotated statistical process control charts. *Infection Control and Hospital Epidemiology* 2002;23:13–18.

Diaz M, Neuhauser D. Pasteur and parachutes: When statistical process control is better than a randomized controlled trial. *Quality and Safety in Health Care* 2005;14:140–143.

Lim TO. Statistical process control tools for monitoring clinical performance. *International Journal of Quality in Health Care* 2003;15:3–4.

Nelson EC, Batalden PB, Huber TP. Microsystems in health care: Part 1. Learning from high-performing front-line clinical units. *Joint Commission Journal for Quality Improvement* 2002;28:472–493.

Nelson EC, Splaine ME, Batalden B, et al. Building measurement and data collection into medical practice. *Annals of Internal Medicine*, 1998;128:460–466.

Neuhauser D, Diaz M. Quality improvement research: Are randomised trials necessary? *Quality and Safety in Health Care* 2007;16:77–80.

Wheeler D J, Chambers D S. *Understanding Statistical Process Control*. 2nd ed. Knoxville, TN: SPC Press; 1992.

Statistical Texts

Hyperstat online statistics textbook. Retrieved November 2008 from http://www.davidmlane.com/hyperstat/

Online statistics: An interactive multimedia course of study. Retrieved November 2008 from http://onlinestatbook.com/

StatSoft electronic statistical textbook. Retrieved November 2008 from http://www.statsoft.com/textbook/stathome.html

Regression Methods

Kahane L. *Regression Basics*. Thousand Oaks, CA: Sage; 2001.

Kleinbaum DG, Kupper LL, Nizati A. *Applied Regression Analysis and Multivariable Methods*. Pacific Grove, CA: Brooks/Cole; 1997.

Skrepnek G. Regression methods in the empiric analysis of health care data. *Journal of Managed Care Pharmacists,* 2005;11:240–251.

Warner RM. *Applied Statistics: From Bivariate Through Multivariate Techniques.* Thousand Oaks, CA: Sage; 2007.

Design of Experiments

Anderson MJ, Whitcomb PJ. *DOE Simplified.* Florence, KY: Productivity Press; 2000.

Box GEP, Hunter WG, Hunter JS. *Statistics for Experimenters—An Introduction to Design, Data Analysis, and Model Building.* New York: John Wiley and Sons; 1978.

Design of experiments. Retrieved November 2008 from http://www.moresteam.com/toolbox/t408.cfm

Kim J, Kalb J. Design of experiments: An overview and application example. Retrieved November 2008 from http://www.devicelink.com/mddi/archive/96/03/011.html

Montgomery DC. *Design and Analysis of Experiments.* New York: John Wiley & Sons; 1984.

Taguchi G. *Introduction to Quality Engineering—Designing Quality into Products and Processes.* Dearborn, MI: Asian Productivity Organization, Distributed by American Supplier Institute Inc.; 1986.

Approaches to Improvement: Standardization and Lean Process Management

■ Standardization: Is It Really a "Four-Letter Word"?

Physicians in particular look upon standardization as anathema. Typical responses to the idea of standardization of medical practice are as follows:

- "My patients are different."
- "Human physiology is too variable to be standardized."
- "I didn't go to school all those years to do cookbook medicine."

Standardization is prevalent throughout clinical medicine, however. For example, laboratory tests are reported in standard units that mean the same regardless of clinical setting. Standard measurements are frequently made to determine specific diagnostic criteria, such as Cobb's angle in scoliosis or the head circumference of an infant to diagnose macrocephaly. Standardized approaches to the measures used for diagnosis and treatment are critical to ensuring that the scientific method can be applied to a physician's work. On the other hand, use of standardized approaches to such tasks as determining which tests to order or selecting a therapeutic regimen stubbornly remain difficult to apply. Most providers have learned standardized algorithms for diagnosis and treatment during training, but many physicians eschew the idea of "cookbook medicine." In situations that require creative thinking (e.g., when a patient is beset with obscure symptoms), algorithms are often inadequate, requiring more advanced thought processes that rely on experience and the ability to change diagnostic and therapeutic approaches as the patient's situation changes. Thus standardization has its place in health care, but it is not a panacea that can be applied in all situations.

Standardized approaches to a number of healthcare processes, however, have become a way for the industry to reduce the probability of errors and improve patient safety. In this chapter we discuss the application of one of the most successful standardization approaches, lean process management, in the contemporary healthcare system.

■ Principles of Lean Management

Producing greater value with less work is the underlying tenet of lean process management. Lean principles come from the Japanese manufacturing industry. Although usually attributed to Japanese automaker Toyota, the roots of lean date to the early 20th century to a mechanical engineer named Fredrick Winslow Taylor. His *Principles of Scientific Management*,[1] first published in 1911, became a popular business tool in the early 1900s and was based on the concept that management could benefit from the application of scientific principles, as he stated in the introduction to the text:

> *To prove that the best management is a true science, resting upon clearly defined laws, rules, and principles, as a foundation. And further to show that the fundamental principles of scientific management are applicable to all kinds of human activities, from our simplest individual acts to the work of our great corporations, which call for the most elaborate cooperation.*

Taylorism, as it was dubbed, proved helpful to early industrial pioneers like Henry Ford, who applied scientific management principles to his assembly lines to create more reliable output in the form of automobiles. Ford's approach to task-oriented optimization of work tasks led to greater standardization of outputs and is found in countless industries in modern societies from assembly lines to produce toothbrushes to fast food restaurants. The tediousness of repetitive work, however, created fatigue and decreased productivity, which Taylor demonstrated was remedied by rest breaks. Interestingly, Henry Ford chose to label these work lapses as a form of malingering he described as "soldiering." Ford's approach to fatigue and lowered productivity was based on his theory that generally workers forced to perform repetitive tasks work at the slowest rate that goes unpunished. Ford observed that equally paid workers in a group tend to do the amount of work that is done by the slowest in the group. Although cynical, this observation confirms that workers must be self-motivated and will not work above the minimal rate unless sufficient performance-based incentives are made available. Ford then proposed that each worker be taught the "one best way" to do a particular task, which led to the relatively extreme level of standardization on early mass production lines. Scientific management became the foundation of industry internationally in the first half of the 20th century and remained the standard into the 1960s, when lean and six sigma programs begin to gain ascendancy. Importantly, however, lean and six sigma extend the tenets of the scientific management approaches developed in the early 1900s.

For many, the lean production system connotes a set of "tools" or approaches to efficient and effective management that focus on identifying and eliminating waste, known in lean terminology as **muda**. These tools include such methods as *value stream mapping, five S* (known in health care as *Six S*), *kanban, poka yoke*, and several others that are the subject of this chapter. By eliminating waste the goals of quality improvement, reduced production time, and decreased costs can be achieved with overall improvements in productivity.

The Toyota Production System (TPS) expanded on these basic principles to include improving workflow to eliminate *mura* (unevenness) in the work system, which has implications for costs incurred for inventory storage, worker fatigue, and other issues that diminish quality output. The techniques used for elimination of mura include *production leveling*, *pull production*, and *heijunka*. These approaches are different from many other improvement methods, but when applied in health care they have been very effective in dealing with such issues as laboratory processing times and patient flow in care settings. Synergy between muda reduction and flow optimization is evident in the way these concepts are applied in practice, often simultaneously, but existing quality problems and wasted work effort are frequently identified as flow optimization is achieved. The major advantage to dealing with process flow initially is the greater focus on considering the entire system, whereas muda elimination typically focuses on specific parts of a process.

Both lean production systems and TPS can be seen as a loosely connected set of potentially competing principles whose goal is cost reduction by the elimination of waste. Several other principles stem from these principles, such as perfect first-time quality, continuous improvement, flexibility, building and maintaining long-term relationships with suppliers, *autonomation* (automation with a human touch), load leveling, and visual control. All these elements of the lean management system are used in health care to improve patient safety and efficiency. The disconnected nature of some of these principles perhaps springs from the fact that the TPS has grown pragmatically since 1948 as it responded to quality problems that arose in production environments. Similarly, the tools have evolved for specific use in health care, such as the addition of a sixth "S" to the 5S concept to represent safety as one of the goals of that approach. Each of the approaches has been refined over the past five decades and in the past few years has been adapted to the healthcare industry. The primary goals remain as follows:

- Reduction in muda ("non–value-adding work")
- Elimination of *muri* ("overburden," or excess work at some points along the production cycle due to uneven flow)
- Eradication of mura ("unevenness," or the lack of uniform flow of process elements to produce an output)
- Systematic determination of the source of these three problems and application of lean tools to ameliorate issues

FIGURE 6.1 shows the lean management system and establishes the relationships between the key concepts in this framework, with the two-pillar concepts of just in time (JIT) and Jidoka that support the goals of increased quality, reduced cost, and faster throughput. These pillar concepts have multiple associated tools that provide

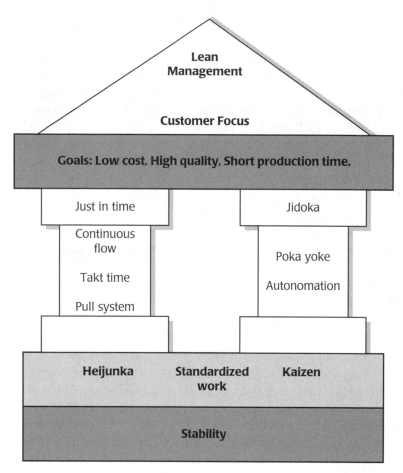

FIGURE 6.1 Lean Management System

the means to achieve each concept's objectives. The pillars list a few of the major approaches that support each of the concepts (e.g., continuous flow, takt time, and pull systems in support of JIT), but the lean toolbox is extensive. A list of the more commonly used tools can be found in TABLE 6.1.

Just in Time

JIT is a crucial element of lean process management and ensures that required process items and resources are available at the right place and at the right time. With all the necessary resources in place, the likelihood of production delays decreases and the probability of achieving smooth process flow increases, achieving the goals of the lean process management framework. Accomplishing JIT performance, of course, requires coordination and application of several other tools in the lean toolbox:

Table 6.1	Lean Tools and Concepts
Tool	Description
5S	A methodology for organizing, cleaning, developing, and sustaining a productive work environment. Improved safety, ownership of work space, improved productivity, and improved maintenance are some of the benefits of the 5S program.
Error proofing	A structured approach to ensure quality and error-free manufacturing environment. Error proofing ensures that defects will not be passed to the next operation.
Current reality trees	A problem-analysis tool that aids in examining cause and effect logic behind the current situation.
Conflict resolution diagram	This is used to resolve hidden conflicts that usually perpetuate chronic problems.
Future reality diagram	A sufficiency-based logic structure designed to reveal how changes to the status quo would affect reality, specifically to produce desired effects.
Inventory turnover rate	The number of times an inventory cycles or turns over during the year. A frequently used method to compute inventory turnover is to divide average inventory level into annual cost of sales.
Kaizen	The Japanese term for improvement; continuing improvement involving everyone—managers and workers. In manufacturing kaizen relates to finding and eliminating waste in machinery, labor, or production methods.
Kanban	Kanban is a simple parts-movement system that depends on cards and boxes/containers to take parts from one workstation to another on a production line. The essence of the kanban concept is that a supplier or the warehouse should only deliver components to the production line as and when they are needed, so that there is no storage in the production area.
Lean metric	Lean metrics allow companies to measure, evaluate, and respond to their performance in a balanced way, without sacrificing the quality to meet quantity objectives or increasing inventory levels to achieve machine efficiencies. The type of the lean metric depends on the organization and can be of the following categories: financial performance, behavioral performance, and core process performance.
Lean performance indicator (LPI)*	LPI is a consistent method to measure lean implementation effectiveness and a key core value metric for motivating performance and rewarding team performance through the PIP plus incentive program. Indicators are real-time performance, continuous improvement implementation, lean sustainment, waste elimination, and profitability. Goal: An LPI monthly goal of 100 equates to 116.3% value-added output performance at level C lean performance. Formula: Value-added sales (total sales minus raw materials, subcontracting, and components) divided by shop rate per hour divided by number of hourly shop floor personnel divided by 2.

(continues)

Table 6.1	Lean Tools and Concepts (continued)
Tool	Description
One-piece Flow	One-piece flow or continuous-flow processing is a concept means that items are processed and moved directly from one processing step to the next, one piece at a time. One-piece flow helps to maximum utilization of resources, shorten lead times, identify problems, and communication between operations.
Overall equipment effectiveness	Measures the availability, performance efficiency, and quality rate of equipment. It is especially important to calculate overall equipment effectiveness for the constrained operations.
Prerequisite tree	A logical structure designed to identify all obstacles and the responses needed to overcome them in realizing an objective. It identifies minimum necessary conditions without which the objective cannot be met.
Process route table	Shows what machines and equipment are needed for processing a component or assembly. These tables aid in creating ordinary lines and grouping work pieces into work cells.
Quick changeover	Quick changeover is a technique to analyze and reduce resources needed for equipment setup, including exchange of tools and dies. Single minute exchange of dies is an approach to reduce output and quality losses due to changeovers.
Standard rate or work	The length of time that should be required to set up a given machine or operation and run one part, assembly, batch, or end product through that operation. This time is used in determining machine requirements and labor requirements.
Takt time	The time required between completion of successive units of end product. Takt time is used to pace lines in the production environments.
Total productive maintenance	Total productive maintenance is a maintenance program concept, which brings maintenance into focus to minimize downtimes and maximize equipment usage. The goal of total productive maintenance is to avoid emergency repairs and keep unscheduled maintenance to a minimum.
Transition tree	A cause and effect logic tree designed to provide step-by-step progress from initiation to completion of a course of action or change. It is an implementation tool.
Value added to non–value added lead time ratio	Provides insight on how many value added activities are performed compared with non–value added activities, using time as a unit of measure.
Value stream mapping	Value stream mapping is a graphical tool that helps to see and understand the flow of the material and information as a product makes its way through the value stream. It ties together lean concepts and techniques.

Table 6.1	
Tool	Description
Value stream costing	Value stream costing methodology simplifies the accounting process to give everyone real information in a basic understandable format. By isolating all fixed costs along with direct labor we can easily apply manufacturing resources as a value per square footage utilized by a particular cell or value stream. This methodology of factoring gives a true picture of cellular consumption to value-added throughput for each value stream company wide. Now you can easily focus improvement kaizen events where actual problems exist for faster calculated benefits and sustainability.
Visual management	A set of techniques that makes operation standards visible so that workers can follow them more easily. These techniques expose waste so that it can be prevented and eliminated.
Workflow diagram	Shows the movement of material, identifying areas of waste. Aids teams to plan future improvements, such as one piece flow and work cells.

*From LPI Copyright © by ShopWerks Software. Jim Warren 2004–2006.

- **Value stream mapping**: A process mapping technique that assists with removal of wasted work effort from a process or group of processes.
- **One piece flow**: Service or product-oriented layout to reduce the time spent moving information, people, materials, and work in progress.
- **Takt time**: Time required for producing specific output (e.g., a specific service).
- **Pull production**: Output based on customer demand rather than producing inventories of products (called "just in case" production).
- **Quality control at source**: Empowers each worker with ensuring the quality of their work and ensuring that defects are not passed on to the next point in the production cycle.
- **Poka yoke**: Error prevention and design of processes to eliminate the likelihood of errors.
- **Preventive maintenance/total productive maintenance**: Ensuring machinery and equipment function perfectly and are continually improved.
- **Elimination of muda**: The seven types of waste include:
  - *Overproduction*: Excess production or capacity for services that are not used.
  - *Waiting*: Time during a process when no value added activity is occurring.
  - *Conveyance*: Movement of process elements from one step in a process to another.
  - *Overprocessing*: Time spent during a process performing non–value added activities.

- *Inventory*: Storage of in-process process elements or end products or services.
- *Motion*: Work activities occurring during process that do not add value (e.g., setup time).
- *Product defects*: Errors in services or products that require rework.
- Some lean practitioners add an eighth form of waste, *knowledge disconnection*, because lack of knowledge at a needed point in a process causes delays in the process (e.g., waiting).
- **6S**: Tidiness in the workplace; the original version of this concept was 5S, and the English equivalents of the "S" are:
  - *Sort*
  - *Set in order*
  - *Shine*
  - *Standardize*
  - *Sustain*

Healthcare workers have added a sixth S in recent years to represent *safety*.

- **Set-up time reduction**: Increases throughput by eliminating non–value added work during setup.
- **Cross training**: A multiskilled work force can be more productive and adds flexibility to the production environment; additionally, job flexibility may add to employee satisfaction.
- **Production leveling**: Methods to even the work load along a process to remove bottlenecks and reduce production delays or overproduction.
- **Kanban**: Simple tools to "pull" products and components through the process.
- **Kaizen events**: Events such as workgroup or task force meetings that bring together owners, managers, and front-line workers to map the existing process, develop improvement strategies, design measures and implementation plans, and start the work of gaining buy in from all process stakeholders.

Jidoka

Taiichi Ohno considered Jidoka to be one of the two pillars of the TPS that he developed in response to the company's desperate financial situation in the 1950s. Jidoka has two interpretations in the lean paradigm. One meaning connotes the practice of stopping a production line if a defect is identified anywhere along the line. Alternatively, Jidoka has been translated as "autonomation," or automation with a human touch. Although originally applied in the manufacturing world, both of these concepts have application to health care.

From Ohno's perspective, automation with a human touch focuses on the need for machines to have sufficient intelligence to notify humans when they need to be adjusted or repaired. On the manufacturing floor this trait can help ensure that a machine does not break down at an inopportune time and shut down a well-functioning production line. However, in a medical environment the need for machines to be "smarter" has led to inventions that reduce errors, like smart intravenous pumps, automated medication dispensing cabinets, and surgical robots that perform precise surgical procedures that exceed human accuracy and reduce the likelihood of errors. These types of intelligent machines allow humans to deal with abnormal situations (sometimes called failure modes or faults), leaving routine tasks to the machines. Not only do machines reduce human work load, but they also reduce fatigue from repetition and thus promote safety and greater accuracy. As computerized decision support systems are increasingly deployed in health care, programs will be used to detect incorrect drug doses or drug interactions at the point of care, decreasing the likelihood that patients receive medications in dosages or with interactions that can cause harm. Ray Kurzweil,[2] famed futurist and inventor of computerized tools like the Moog synthesizer and speech recognition, posits the ultimate merging of human and machine intelligence to produce a "singularity" (i.e., a melding of human and machine intelligence to the benefit of civilization). In this situation machines will be perfectly harmonized to ensure optimized safety and effectiveness of the machine/human interface.

The other meaning of Jidoka, stopping the production line to prevent a defect from moving along the production process, is already applied in health care in places like the surgical suite. The mandatory preoperative stop verifies the patient's identity, procedure, surgical site, and so on with the goal of preventing errors and increasing safety. Although data regarding efficacy of the approach are indeterminate at this point, the practice has been widely adopted as one of The Joint Commission's standards. Some healthcare organizations have begun empowering staff to address potential errors by halting a care process if a patient's safety is in jeopardy. These organizations are adopting the crew resource management technique popularized by the military and is being disseminated in health care through training programs around the United States.

The lean approach is therefore focused on getting the right things to the right place at the right time in the right quantity to achieve perfect workflow while minimizing waste and being flexible and able to change. The result of this flexibility and change is production leveling, which ensures smooth process flow and reduces the need for work system adaptations to accommodate variation in process capacity requirements. These concepts must be understood and embraced by the staff members who actuate the processes and provide care that delivers value to customers. The cultural and managerial aspects of lean implementation are thus at least as important as the actual tools or methods of process improvement. In fact, application of lean tools will likely fail if appropriate cultural change is not effectively deployed along with lean improvement efforts.

■ Lean Improvement Cycle

The two pillars of lean management, JIT and Jidoka, form the basis of the lean improvement cycle. Implementation of a lean improvement strategy should be undertaken methodically. The steps in lean deployment involve the following:

1. Gaining senior management buy-in for the approach.
2. Promoting the approach among staff members involved in implementation.
3. Selecting a project for which lean improvement strategies will work.
4. Conducting a kaizen event with a select team.
5. Developing plans for implementing the lean strategies developed in the kaizen event.
6. Measuring results and reporting and celebrating successes.

Gaining Senior Management Buy-In

Like any quality improvement program, senior management support is critical for ensuring that necessary resources are allocated for the project. As discussed in Chapter 2, gaining senior management support usually depends on a compelling business case, and several factors in the lean approach are helpful as persuaders:

- Reduction in non–value added work, which eliminates unnecessary costs.
- Reduction in nonproductive inventories, both for in-process items and for end products.
- Engagement of staff in improvement efforts through kaizen events, leading to increased likelihood of success.
- The lean philosophy of improving both quality and throughput with little or no increase in resources required, leading to a higher return on investment.

Once senior leaders have bought into the lean approach, promoting the concept among staff members can take a number of directions. In many cases staff members can be enticed by the lean approach though assurances that "lean" does not equate with "fewer employees" but rather realignment of work and elimination of non–value added work (what we in health care sometimes call "scut work").

Promoting the Approach Among Staff Members

Most workers are concerned about their jobs, and lean always seems to evoke the idea that jobs will be eliminated. One approach that ensured the TPS was successful was the cultural norm that ensured workers' jobs. Thus one of the more important tasks of every lean cultural change is ensuring workers of the security of their jobs, or at least being honest with employees about reductions that must be made. Workers should be quickly involved in the transformation, and educational programs should be deployed to help staff members understand the goals and objectives of the lean approach. Didactic programs can culminate in the initial lean kaizen events that begin to teach lean tools and develop initiatives to improve processes and demonstrate the efficacy of the approach.

Selecting Projects That Demonstrate the Value of Lean

After the introduction of the lean approach, teams should be empowered to develop projects that are most amenable to the application of lean tools. The approaches to choosing projects outlined in Chapter 2 apply to selection of lean projects, including Goldratt's Theory of Constraints and the Pareto Principle, but in clinical settings the "three highs"—high cost, high risk, high volume—may also be used as criteria. In other words, clinical processes that could be considered for lean process management are those that involve high cost from material or manpower aspects, or entail a high degree of risk for patient harm or environmental damage, or consume substantial resources due to high volume. These types of projects usually have the greatest likelihood of success when the lean process management approach is used.

Conducting a Kaizen Event

A kaizen event is the organized framework for implementing lean principles by focusing on eliminating waste, improving productivity, and achieving sustained continual improvement in targeted processes. This philosophy is based on routine, sustained application of incremental changes over a long period by involving workers who use analytic techniques from the lean toolbox, such as value stream mapping and "the 5 why's" (discussed in Chapter 3), to identify opportunities, develop measures and interventions, and create an implementation plan that is followed through to completion. The corrective action is deployed quickly, usually within 72 hours of the completion of the kaizen planning sessions. One key goal of a kaizen event is to focus on solutions that do not require substantial increases in resources to achieve success.

Subsequent follow-up events review the metrics to evaluate the effectiveness of the interventions and to make any necessary midcourse corrections. In some cases kaizen teams change during implementation, but most of the time the teams remain intact until the project is completed.

Several important principles underlie a kaizen event. First, workers become empowered to evaluate and improve a process or a value stream. Although managers or facilitators often lead the event, staff members perform all the key steps in the kaizen process. Second, workers learn to use and critique data as an improvement paradigm. In many cases finding fault with the data available for the improvement effort prompts employees to take greater care in collecting and reporting data for this and future projects. Another principle that is practiced in a kaizen event is the concept of rapid improvement. Most lean interventions are applied as rapid cycle improvements, with measures and reviews conducted frequently, sometimes as often as weekly.

Additionally, the principle of JIT is evidenced by providing training on specific lean principles and tools as part of the event so they can be applied immediately, which not only ensures the right information is available at the right time, but also uses principles of adult learning to enhance the learning process. Finally, Jidoka becomes a central factor in the implementation of the interventions developed in the kaizen event, because any improvement efforts must be monitored closely with rapid intercession by staff members if the intervention makes the process worse. The other interpretation of Jidoka—autonomation—also becomes important as the team considers how to effectively apply automation to enhance human performance.

The following steps are used in a kaizen event:

1. *Planning and preparation*: Selection of a target process or value stream. Using techniques like the Goldratt Theory of Constraints and Pareto Principle (see Chapter 3), the team develops a list of potential target areas for investigation. Process points for consideration often involve those that are subject to the "three highs" (high risk, high cost, high volume), because those points typically have constraints such as extra inspection, waiting times, and bottlenecks that impede process flow. Some other areas that attract attention might include those that have substantial disorder (e.g., the flow in an emergency department).

2. *Identification of waste (muda)*: Once a process is selected, a value stream map exercise helps the team understand the potential targets for eliminating one or more of the seven deadly wastes. The targeted problem becomes the subject of the kaizen event. This step is particularly dependent on in-depth understanding of the process that only process owners and workers may know, and so inclusion of these staff members is important for success. However, addition of other staff members from different departments prevents the team from perseverating on long-standing habits ("But we've always done it this way..."). Kaizen events usually take from 1 to 7 days, depending on the complexity of the problem, and team members are expected to shed most of their operational responsibilities during this period to ensure adequate focus on the kaizen event.

3. *Creation of a plan to eliminate targeted waste*: The team next sets out to create initiatives to eliminate the areas of waste that need to be eradicated. Using the teamwork approaches and tools outlined in Chapter 2, multifunctional teams can conduct kaizen events to develop interventions and implementation plans that can be immediately put into effect to achieve a rapid cycle improvement program. In fact, many lean improvement programs are designed for fast implementation and evaluation so that the system may achieve greater efficiency as quickly as possible. The elements of the plan must include:
   ○ Time frame for intervention
   ○ Detailed current process design
   ○ Details of planned changes

- Expected outcomes of the intervention
- Metrics to be used to determine effect
- Celebration at conclusion of the project

Each of these elements is important for the success of the planned change, and the celebration is a key element of the program. Workers must be rewarded not just for success but also for hard work and creativity, even if the project did not achieve the desired outcome.

4. *Implementation of the plan*: The kaizen team not only designs the intervention, but the group is typically involved in implementing the plan as well. Beginning with educating other affected workers and extending through process change management and measurement, the team manages implementation through the final report. Workers must have a common understanding of the process and suggested improvements, and so frequent interaction between team members and other workers involved in the implementation phase is crucial for success. A lean implementation team often uses the technique of visual management, in which the team "sees as a group, knows as a group, and acts as a group" (see FIGURE 6.2). Visual management is one of the lean tools described later.

The implementation phase leverages the value stream map to help everyone involved in the project better understand the targets for intervention as well as the key metrics to determine success. Metrics should be directly related to specific process steps or outcomes of the process and thus directly linked to the value stream map. The implementation plan includes a communication plan to report progress and results to senior managers and relevant stakeholders, connected to a strategy to sustain the gains achieved during the project and institutionalizing the changes to ensure long term control of the process.

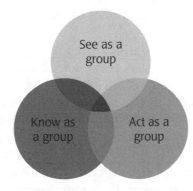

FIGURE 6.2 **Principles of Visual Management**

The lean cycle depends extensively on the tools discussed in Chapter 2, but this approach has spawned a number of other tools (i.e., the lean toolbox).

■ The Lean Toolbox

Over the past six decades the TPS has been widely applied to a number of industries, particularly in manufacturing, and the lean toolbox has been extended with new approaches and modifications to enhance effectiveness. Some techniques, such as the "5 why's" discussed in Chapter 3, have been adopted for other applications, like root-cause analysis. On the other hand, some techniques are unique for the lean management, like value stream mapping.

Value Stream Mapping

This technique involves flowcharting the steps, activities, material flows, communications, and other process elements that are involved with a process or transformation (e.g., transformation of raw materials into a finished product, completion of an administrative process, or completion of a surgical procedure). Value stream mapping (VSM) helps an organization identify the non–value added work in a process. The approach is similar to process mapping or flowcharting, as described in Chapter 3, but there are a number of important nuances.

During a kaizen event the team collects information on the targeted process, like measurements of overall service quality, waste, patient flow through the process (which may include distances in transit for patients and staff), footprint of the process, transitions, bottlenecks, inventories used in the process, and staffing levels. The composition of the team is important to ensure that all these issues are addressed. Team members are assigned specific roles for research and analysis based on their experience. As more information is gathered, team members add detail to value stream maps of the process and conduct time studies of relevant operations (e.g., takt time, lead time).

Value stream mapping is used to find areas for improvement, which in lean are often defined as those points in the process that are bottlenecks. Team members use the value stream map to identify and record all observed waste by evaluating whether each step or element adds value toward meeting the goal of the process. Once waste or non–value added activity is identified and measured, team members then brainstorm improvement options. Using an idealized value stream map without the muda, the team then can test the proposed improvements to determine if the process benefits from the changes. To fully realize the benefits of the kaizen event, team members observe and record new cycle times and calculate overall savings from eliminated waste, unnecessary motion, conveyance, improved flow, and throughput time.

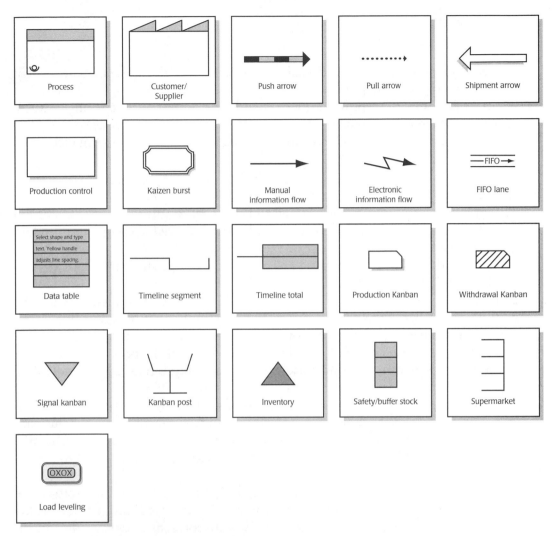

FIGURE 6.3 VSM Flow Charting Symbols

Value stream mapping uses specialized symbols (see FIGURE 6.3), but the approach still focuses on describing the process accurately. However, the goal of a lean process review is to eliminate non–value added steps, which are those steps that do not add any features to a service or product for which a consumer might be willing to pay. Non–value added work that is performed in those steps adds cost, either in time, materials, or other expenditures, but does not increase the value of the service or product to the customer. Thus the value stream map is a key tool to identify the non–value added steps in a process that become targets for improvement efforts.

When To Use

Value stream maps are used:

- To help the improvement team describe the process and calculate lean management statistics at appropriate points.
- To identify points or steps in the process with one or more of the forms of waste identified in the lean management philosophy.
- To guide the team in methods to correct substandard process performance.

Procedure

1. Outline process flow as for a standard flowchart. Capture the major steps in the process as well as any subprocesses that are required to complete a product or service.
2. Create a flowchart with the essential steps in the process to guide the next stage of the analysis.
3. Perform a "walk through" of the process. In this step team members use the flowchart as a rough guide to observing the process in action, recording deviations from the expected flow, time for each step, and any additional staff, vendors, or consultants involved in the completion of the process.
4. At this stage many teams find it useful to put each step and its time on individual sticky notes and arrange the notes in order on the wall, grouped according to steps in the process, as in FIGURE 6.4. Each of the rectangles in FIGURE 6.4 would have a brief description of the step activities and the time for that step. The team then determines if the step is a value added or non–value added step and puts a notation, such as the dots on the cards in the example in FIGURE 6.4 to denote the step's status.
5. The team then rearranges the steps, using only the value added steps, to create an ideal process flow (no muda), which then is converted into the ideal value stream map with associated time metrics that represent only the value added steps in the idealized process.
6. Once the team and stakeholders agree on the new value stream map, the team works to identify gaps between the current and ideal process flow using a spreadsheet such as that in TABLE 6.2. Each of the remedial actions is further fleshed out with a project plan and timeline for completion.
7. As the team and other stakeholders put the corrective actions into place, progress should be monitored by metrics or milestones in process performance that demonstrate the effects of the improvements. The rate of implementation of corrective actions depends on a number of factors, such as human and financial resources, timelines required for changes, and, in some cases, the need for sequential execution of action plans.

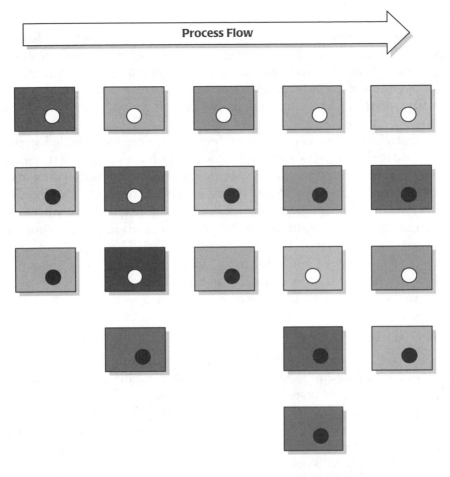

Process Flow

Legend: Open circles = Value added work
Black circles = Non–value added work

FIGURE 6.4 Sticky Notes Example

Table 6.2	Template for Gap Analysis		
Current State	Optimized State	Identified Gap	Remedial Action(s)
Emergency Department support staff must call three departments to arrange for a bed for admission	One telephone call or a computer entry screen to request an inpatient bed for admission	Excessive time spent arranging for bed	Admissions office arranges for inpatient bed for admitted patient Single screen entry for inpatient bed request immediately routed to admissions office

Tips and Tricks
1. Use different colored sticky notes for different participants or departments involved in the process. For example, in an evaluation of an emergency department flow, the physician could be represented by one color, the nurse by another, and the support person by yet another color. In this way the team can readily identify the time commitments and value added by each team member.
2. In general, inspection steps are considered to be non–value added steps, but in some situations inspections may be necessary. For example, if an accrediting agency requires an inspection at specific points in the process, then inspection steps may be required and should be retained in the process. Additionally, some customers may find an inspection step reassuring (e.g., when a nurse performs a second check at the patient's bedside on a medication before administration of drug that may be subject to harmful side effects). These "prudent consumer" steps may not seem to add value for a "value consumer" (i.e., one who would not pay for non–value added inspection steps), but for a prudent consumer these extra steps may warrant an extra cost.

Continuous Flow Process Box

Any process that has continuous flow is depicted by the simple symbol of a process box (see FIGURE 6.5). Although the box may represent highly complex subprocesses involved, as long as the involved work in progress (e.g., information or individual patients) does not stop at any point in this process step, the entire process step and its associated subprocesses are depicted as a single continuous flow process box. In essence, this symbol can represent a "black box" that does not impede process flow but in which value added work is performed. For example, the black box could represent a highly efficient laboratory process in which a specimen is sent from a patient care area, testing performed, and a result returned. The ultimate goal is to design a process for continuous flow so that a patient or packet of information or inventory item can flow through the process without any stops. Thus the ultimate value stream map consists of a single process box, because no interruptions to flow would ever occur.

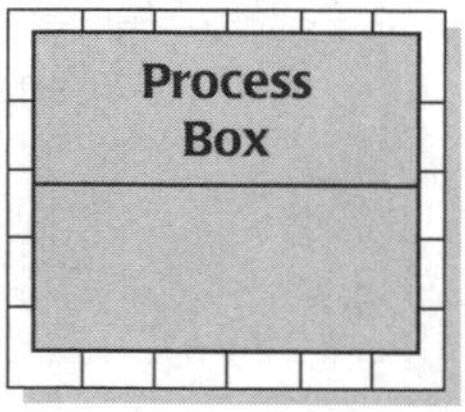

FIGURE 6.5 Process Box

Supermarket

A supermarket (see FIGURE 6.6) is a storage space usually located between two or more processes where a fixed amount of work in progress or value added inventory is stored to supply a downstream process without interruption due to product or process variability. For example, a hospital laboratory may store blood-drawing supplies in an emergency department triage room so that a blood specimen can be obtained more efficiently during the emergency department intake and sent for processing in the laboratory. This practice eliminates the need for the lab technician to carry materials to the emergency department to obtain the specimen and enables emergency department staff to perform the blood draw and eliminate the need for a phlebotomist to travel to the emergency department to perform the service.

A value stream mapping supermarket may also be used to control the flow of production between two processes that cannot be integrated into a single continuous flow process box, because cycle times may be different (such as in the example above for emergency department blood drawing), and the transition between two distinct processes may require a change in the flow rate. Additionally, as noted in the emergency department blood drawing example, the placement of blood drawing supplies at the point of care also eliminates travel time for the phlebotomist (one of the seven deadly sins of lean). Although some of these issues might change with process improvements, the supermarket can help temporize while processes are being coordinated and streamlined. In the value stream map the supermarket symbol always faces the upstream supplier, as in FIGURE 6.7.

FIGURE 6.6 **Supermarket**

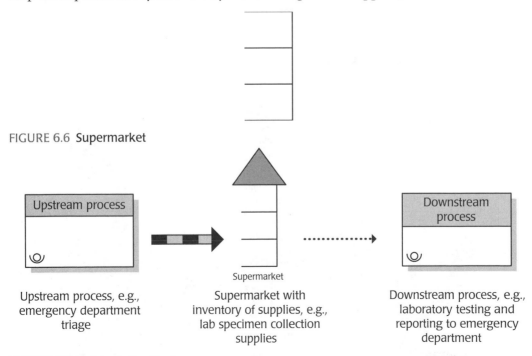

Upstream process, e.g., emergency department triage

Supermarket with inventory of supplies, e.g., lab specimen collection supplies

Downstream process, e.g., laboratory testing and reporting to emergency department

FIGURE 6.7 **Safety Buffer Stock**

A safety buffer stock (see FIGURE 6.8) may be viewed as a specialized kind of supermarket that maintains an inventory of supplies that are critical for maintaining a safe environment. A prime example of a safety buffer stock might be the crash cart found on most hospital patient care units. The crash cart contains all the supplies needed to perform emergency resuscitation in the event of a cardiac or respiratory arrest, kept at the point of care where they may be needed immediately. This type of inventory must be kept at the point in the process flow where it is most likely to be needed to create a safe environment for patient care.

Kanban

A kanban (see FIGURE 6.9) is any signaling device that gives authorization and the minimal instructions needed for a supplying process to know what to produce or for a process manager to know what inventory to replenish. A kanban can be as simple as a paper card physically placed in a container of supplies, or it could be more sophisticated like a radiofrequency identification chip placed in a patient's identification bracelet to indicate next steps in the patient's care on a computer screen. In the

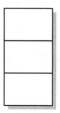

FIGURE 6.8 Use of Supermarket Symbol in VSM

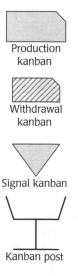

Production
kanban

Withdrawal
kanban

Signal kanban

Kanban post

FIGURE 6.9 Kanban

manufacturing world where lean was born, as inventory is depleted a kanban card is "freed" or becomes visible (e.g., a card at the bottom of a box of parts that is hidden until the parts are almost gone) and then gets put back into a **kanban post** where the kanban "requests" are fulfilled. In a medical setting, many medical offices have signal "flags" outside exam rooms (see FIGURE 6.10) to indicate the need for a specific service or staff person to provide services for the patient.

A **signal kanban** is denoted by an inverted triangle (an upright triangle is the symbol for inventory) and is used in processes that are not designed for continuous flow. An example of a signal kanban in a medical office would be a signal from a nurse or medical assistant to the staff at the reception desk that more patients can be accommodated in empty exam rooms. A simple way to signal would be to send a message through interoffice messaging, but another method using lean process management might be to place a triangular signal kanban in a stack of paper charts (in the pre-EMR era) that indicates to the reception staff that more charts can be added to the stack for processing. The stack of paper charts represents a supermarket for the clinical staff with an inventory of charts to be processed.

A **production kanban** indicates the need for more parts to be sent from the upstream part of the process. Used for the office chart scenario, a production kanban could be used by the clinical staff to signify that more patients could be sent for examination. Thus a production kanban might be a message on an interoffice system to send more charts back for processing, or it might be a card that is placed at a certain point in a

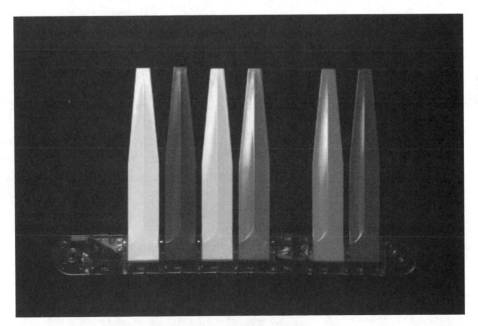

FIGURE 6.10 Exam Room Flags as an Example of Kanban

© Jones and Bartlett Publishers. Exam room signals courtesy of Kull Industries, LLC.

stack of charts to indicate that more charts can be added to the stack for processing. In the manufacturing environment the production kanban often includes some information about what needs to be produced (e.g., some specific parts that are to be used by the downstream process). In the office chart case, it could simply involve a listing of the patient's chief complaint or reason for coming to the clinic.

A **withdrawal kanban** indicates when a particular item has been taken from the supermarket or other inventory resource and signals the need to replenish the stock. This kanban can be used to signal a vendor that a particular stock item is low and needs to be replaced. For example, a hospital central supply system might have a card or other device that signals managers when a certain medical supply reaches a critical level and needs to be replenished. The withdrawal kanban keeps track of the stock and then notifies workers when an item needs to be ordered and restocked.

FIFO Lane

FIFO ("first in, first out") lanes (see FIGURE 6.11) are used when it is not practical to keep a supermarket full of items between processes. Some reasons might include the following:

- Too many variations (custom items)
- Usage volumes are too low
- Short shelf life
- Too fragile to risk storage
- Very expensive

Between two processes there is sometimes both a supermarket and a FIFO lane for different types of items. In health care this concept can be applied particularly when certain items are very expensive, such as the hardware used in spinal surgery, which can cost many thousands of dollars. In these cases specialized procurement processes may be necessary, such as special arrangements with vendors to supply such expensive supplies "just in time" for the surgical procedure to limit a hospital's

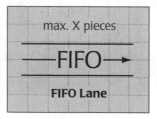

FIGURE 6.11 FIFO Lanes

investment in an inventory of these types of items. Although a FIFO lane may use a kanban signal, many of these items are subject to distinct supply chain systems to limit cost and improve cash flow.

Load Leveling

So many healthcare processes are configured in batches because input into the system may occur in waves. Emergency departments see such surges of demand and must accommodate patient flow that can be somewhat unpredictable. Some of the methods used by the emergency department to deal with the uneven flows include increasing staffing at peak periods, offloading nonemergency cases to urgent care clinics near the department, and triage systems to ensure that the most critical cases are handled expeditiously. Such approaches are examples of load leveling (see FIGURE 6.12), which is an important cornerstone of the lean process management approach. Load leveling is usually applied in the following ways:

- Releasing only enough upstream work in a time period to meet takt time demand, thereby leveling demand spikes.
- Spreading the types of work in progress throughout the work time as much as possible; this technique is used in many medical offices by grouping specific types of patient visits (e.g., well child exams) to ensure that resources meet patient needs and waiting times are reduced.

Load leveling is particularly helpful in reducing variation in a process flow that can lead to increased costs. Changing volumes of work during a time period require special planning to ensure resources are available at appropriate levels and at specific times, which often adds to complexity and cost.

Lean Is the Road to Efficiency

Lean process management focuses on attaining maximum efficiency through elimination of non–value added work using the tools that have evolved over many years in the manufacturing sector. Designing systems and processes using lean principles like customer pull production, continuous flow, 6S, and use of analytics helps to identify opportunities for eliminating non–value added work. Appropriate application of these well-established approaches in health care holds great promise for finding new ways of meeting the Institute of Medicine goals of a more responsive, value-driven healthcare delivery system.

FIGURE 6.12 Load Leveling Step

■ Application of Standardization: Clinical Practice Guidelines

Although medicine is practiced in the environment of a single practitioner and a single patient, the inexorable move toward industrialization has increasingly influenced the doctor–patient relationship as the cost of health care has risen to consume a larger proportion of personal and national income. Not only is the individual encounter more closely scrutinized by payers like insurance companies and federal and state governments, but consumers are viewing health care through a different lens as well. Where the physician of 20 or 30 years ago was the "captain of the ship," today's providers are increasingly recognized as members of a team providing care in the context of an organized delivery system. Progressive payers and providers are moving toward greater integration and a more collaborative relationship to optimize the experience for their mutual customer (for the insurer the member or beneficiary, for the provider the patient).

One sign of this confluence in the delivery system is the effort to standardize care in some circumstances and to bring the most currenmt information from research studies and best practices to improve outcomes of care. Clinical practice guidelines (CPGs) were proposed by the Agency for Health Care Policy and Research (AHCPR) in the 1980s and 1990s as a way of bringing evidence-based care to the provider–patient encounter. AHCPR developed 19 guidelines as a model during the first half of the 1990s, but since that time the number of CPGs has exploded to several thousand. Nearly every professional medical society has developed guidelines within its area of expertise, many of which overlap with those in other societies. Additionally, healthcare delivery systems, payers, and health consortia have devoted efforts at creating CPGs for patient management and payment purposes or to evaluate the quality of care. The focus of the CPG often determines the nature of recommendations, particularly where evidence is scant and consensus recommendations must be used.

Evolution of CPGs

Clinical guidelines evolved from the need of multiple stakeholders in the healthcare system to work from a standard set of criteria to improve the value proposition in health care (i.e., to improve quality and reduce cost). Practitioners need the most current evidence for care to ensure the highest quality for patients, and healthcare planners and payers require information about the best patterns of care to determine where to allocate resources to achieve the best outcomes. As new treatment modalities are created, administrators in hospitals and medical practices need to understand how these innovations impact care to ensure that scarce resources are used appropriately. To address these various needs, Congress passed Public Law 101-239 in 1989 to create the AHCPR, with a mandate to improve the quality, appropriateness, and effectiveness of health care by supporting research and improving access to health care. To accomplish this mission, AHCPR worked with the Institute of Medicine to create the concept of CPGs that would be clinically relevant and useful to health professionals, planners, and administrators in determining how health conditions could be managed in the most effective manner. Thus CPGs were designed as a method of standardizing certain aspects of health care and bringing evidence to the diagnosis and treatment of disease.

The definition of CPGs that arose from this collaboration was included in a text by Field and Lohr: "systematically developed statements to assist practitioner and patient decisions about appropriate health care for specific clinical circumstances."[3] It is particularly notable that the definition mandates a rigor and systematic approach to development of CPGs as well as an inference that guidelines must be based on solid medical evidence. Since those early stages of development CPGs have risen to the forefront of the healthcare industry and now represent a major factor in quality and performance improvement. The National Guideline Clearinghouse was established by the successor to AHCPR, the Agency for Healthcare Research and Quality (AHRQ), and now serves as a primary source of clinical guidelines from many organizations in the United States and throughout the world. Clinical guideline sources have been developed by other countries as well, and a number of these resources are shown in TABLE 6.3.

Table 6.3	International Sources for Clinical Practice Guidelines
Resource	Web address
National Guideline Clearing House™ (USA) (a public resource for evidence-based clinical practice guidelines)	http://www.guideline.gov/
Clinical Practice Guidelines Online, Agency for Healthcare Research and Quality (AHRQ)	http://www.ahrq.gov/clinic/cpgonline.htm
Canadian Medical Association Clinical Practice Guidelines	http://www.cma.ca/
Centres for Health Evidence, Canada	http://www.cche.net/
Guideline Advisory Committee ("a joint body of the Ontario Medical Association and the Ontario Ministry of Health and Long-Term Care")	http://www.gacguidelines.ca/
Danish Secretariat for Clinical Guidelines, National Board of Health	http://www.sst.dk/Planlaegning_og_behandling/SfR.aspx?lang=en
French National Agency for Accreditation and Evaluation in Health, la Haute Autorité de santé, formerly ANAES: l'Agence Nationale d'Accréditation et d'Évaluation en Santé (ANAES)	http://www.has-sante.fr/

(continues)

Table 6.3	International Sources for Clinical Practice Guidelines (continued)
Resource	Web address
Agence Francaise de Sécurité Sanitaire et des Produits de Santé (AFSSAPS)	http://agmed.sante.gouv.fr/htm/7/7000.htm
Fédération Nationale des Centres de Lutte Contre le Cancer (FNCLCC) - Recommandations pour la pratique clinique en cancérologie en accés libre	http://www.fnclcc.fr/sor/structure/index-sorspecialistes.html
German Guidelines Information Service, German Agency for Quality in Medicine (AQuMed)	http://www.leitlinien.de/
Piano Nazionale Linee Guida (PNLG)	http://www.pnlg.it/
Kwaliteitsinstituut voor de Gezondheidszorg (CBO), Dutch Institute for Healthcare Improvement	http://www.cbo.nl/
Scottish Intercollegiate Guidelines Network	http://www.sign.ac.uk/
NICE published guidelines (National Institute for Clinical Excellence, England and Wales)	http://www.nice.org.uk/catrows.asp?c=20034
NICE Guidance, published appraisals	http://www.nice.org.uk/catrows.asp?c=153
Guidelines Finder, index to over 1.200 UK national guidelines. National electronic Library for Health in collaboration with Sheffield Evidence for Effectiveness and Knowledge (SEEK)	http://libraries.nelh.nhs.uk/guidelinesFinder/
PRODIGY guidance (NHS England and Wales)	http://www.prodigy.nhs.uk/guidance
Royal College of Nursing (UK), Clinical Guidelines	http://www.rcn.org.uk/resources/guidelines.php
Clinical Effectiveness and Evaluation Unit (CEEU), of the Royal College of Physicians, UK	http://www.rcplondon.ac.uk/college/ceeu/ceeu_guidelinesdb.asp
Guidelines (types) from the Ministry of Health, Singapore	http://www.moh.gov.sg/corp/publications/list.do?id=pub_med_guidelines
Individual guidelines from the Ministry of Health, Singapore	http://www.moh.gov.sg/cpg
Kementerian Kesihatan Malaysia, Malaysia Ministry of Health	http://www.moh.gov.my/
Japan Council for Quality Health Care	http://jcqhc.or.jp/
Academy of Medicine of Malaysia, guidelines	http://www.acadmed.org.my/

Table 6.3	
Resource	Web address
Australian National Health and Medical Research Council	http://www.health.gov.au/nhmrc
The Medical Journal of Australia (Australian Medical Association)	http://www.mja.com.au/public/guides/guides.html
New Zealand Guidelines Development Group	http://www.nzgg.org.nz/index.cfm
klinrek.ru, clinical guidelines in Russian	http://www.klinrek.ru/

CPGs have assumed increasing importance in health care as the industry tries to reach the so-called STEEEP aims set by the Institute of Medicine for care:

- Safe
- Timely
- Effective
- Efficient
- Equitable
- Patient-centered

Payers and providers alike view CPGS as one method of achieving these goals as well as providing a framework for evaluating variation in care provided to individuals. The fact that CPGs have been developed by medical and surgical specialty societies, as well as numerous other organizations with expertise in specific disease entities, adds to their validity, as long as a few important principles are followed. One example of the value of CPGs to payers in particular was the creation of the Healthcare Employer Data and Information Set (HEDIS) in the 1990s for use in evaluating health plans. Using criteria derived from clinical guidelines and best practices, expert panels regularly update the HEDIS measures through the National Commission on Quality Assurance. Similarly, other organizations that create and implement CPGs must have a mechanism for updating the guidelines as medical knowledge changes.

Although CPGs are based on the best contemporary recommendations from medical literature and expert consensus, they should not usually be construed as medical policy or legal standards of care. CPGs are best used to seek variation in clinical processes by comparing current patterns of care with the evidence-based approaches outlined in the guideline. In some cases a step or section of a CPG might be supported with enough evidence to be adopted as a medical policy (e.g., use of beta blockers after myocardial infarction or the annually updated immunization schedule from the Advisory Committee for Immunization Practices). In general, though, CPGs are used to examine and reduce variation, using techniques similar to value stream mapping to create recommended patterns of care. The application of continuous quality improvement approaches that were pioneered by AHRQ now can be supplanted with some of the lean approaches used for decades by other industries to create highly effective guides that can combine customer value with effective medical practice.

CPGs are applied in a number of different situations by nearly all sectors of the healthcare industry:

- Providers
  - Standardizing care for certain clinical conditions (e.g., development of critical path in hospitals or clinics)
  - Comparison of practice patterns for outcomes research and management
  - Algorithms for electronic record and decision support systems
  - Development of metrics to assess quality of care
  - Framework to continually improve care by using evidence to examine and change clinical recommendations that constitute the steps of CPGs
- Payers
  - Guide for care management staff to ensure appropriate services are available and rendered
  - Basis for clinical coverage guidelines that determine which services are reimbursable
  - Use for credentialing and recredentialing providers based on adherence to evidence-based practice
  - Development of metrics to assess quality of care to satisfy accreditation and other oversight agencies
- Consumers
  - Information on current practice recommendations as a means of evaluating their own care
  - Basis for discussing care with providers and participating in planning clinical interventions

Clinical guidelines thus have numerous uses, and ensuring that the guidelines are of the highest quality becomes especially important. The CPG development cycle designed by AHRQ and refined over the past two decades can provide a framework to continually improve health care.

CPG Development and Maintenance Cycle

When clinical guidelines were first suggested as the basis for improvement strategies, AHCPR also published recommendations for development and maintenance.[4] A current version of the guideline framework is shown in FIGURE 6.13. Evident in the diagram is the cyclical nature of the life of a CPG. A number of factors contribute to the creation

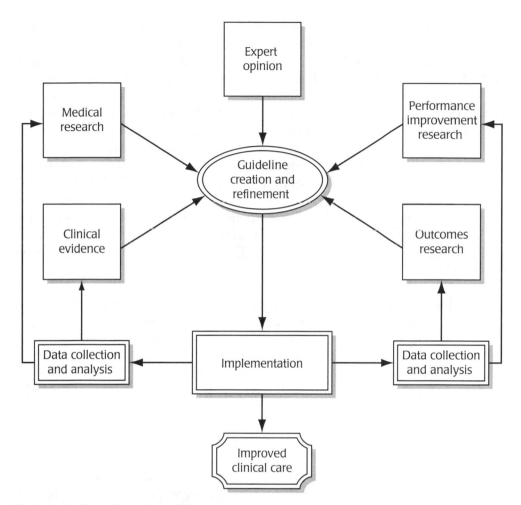

FIGURE 6.13 Clinical Practice Guideline Cycle

of a CPG, but after its birth data collected from the CPG contributes to the improvement cycle, along with new medical knowledge.

The need for a CPG can be established in one of many ways. Frequently, a payer determines that a CPG is needed for determining coverage for services, leading to the impetus to create a clinical guideline that directs payment policies for medical services. On the other hand, guidelines are now proactively developed by medical professional organizations to enlighten other sectors of the healthcare industry with the most credible evidence and expert opinions for diagnosing and treating a clinical condition that falls within the professional society's area of expertise. In this way medical professionals can exert some control over approved and reimbursed practice patterns as well as inform the public of their recommendations. Finally, CPGs may also be established by other sectors of the healthcare industry (e.g., pharmaceutical companies or technology companies) to establish the criteria for using a new drug or other technology.

Selection of a clinical condition for a clinical guideline usually corresponds to the "three highs": high cost, high volume, or high risk. Payers often select high cost clinical conditions for intervention, because a clinical guideline can help reduce inappropriate variation that adds cost to the care model. Additionally, reducing variation also decreases complications and untoward outcomes that only boost costs. In some cases high volume conditions, like cardiovascular disease, are targeted simply because variation in care for these conditions adds both to cost and poor outcomes. Even a relatively small change in rates of inappropriate care for high volume conditions can have a pronounced effect on the overall cost and number of patients who suffer complications. Finally, high risk conditions are often subject to CPGs to reduce the risk of patient harm and improve patient safety.

Several other factors may influence which clinical conditions are selected for guideline development:

- The condition and/or patterns of care can be improved through interventions.
- Current performance in care for the condition is suboptimal.
- Patients with the target disease or condition can be clearly identified.
- The condition's underlying cause and course is well understood.
- Interventions are inexpensive and/or easy to implement.
- Payers, regulators, and consumers will value improvements in the care provided for the condition.
- Data for metrics are accessible and can be collected easily.
- Validated performance indicators are available.

Although many of these factors (e.g., understanding a condition's underlying causes and clinical course) are often missing, they are of great importance in predicting a successful outcome to CPG development and implementation.

FIGURE 6.13 demonstrates multiple sources of input into the developing CPG. The most robust resource used in CPG creation is established evidence in the medical literature, usually through the gold standard double-blind, randomized, controlled trial (RCT). Unfortunately, RCTs are very expensive to conduct and take many years to complete. For example, research supported by the National Institutes of Health may cost several million dollars and take many years to finish. Thus other types of evidence are considered in defining the steps and clinical recommendations. Increasingly, data from quality improvement studies has become important as a resource for CPGs.

Quality improvement studies are scientific studies, much like the RCT, but they usually involve smaller sample sizes. The quality improvement study usually is focused on a series of interventions in a process over a period of time, called the improvement cycle. Using techniques like design of experiments, quality improvement studies can provide statistically valid information about the effects of these interventions in the process, allowing some degree of generalization to other systems. Unlike the RCT, however, the sample size or specificity of the process may limit the degree of generalization to other processes or populations. For example, if a hospital improves a process for delivering emergency department services through multiple interventions, those same improvements may not be readily transferable to other situations without some modification to accommodate different patient populations or work environments. Thus although quality improvement studies may provide statistically valid information about a process of care, they might have some limitation in applicability to processes in other systems of care.

Another important source of information for CPG developers is expert opinion. In many cases this expertise may come from a variety of sources, such as specialists on a medical staff or within a health plan's network or perhaps from a medical specialty society. For example, guidelines on diabetes often rely on expertise from clinical endocrinologists or the endocrinology specialty societies. In general, though, expert panels usually are composed of specialists from multiple disciplines to ensure the broadest possible input into the guideline process. These experts convene to review pertinent literature and engage in discussions of guideline recommendations that lack sufficient evidence for adoption. One effective approach to these reviews was advanced by Oxman, Sackett, and Guyatt and the Evidence Based Medicine Working Group 1993.[5] The principles developed by the Working Group have been translated into a literature review technique known as the matrix method,[6] which provides a framework for literature searches and reviews that is helpful in finding appropriate articles and evidence for a CPG project. The results of the literature review are often divided into three categories:

- **Category A:** This highest ranking defines RCTs with consistent results and unimpeachable methods, such as effective randomization and a sufficiently large sample size or a study that encompasses an entire population.
- **Category B:** This classification is reserved for RCTs with methodological flaws or inconsistent results (e.g., studies that have incomplete randomization or potential shortcomings in the randomization process). Additionally, these types of studies might have borderline sample sizes or high dropout rates that can bias the results.
- **Category C:** This class generally comprises observational studies or extending results from an RCT with specific criteria to another population or sample of subjects that have similar characteristics but are not exactly the same as the original study group. Some classifications might be classified as C+ if experts reviewing a study find compelling evidence that the observational study presents overwhelming evidence of efficacy.

Using the lean framework and standardization as a framework for development of CPGs, the expert working group often assumes responsibility for working with a dedicated staff to create the guideline and developing the recommendations for implementation in clinical practice. Experts review the literature and assign weights to the evidence based on the categories listed above, and then the evidence in the articles is used to craft the guideline in the format best suited to the users of the information. The AHCPR (now AHRQ) formulation for CPGs has been widely used, but clinical guidelines now have a number of different formats, from review articles to complete clinical guidelines as described in TABLE 6.4. The format in TABLE 6.4 follows the original AHCPR form with a few modifications, and although CPGs may be redacted in multiple ways to suit particular end users, the primary users, clinicians and consumers ("patients"), are best served by the format noted in TABLE 6.4.

Table 6.4	Clinical Practice Guideline Components	
Intended Audience	Guideline Element	Description
Clinicians	Definition	Identification of the clinical condition to which the guideline applies, usually including ICD codes to specifically denote the clinical condition.
	Narrative	Description of the guideline development process, including a list of development and advisory groups. Additionally, the narrative section should include the timetable for review and updating the guideline.
	Literature review and grading	A detailed description of the literature review and grading performed by the expert panel to support the recommendations in the guideline.
	Flowchart	Detailed flowchart of the guideline recommendations to represent the processes of care to be implemented. The flowchart may also include exit points from the CPG, when appropriate.
	Notes	Explanatory notes for steps in the CPG that may expand on specific recommendations, e.g., an explanation of the group's recommendation when several options were available or when controversy may exist about a particular suggested course of diagnosis or treatment.

Table 6.4

Intended Audience	Guideline Element	Description
	Performance indicators	Listing of all performance indicators defined for the process with details of what data are collected, frequency of collection and reporting, methods of analysis, and benchmarks used in determining performance standards.
	Multimedia sources	Some guidelines include a media section that may have video or audio files for better explaining a process or procedure in the guideline. For example, a surgical procedure may be videotaped and placed in the CPG for clinicians to view the surgical method.
	Bibliography	A list of sources used for the CPG and any other potential resources that may be helpful in understanding the recommendations
	Practice aids	Resources such as care paths, order sets, automated systems for process implementation, and diagrams for staff and patient education.
Consumers	Definition	Situations in which the guideline can be applied as well as times when it should not be applied. This section involves a description of the clinical condition and signs and symptoms related to the condition.
	Care plan	What to expect for diagnostic tests and treatments, including an approximate time frame for the events to occur. In some cases an easily understood flowchart may be helpful to improve understanding.
	Alerts	How to detect problems in care or diagnosis that indicate a deviation from the expected course of care.
	Performance indicators	Basic description of methods of measuring the process with layperson definitions of terms and established benchmarks that indicate expected results of diagnosis and treatment.
	Contact information	If the guideline is being promulgated by a medical practice or other provider, this section might include appropriate contact information for any questions or problems.

As in any lean implementation, CPG development is overseen by a multidisciplinary team that optimally includes representatives of diverse stakeholder groups from the payer, provider, and consumer communities. For example, a team for developing a CPG for attention deficit disorder might include pediatricians, developmental specialists, child psychiatrists, psychologists, educators, parents of children with the disorder, and adults with the disorder. As the guideline is being crafted, perspectives from each of these stakeholder groups are incorporated into the final product, so that all stakeholders involved in the condition may influence the CPG. Ensuring multiple sources of input usually requires more time and willingness to compromise, but the final guideline will likely be more widely accepted and more readily adopted by practitioners and those affected by the condition as well as being supported by payers.

As the process in FIGURE 6.13 evolves, the multidisciplinary oversight panel provides insight into steps in the process of care that may present problems for clinicians or consumers according to the STEEEP criteria. The AHCPR termed these issues "medical review criteria," and they represent steps in the process of care at which nonconformities, such as errors or problems with access to care, might occur. These issues are prioritized according to an appropriate schema that relates to the STEEEP criteria and conforms to the emphasis that stakeholders place on each of the issues in the delivery of care. For example, a consumer advocate might emphasize access to care, whereas a payer might be concerned with the cost of a particular step that is related to excessive variation. On the other hand, providers might be concerned with safety issues, and governmental oversight bodies may focus on equity in the way care is provided. Regardless of the driving factors, the CPG team must create a prioritization approach that accounts for the important issues related to a care path, and tools like the decision matrix described in Chapter 3 may help establish the priorities more systematically.

When medical review criteria have been identified, the team can then start to focus on performance indicators to assess each criterion. Definition of performance indicators is an important part of the CPG development process, and these metrics consist of both process and outcome measures. Process measures assess the efficiency of the process and might include takt time or other lean metrics, whereas outcome measures allow evaluation of the effectiveness of the care program, such as cure rates, mortality rates, or complication rates. The CPG now conforms to the lean process management approach to process standardization, complete with measures to determine how the system functions with the standardized approach.

Performance indicators may be subject to outside influence. For example, many payers now are accountable for HEDIS (Health Effectiveness Data Information Set) measures, and as clinical guidelines are created, the use of HEDIS measures as performance indicators helps satisfy the payer's need for compliance with regulatory and accreditation standards, while providing the metrics to evaluate a clinical guideline. Other measurement sets have also become more important in pay for performance, pay for reporting, and pay for quality arrangements (see Chapter 4 for a discussion of the Physician Quality Reporting Initiative). Many quality initiatives are thus directed at improving these types of measures, but they are most effective when applied in the context of standardized processes defined by CPGs.

Many organizations use CPGs to direct improvement activities. Once the CPG is defined and medical review criteria identified, improvement teams can work to enhance the efficiency and effectiveness of the process using the performance indicators defined by the CPG team. For example, an improvement team might focus on ensuring that each person admitted to a hospital with myocardial infarction receives a beta-blocker medication (unless contraindicated) and continues on the medication after discharge. This measure is one of the HEDIS indicators for which the patient's insurer is likely accountable, but it also improves the clinical outcome for the patient. Thus the improvement team can develop interventions to ensure that the standardized approach to care includes appropriate prescription of a beta blocker and continuation on discharge. In fact, some organizations have published their improvement programs for others to use, like the Cardiovascular Hospitalization Atherosclerosis Management Program (CHAMP) developed by the University of California Los Angeles.[7] Using data gathering, analysis, and reporting approaches that leverage the power of medical informatics and statistical techniques like control charts, improvement teams can effect substantial changes in the care of complex medical conditions.

The improvement cycle for interventions usually conforms to the Shewhart cycle, plan-do-study-act (PDSA; see FIGURE 6.14). As we shall see in Chapter 7, a variation of PDSA used in six sigma programs is define-measure-analyze-improve-control, but the basic approach is the same. The four phases of the PDSA cycle are important to ensuring that an improvement initiative is completed and is based on evidence rather than supposition and presumption. The "plan" phase sets the stage by thoroughly describing the system and process(es) to be scrutinized. During this phase the team performs the lean process management steps of:

- Creating a value stream map
- Performing a walk-through
- Developing performance indicators
- Developing a project plan

The "do" phase entails the implementation of the improvement plan with a defined schedule and checkpoints during the project. As data are collected, the team continuously analyzes information to ensure that the process improvements are performing as expected; if not, mid-course corrections may be made to enhance the improvement project and increase the likelihood of success. At the conclusion of the intervention, the team formally analyzes the effect of the project during the "study" phase. Ideally, preparation for this step makes the study phase a relatively short period so that the team does not get bogged down in over-analyzing the data. If the intervention has demonstrated success through the data analysis, then the improvement can be incorporated into the process and disseminated throughout the organization, sometimes called "institutionalized," during the "act" phase. The goal of this institutionalization

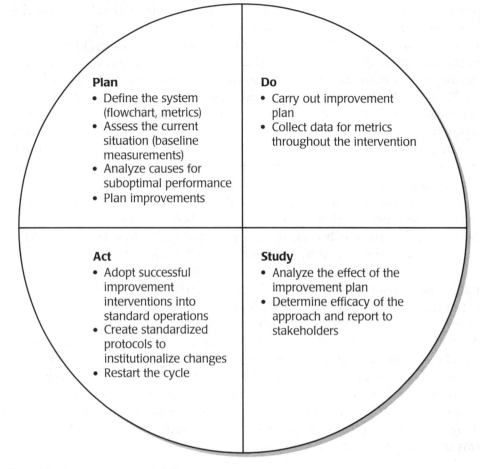

Plan
- Define the system (flowchart, metrics)
- Assess the current situation (baseline measurements)
- Analyze causes for suboptimal performance
- Plan improvements

Do
- Carry out improvement plan
- Collect data for metrics throughout the intervention

Act
- Adopt successful improvement interventions into standard operations
- Create standardized protocols to institutionalize changes
- Restart the cycle

Study
- Analyze the effect of the improvement plan
- Determine efficacy of the approach and report to stakeholders

FIGURE 6.14 Plan–Do–Study–Act Cycle

of the improvement is to sustain gains made by the initiative. For a CPG improvement, this new process step may also be useful for other practitioners who treat the same clinical conditions. In fact, many of these improved CPGs are published in the AHRQ Clinical Guideline Clearinghouse for use by other practitioners.

The difference between the older quality assurance approach and the continuous quality improvement approach codified in the PDSA cycle is the last step in the act phase: restart the cycle. If performance indicator targets have been met, a typical quality assurance project will stop at this point, but a continuous quality improvement project using PDSA simply starts at the plan phase again to identify the next process improvement target. For example, an organization wishing to improve performance in treating patients with coronary artery disease might use the interventions in the CHAMP program, but in most cases all the interventions cannot be implemented at the same time. Thus, after an intervention has shown success, other interventions in the CHAMP toolkit may be considered in the PDSA cycle to continuously improve performance and increase the value of the providers' services for all stakeholders. A cogent approach to implementation involves monitoring other process measures during the improvement project to determine the effect that a single intervention might have on other steps in the process. That information can be used to inform the team as the plan phase starts again.

Once the CPG has been through several cycles of refinement, the team may consider converting some elements of the guideline into medical policy. Many elements of guidelines have become medical policy, such as the use of beta blockers in myocardial infarction, angiotensin-converting enzyme inhibitors in congestive heart failure, immunizations in primary care preventive practice, and many others. Medical policies are useful in providing direction to providers on best practices, to payers for creating rules for payment for medical services, and for administrators and leaders to direct resource allocation. When policies are available, a great deal of debate on where or not to perform or pay for a service is avoided. Thus, as evidence accumulates from improvement projects, it has potential for supporting medical policies that can lead to more efficient and effective medical care.

One major challenge that teams encounter when trying to initiate quality improvement projects using CPGs is the difficulty in measuring healthcare quality, because physicians and analysts may disagree on valid metrics. Additionally, current systems for collecting clinical data are immature at best and often require substantial effort and cost to recover data for analysis. CPGs have proven to be one method for understanding and measuring health care through the framework that promotes the development of measures that are acceptable to clinicians and amenable to statistical validation. Every quality improvement professional is familiar with one of the laws of quality that is often ascribed to W. Edwards Deming, one of the icons of quality improvement: "You can't manage what you can't measure." CPGs help remedy that deficiency in the healthcare industry.

The maintenance phase of CPGs is important because medical knowledge continues to advance at an exponential rate. Diagnostic and treatment modalities for some conditions, particularly those like cardiovascular disease that are the focus of extensive research, can change care recommendations and require modifications in CPGs. A systematic review process for CPGs helps prevent the guideline from becoming obsolete, and every guideline must have an established schedule for review and updating. In most cases annual reviews are sufficient to ensure that the guideline contains the most up-to-date information, but those that may involve rapidly changing knowledge may require a surveillance system to quickly detect an important change to diagnostic or treatment recommendations due to newly published medical evidence. As a new modality is published and validated, a mechanism must be in place to reconvene the expert team to vet the new information and determine if the guideline should be modified before the annual review. For example, the Advisory Committee on Immunization Practices publishes the vaccine schedule for children and adults annually, but if a new vaccine becomes available in the middle of the year, a process is in place to ensure that the vaccine schedule is modified accordingly.

Challenges in CPG Implementation

At the start of this chapter we noted that some clinicians view attempts at standardization as anathema for the medical profession. Anything that removes clinician autonomy or creates expectations and accountability for independent practitioners is considered by these practitioners as invasive and to increase the cost of care and the "hassle factor." Although that view is changing, it still creates a barrier to implementation that is difficult to surmount. Until providers see the value of CPGs as a way to improve the quality of care, this view is likely to persist, at least in some circles. However, CPG teams can deal with these objections in a number of ways. First, involving clinicians in the multidisciplinary teams that develop guidelines can allow input into the process of guideline creation and defuse objections that the review of medical knowledge was somehow inadequate. Many of these professionals assume ownership of the CPG and can even assist in convincing their peers to adopt the guideline. The second approach to gaining clinician support leverages this involvement to cultivate physician champions, who are respected by their peers and who are committed to guideline implementation. These physician champions become the spokespersons for the implementation team and often help with data collection and analysis, further validating the CPG. Physician champions lead by example, but they also can help their peers understand the nature of the guideline and value to its adoption. Finally, many organizations are aligning incentives with those physicians who follow CPG recommendations. Additionally, payers like Centers for Medicare and Medicaid Services are beginning to penalize providers for not following recommendations and ending up with "never event" complications such as:[8]

- Surgical events
  - Surgery performed on the wrong body part
  - Surgery performed on the wrong patient
  - Wrong surgical procedure on a patient
  - Retention of a foreign object in a patient after surgery or other procedure
  - Intraoperative or immediately postoperative death in a normal health patient (defined as a Class 1 patient for purposes of the American Society of Anesthesiologists patient safety initiative)
- Product or device events
  - Patient death or serious disability associated with the use of contaminated drugs, devices, or biologics provided by the healthcare facility
  - Patient death or serious disability associated with the use or function of a device in patient care in which the device is used or functions other than as intended

- Patient death or serious disability associated with intravascular air embolism that occurs while being cared for in a healthcare facility
- Patient protection events
  - Infant discharged to the wrong person
  - Patient death or serious disability associated with patient elopement (disappearance) for more than 4 hours
  - Patient suicide, or attempted suicide resulting in serious disability, while being cared for in a healthcare facility
- Care management events
  - Patient death or serious disability associated with a medication error (e.g., error involving the wrong drug, wrong dose, wrong patient, wrong time, wrong rate, wrong preparation, or wrong route of administration)
  - Patient death or serious disability associated with a hemolytic reaction due to the administration of ABO-incompatible blood or blood products
  - Maternal death or serious disability associated with labor or delivery on a low-risk pregnancy while being cared for in a healthcare facility
  - Patient death or serious disability associated with hypoglycemia, the onset of which occurs while the patient is being cared for in a healthcare facility
  - Death or serious disability (kernicterus) associated with failure to identify and treat hyperbilirubinemia in neonates
  - Stage 3 or 4 pressure ulcers acquired after admission to a healthcare facility
  - Patient death or serious disability due to spinal manipulative therapy
- Environmental events
  - Patient death or serious disability associated with an electric shock while being cared for in a healthcare facility
  - Any incident in which a line designated for oxygen or other gas to be delivered to a patient contains the wrong gas or is contaminated by toxic substances
  - Patient death or serious disability associated with a burn incurred from any source while being cared for in a healthcare facility
  - Patient death associated with a fall while being cared for in a healthcare facility
  - Patient death or serious disability associated with the use of restraints or bed rails while being cared for in a healthcare facility

These preventable errors can be avoided through the use of guidelines and some of the other lean approaches discussed in this chapter, and because providers will no longer be paid for treating these complications, impetus may build to adopt CPGs to preclude these costly events. In short, clinicians will increasingly be provided with both incentives and disincentives to adopt standardized approaches to care.

As discussed in Chapter 1, the business case for quality involves a number of gains as well as potentially reduced costs. Unfortunately, the payoff for quality improvement efforts may not be immediate in a financial sense. For example, implementing a CPG for diabetes that includes eye exams for early detection and treatment of diabetic retinopathy may not show a return in the current fiscal year, but over a period of several years of high performance on this measure the rate of blindness from diabetes will decrease, thereby reducing the cost of care and improving the lives of diabetics.[9] However, some interventions demonstrate almost immediate as well as long-term benefits. Many vaccinations in children exhibit this pattern (e.g., the varicella vaccine, which prevents the disease starting shortly after the vaccination and for several years into the future). Those types of rewards are generally much easier to sell to a payer than a longer term prospect of preventing blindness in diabetics many years in the future. These challenges are often met by gaining industry-wide support for the guideline. In the case of diabetic eye exams, the Centers for Medicare and Medicaid Services and the National Commission on Quality Assurance have adopted a HEDIS measure for dilated diabetic eye exams that not only provides incentives for health plans but also for providers.

A major dissatisfier in healthcare systems around the world, including the United States, is the perceived poor quality of care. Several studies have shown a correlation between quality of care and patient satisfaction in a variety of conditions, such as HIV/AIDS,[10] liver disease,[11] and dermatologic conditions.[12] Although many factors contribute to customer satisfaction with care, factors like waiting time in the outpatient clinic and pain control in the hospital are important and amenable to performance improvement approaches. As the quality of care improves, patient satisfaction with care should also increase. As patient surveys become increasingly important in evaluating healthcare services, from health plans to primary care providers, the case for creating a more efficient and effective system of care has never been more compelling. Customer satisfaction has become a major reason for implementing tools like CPGs and can serve to support the business case for adopting CPGs and other types of interventions to create value.

Another barrier to implementing CPGs is the extraordinary complexity of care for many diseases. The lean approach to this conundrum is to break the process into smaller subprocesses that can be analyzed and improved. The concept of "episodes of care" has been operational in health care for several decades, but with the increasing need for standardization, this model is expected to become more important. An episode of care may be somewhat specific by clinical condition (e.g., an acute exacerbation of asthma [status asthmaticus] or decompensation of a patient with congestive heart failure requiring hospitalization). CPGs can be developed for these specific episodes rather than for an entire clinical course of a chronic disease, which may be too complex for a manageable guideline. Using episodes of care has been especially useful in evaluating high cost or high risk subprocesses for opportunities for intervention and in defining performance indicators using available data sources.

As noted previously, the proliferation of CPGs has also created some redundancy and in some cases contradictory recommendations, particularly for high cost diseases like congestive heart failure. Additionally, some CPGs may incorporate the use of specific resources (e.g., positron emission tomography) that may not be available at all facilities. Although this plethora of CPGs may help a development team, in some cases it can create increased work to determine which CPG is most germane to a particular setting.

Finally, the full CPG is often not useful in real time for providers trying to use the recommendations in practice. Thus abbreviated versions of the guideline that can be put into a computer algorithm or a short description on a personal digital assistant (PDA) can improve adoption and use of guidelines in daily practice. Decision support systems rely on use of electronic health records, as described in Chapter 4, and so they have been minimally deployed as of this writing. However, the use of guidelines and references on PDAs has become commonplace among many physicians and advance practice nurses, and numerous guideline resources can now be found on the World Wide Web. These short versions of guidelines are sometimes called clinicians' guides and generally consist of the following components of the CPG:

- Definition of patient characteristics or diagnoses covered by the guideline
- Flowchart of the recommended clinical pathway
- Footnotes for the CPG to clarify any steps that may require more information
- Forms or tables that may be used to properly implement the CPG

PDA guidelines have these characteristics, and AHCPR provided a format for clinicians' guides in paper format that is still used in some applications where electronic guidelines may not be practicable.

■ Summary

CPGs are a prime example of the move toward standardization in health care. Appropriately applied, standardization of healthcare processes using the lean process management approach can improve performance by reducing variation and the risk of errors. By taking the process of guideline creation to its next logical level using lean management, the healthcare industry can achieve higher performance and improve value for all stakeholders.

■ Discussion Questions

1. Describe the evolution of the lean process management system in the healthcare industry. How does the lean management system complement healthcare performance improvement efforts?
2. Why do practitioners resist efforts at standardization? Can standardization cure the problems facing the healthcare system of high cost and poor quality?

3. Describe Taylorism. How does the work of F. W. Taylor apply to modern industries like health care?

4. What characteristics of the TPS are germane to the healthcare delivery system? Give examples of how the TPS can be implemented in health care.

5. Describe three tools from the TPS that can be applied in health care. Give examples of how they might be beneficial.

6. What is autonomation? How can it be applied to improve health care?

7. Name the seven forms of muda. Give examples of each in the healthcare industry.

8. What is a kaizen event? How can it be leveraged to improve performance?

9. Describe 6S. How can it improve the risk of patient injury?

10. Describe the lean improvement cycle. Give an example of how the cycle would be applied in a hospital system.

11. What is value stream mapping? How is this tool used in a lean improvement cycle?

12. Define kanban. How is it applied in the healthcare industry at the present time?

13. Why is load leveling important in a process? How can the concept be applied in health care?

14. How are CPGs examples of standardization? Discuss three benefits of CPGs in the healthcare delivery system.

15. Define STEEEP. Why are these concepts important for healthcare practitioners?

16. How are CPGs used by each of the major stakeholders? Why is the quality of CPGs important?

17. Describe the CPG development and maintenance cycle. Why is the maintenance phase important?

18. What are the major factors in selecting a condition for CPG development? Explain why each one is important to selecting a target condition.

19. How are quality improvement studies different from randomized controlled trials? Which of these approaches provides the best evidence for care?

20. What are the three categories for literature review in support of a CPG? Explain how the categories are important to clinicians interpreting the CPG.

21. What are medical review criteria? How are they used in development of a CPG?

22. Describe Shewhart's PDSA cycle. How is it applied to quality improvement in health care?

23. What are the major steps in the plan phase of PDSA? Which lean tools might be involved in this phase?

24. Name three challenges to CPG implementation and describe how they create barriers to implementation.

25. What are "never events"? How are they being used in health care to promote quality care?

26. What is an "episode of care"? How does this concept apply to CPG development?

References

1. Taylor FW. *Principles of Scientific Management*. New York: W. W. Norton & Company; 1967. Retrieved December 2008 from http://www.eldritchpress.org/fwt/ti.html

2. Kurzweil R. *The Singularity Is Near*. New York: Penguin; 2005.

3. Field MJ, Lohr KN, eds. *Clinical Practice Guidelines: Directions for a New Program*. Institute of Medicine, Washington, DC: National Academy Press; 1990.

4. U.S. Department of Health and Human Services, Public Health Service, Agency for Health Care Policy and Research. *Using Clinical Practice Guidelines to Evaluate Quality of Care*. AHCPR Pub. No. 95-0045; 1995.

5. Oxman AD, Sackett DL, Guyatt GH. Users' guides to the medical literature: I. How to get started. *Journal of the American Medical Association*, 1993;270:17.

6. Garrard J. *Health Sciences Literature Review Made Easy: The Matrix Method*. Sudbury, MA: Jones and Bartlett; 2007.

7. UCLA Medical Center. Cardiovascular Hospitalization Atherosclerosis Management Program (CHAMP). Retrieved March 2009 from www.med.ucla.edu/champ

8. CMS Office of Public Affairs. Eliminating serious, preventable, and costly medical errors—Never events. Retrieved March 2009 from http://www.cms.hhs.gov/apps/media/press/release.asp?Counter=1863

9. Fong DS, Aiello LP, Ferris FL, Klein R. Diabetic retinopathy. *Diabetes Care*, 2004;27:2540–2553.

10. Tsasis P, Tsoukas C, Deutsch G. Evaluation of patient satisfaction in a specialized HIV/AIDS care unit of a major hospital. *AIDS Patient Care and STDs*, 2000;14:347–349.

11. Gutteling JJ, de Man RA, Busschbach JJ, Darlington AE. Quality of health care and patient satisfaction in liver disease: The development and preliminary results of the QUOTE-Liver questionnaire. Retrieved March 2009 from http://www.biomedcentral.com/1471-230X/8/25

12. Poulos GA, Brodell RT, Mostow EN. Improving quality and patient satisfaction in dermatology office practice. *Archives of Dermatology*, 2008;144:263–265.

Additional Reading

Carlino A, Flinchbaugh J. *The Hitchhiker's Guide to Lean*. Dearborn, MI: Society of Manufacturing Engineers; 2005.

Chalice RW. *Improving Healthcare Using Toyota Lean Production Methods—46 Steps for Improvement* Milwaukee, WI: ASQ Quality Press; 2007.

George ML. *Lean Six Sigma for Service*. New York: McGraw-Hill; 2003.

Graban M. *Lean Hospitals: Improving Quality, Patient Safety, and Employee Satisfaction*. New York: Productivity Press; 2008.

Hirano H, Furuya M. *JIT Is Flow: Practice and Principles of Lean Manufacturing*. Vancouver, WA: PCS; 2006.

Levinson WA. *Henry Ford's Lean Vision: Enduring Principles from the First Ford Motor Plant*. New York: Productivity Press; 2002.

Liker J. *The Toyota Way: 14 Management Principles from the World's Greatest Manufacturer*. New York: McGraw-Hill; 2003.

Norwood EP. *Ford: Men and Methods*. New York: Doubleday; 1931.

Ohno T. *Toyota Production System: Beyond Large-scale Production.* New York: Productivity Press; 1988.

Womack JP, Jones DT. *Lean Thinking.* Tanupa, FL: Free Press; 1998.

Womack JP, Jones DT, Roos D. *The Machine that Changed the World: The Story of Lean Production.* New York: Harper Perennial; 1991.

Articles From the Evidence Based Medicine Working Group on Classification of Evidence in the Medical Literature

Barratt A, Irwig L, Glasziou P, et al. Users guide to medical literature. XVII. How to use guidelines and recommendations about screening. *Journal of the American Medical Association,* 1999;281:2029.

Bucher HC, Guyatt GH, Cook DJ, Holbrook A, McAlister FA. Users' guides to the medical literature. XIX. Applying clinical trial results: A. How to use an article measuring the effect of an intervention on surrogate end points. *Journal of the American Medical Association,* 1999;282:771–778.

Dans AL, Dans LF, Guyatt GH, Richardson S. Users' guides to the medical literature. XIV. How to decide on the applicability of clinical trial results to your patient. Evidence Based Medicine Working Group. *Journal of the American Medical Association,* 1998;279:545–549.

Drummond MF, Richardson WS, O'Brien BJ, Levine M, Heyland D. Users' guides to the medical literature. XIII. How to use an article on economic analysis of clinical practice: A. Are the results of the study valid? Evidence-Based Medicine Working Group. *Journal of the American Medical Association,* 1997;277:1552–1557.

Giacomini MK, Cook DJ. Users' guides to the medical literature. XXIII. Qualitative research in health care: A. Are the results of the study valid? *Journal of the American Medical Association,* 2000;284:357–362.

Giacomini MK, Cook DJ. Users' guides to the medical literature. XXIII. Qualitative research in health care: B. What are the results and how do they help me care for my patients? *Journal of the American Medical Association,* 2000;284:478–482.

Guyatt G, Rennie D, the Evidence Based Medicine Working Group. Why users' guides? EBM Working Paper Series no. 1. Retrieved March 2009 from http://www.cche.net/principles/content_why.asp

Guyatt GH, Haynes RB, Jaeschke RZ, et al. Users' guides to the medical literature. XXV. Evidence-based medicine: Principles for applying the users' guides to patient care. *Journal of the American Medical Association,* 2000;284:1290–1296.

Guyatt GH, Naylor CD, Juniper E, et al. Users' guides to the medical literature. XII. How to use articles about health-related quality of life. Evidence-Based Medicine Working Group. *Journal of the American Medical Association,* 1997;277:1232–1237.

Guyatt GH, Sackett DL, Cook DJ. Users' guides to the medical literature. II. How to use an article about therapy or prevention: A. Are the results of the study valid? *Journal of the American Medical Association,* 1993;270:2598–2601.

Guyatt GH, Sackett DL, Cook DJ. Users' guides to the medical literature. II. How to use an article about therapy or prevention: B. What were the results and will they help me in caring for my patients? *Journal of the American Medical Association,* 1994;271:59–63.

Guyatt GH, Sackett DL, Sinclair JC, Users' guides to the medical literature. IX. A method for grading health care recommendations. *Journal of the American Medical Association,* 1995;274:1800–1804.

Guyatt GH, Sinclair J, Cook DJ, Glasziou P. Users' guides to the medical literature. XVI. How to use a treatment recommendation. *Journal of the American Medical Association,* 1999;281:1836–1843.

Hayward RSA, Wilson MC, Tunis SR, Bass EB, Guyatt G. Users' guides to the medical literature. VIII. How to use clinical practice guidelines: A. Are the recommendations valid? *Journal of the American Medical Association*, 1995;274:570–574.

Hunt DL, Jaeschke R, McKibbon KA. Users' guides to the medical literature. XXI. Using electronic health information resources in evidence-based practice. Evidence-Based Medicine Working Group. *Journal of the American Medical Association*, 2000;283:1875–1879.

Jaeschke R, Gordon H, Guyatt G, Sackett DL. Users' guides to the medical literature. III. How to use an article about a diagnostic test: B. what are the results and will they help me in caring for my patients? *Journal of the American Medical Association*, 1994;271:703–707.

Jaeschke R, Guyatt G, Sackett DL. Users' guides to the medical literature. III. How to use an article about a diagnostic test: A. Are the results of the study valid? *Journal of the American Medical Association*, 1994;271:389–391.

Laupacis A, Wells G, Richardson S, Tugwell P. Users' guides to the medical literature. V. How to use an article about prognosis. *Journal of the American Medical Association*, 1994;272:234–237.

Levine M, Walter S, Lee H, Haines T, Holbrook A, Moyer V. Users' guides to the medical literature. IV. How to use an article about harm. *Journal of the American Medical Association*, 1994;271: 1615–1619.

McAlister FA, Laupacis A, Wells GA, Sackett DL. Users' guides to the medical literature. XIX. Applying clinical trial results: B. Guidelines for determining whether a drug is exerting (more than) a class effect. *Journal of the American Medical Association*, 1999;282:1371–1377.

McAlister FA, Straus SE, Guyatt GH, Haynes RB. Users' guides to the medical literature. XX. Integrating research evidence with the care of the individual patient. *Journal of the American Medical Association*, 2000;283:2829–2836.

McGinn TG, Guyatt GH, Wyer PC, Naylor CD, Stiell IG, Richardson WS. Users' guides to the medical literature. XXII. How to use articles about clinical decision rules. *Journal of the American Medical Association*, 2000;284:79–84.

Naylor CD, Guyatt GH Users' guides to the medical literature. X. How to use an article reporting variations in the outcomes of health services. Evidence-Based Medicine Working Group. *Journal of the American Medical Association*, 1996;275:554–558.

Naylor CD, Guyatt GH. Users' guides to the medical literature. XI. How to use an article about a clinical utilization review. Evidence-Based Medicine Working Group. *Journal of the American Medical Association*, 1996;275:1435–1439.

O'Brien BJ, Heyland D, Richardson WS, Levine M, Drummond MF. Users' guides to the medical literature. XIII. How to use an article on economic analysis of clinical practice: B. What are the results and will they help me in caring for my patients? Evidence-Based Medicine Working Group. *Journal of the American Medical Association*, 1997;277:1802–1806.

Oxman AD, Cook DJ, Guyatt GH. Users' guides to the medical literature. VI. How to use an overview. Evidence-Based Medicine Working Group. *Journal of the American Medical Association*, 1994;272:1367–1371.

Oxman A, Sackett DL, Guyatt GH. Users' guides to the medical literature. I. How to get started. *Journal of the American Medical Association*, 1993;270:2093–2095.

Randolph AG, Haynes RB, Wyatt JC, Cook DJ, Guyatt GH. Users' guide to medical literature. XVIII. How to use an article evaluating the clinical impact of a computer-based clinical decision support system. *Journal of the American Medical Association*, 1999;282:67–74.

Richardson WS, Detsky AS. Users' guides to the medical literature. VII. How to use a clinical decision analysis: A. Are the results of the study valid? *Journal of the American Medical Association*, 1995;273:1292–1295.

Richardson WS, Detsky AS. Users' guides to the medical literature. VII. How to use a clinical decision analysis: B. What are the results and will they help me in caring for my patients? *Journal of the American Medical Association,* 1995;273:1610–1613.

Richardson WS, Wilson MC, Guyatt GH, Cook DJ, Nishikawa J. Users' guides to the medical literature. XV. How to use an article about disease probability for differential diagnosis. *Journal of the American Medical Association,* 1999;281:1214–1219.

Richardson WS, Wilson MC, Williams JW, Moyer VA, Naylor CD. Users' guides to the medical literature. XXIV. How to use an article on the clinical manifestations of disease. *Journal of the American Medical Association,* 2000;284:869–875.

Wilson MC, Hayward RSA, Tunis SR, Bass EB, Guyatt G. Users' guides to the medical literature. VIII. How to use clinical practice guidelines: B. What are the recommendations and will they help you in caring for your patients? *Journal of the American Medical Association,* 1995;274:1630–1632.

■ Lean Glossary and Concepts

Agile Management: The ability to thrive under conditions of constant and unpredictable change by seeking to achieve rapid response to customer needs. Agile management also emphasizes the ability to quickly reconfigure operations—and strategic alliances—to respond rapidly to unforeseen shifts in the marketplace, which in the healthcare industry of the 21st century is critical to survival. Healthcare leaders now recognize the need for applying other principles, like "mass customization," to satisfy unique customer requirements but maintaining the efficiencies of a mass production operation.

Andon (Lantern): A signal, light, bell, or music alarm triggered by an operator confronted with a nonstandard condition. In a manufacturing setting these conditions may include tool failure, machine failure, bad part, lack of parts, or the inability to keep up. In health care any evidence of impending patient or worker harm may trigger Andon, and, most recently, high performing organizations are empowering all employees to signal if any evidence of a harmful situation arises. The Andon is a useful tool for implementing poka yoke.

Andon Board: The Andon board is a visual control device in a production area, such as an operating theater or an emergency department, which is typically a light display or a computer screen, giving the current status of the system and alerting team members of emerging problems. These displays may help identify bottlenecks in patient flow that require intervention.

Annual Inventory Turns: A measure that is calculated by dividing the value of annual plant shipments at plant cost (for the most recent full year) by the total current inventory value at plant cost. Total current inventory includes raw materials, work in process, and finished goods. Plant cost includes material, labor, and plant overhead.

Autonomation (English translation of Jidoka): "Automation with a human touch"; design of a process so that machines automatically inspect items as they are produced, with the ability to notify humans if a defect is detected and stop production of the item or service. In the Toyota Production System this concept is extended to include all workers on the production line or involved in the process. Each worker is empowered to stop production if a defect is discovered, which has particular applicability in the healthcare delivery system to prevent harm to patients.

Baka-yoke: Literally to design a process to be foolproof; a process or a machine is designed so that the only way it can be performed or used is the correct way. This type of process design generally involves a warning (Andon) if the process or machine produces a nonstandard condition. Healthcare applications have been concentrated on Failure mode and effects analyses, using such tools as Pareto analysis.

Cellular Manufacturing: A process design approach in which equipment and workstations are arranged to facilitate small-lot, continuous-flow production. In a manufacturing context a "cell" is designed so that all operations necessary to produce a component or subassembly are performed in close proximity, thus allowing for quick feedback between operators when quality problems and other issues arise. Cross-training workers in a manufacturing cell ensures that each worker in the cell can assume responsibility for any step.

Chaku-chaku: "Load-load" in Japanese. A method of implementing single-piece flow in which the operator proceeds from machine to machine, taking a part from the previous operation and loading it in the next machine, then taking the part just removed from that machine and loading it in the following machine.

Continuous flow production: Implementation of "just in time" techniques to reduce setup times, slash work-in-progress inventory, reduce waste, minimize non–value added activities, improve throughput, and reduce cycle time. Continuous flow production typically involves use of "pull" signals to initiate production activity, in contrast to work-order ("push") systems in which production scheduling typically is based on forecasted demand rather than actual demand. In many pull systems a customer order or delivery date triggers completion of the process, which in turn cascades messages backward in the process to force replenishment of components required for upstream inventory to prepare for subsequent production.

Cpk: A statistic that indicates how well a design tolerance compares with the normal process variation (defined as ±3) that also accounts for the difference between the process target and the actual process mean. Cpk values vary between 0 and 2, with higher values being desirable. Cpk values of 1.33 are considered a minimum acceptable process capability, indicating a sigma level of 3; higher Cpk values approach six sigma capabilities of 3.4 defective units per million opportunities.

Cross-functional teams: Multidisciplinary and interdepartmental teams of employees who represent a cross-section of disciplines and/or different process segments who participate on ad hoc teams to deal with a specific problem or perform a specific task.

Cycle time: In industrial engineering, the time between completion of two discrete units of production. For example, in health care the cycle time of a surgical unit is the number of cases performed per hour or some other time unit. The goal of a process is for cycle time to equal takt time, which indicates single piece flow.

Defects per million opportunities (DPMO): The ratio of defects found per unit of production to the average opportunities for error in one unit and then multiplied by 1,000,000. DPMO is frequently used in benchmarking as a normalized value to compare products or services of varying complexity.

Design for quality: Designing quality assurance and customer perception of product quality into a process being newly created or improved.

Failure modes and effects analysis: A procedure used to identify and assess risks associated with potential product or process failure modes.

First-pass yield: The percent of finished product or service units that meet all quality-related specifications at a critical test point in the process. This metric assesses the yield that results from the first time through the process, before any rework, and it is calculated as the percent of output that meets target-grade specifications after the first time through the process.

Five (5) S's:

> **Sort:** to clearly distinguish the needed from the unneeded
>
> **Straighten:** keeping needed items in the correct place to allow for easy and immediate retrieval
>
> **Shine:** keeping the workplace swept and clean
>
> **Standardize:** consistency applying 6S methods in a uniform and disciplined manner
>
> **Sustain:** making a habit of maintaining established procedures

Or 5S in Japanese:

> **seiri:** eliminating everything not required for the work being performed
>
> **seiton:** efficient placement and arrangement of equipment and material
>
> **season:** tidiness and cleanliness
>
> **seiketsu:** ongoing, standardized, continually improving seiri, seiton, seison
>
> **shitsuke:** discipline with leadership

Five (5) why's: Taiichi Ohno's practice of asking "why" five times whenever a problem was encountered to identify the root cause of the problem.

Flexible manufacturing systems: Automated manufacturing equipment and/or cross-trained work teams that can accommodate small-lot production of a variety of product or part configurations. In a service environment flexible manufacturing systems connotes cross-training for improved productivity and use of small teams in "microsystems."

Flow: The progressive achievement of tasks along the value stream so that a product or service proceeds through each step of the process with no stoppages, waste, or back flows.

Heijunka: A Japanese word that means "make flat and level," referring to production smoothing, which is a technique used to adapt production to naturally fluctuating customer demand. Customer demand must be met within preferred delivery times, but customer demand is uneven, necessitating interventions on the part of managers to smooth demand as much as possible.

Hoshin kanri (policy deployment): Alignment of strategy with improvement initiatives to achieve strategic objectives. Visual matrix diagrams are used to select three to five key objectives and translate them into specific projects deployed at the front line customer level. Targets for these objectives are established and used to measure progress toward goals.

Improvement: In the lean process management system, improvement is a philosophy of maintaining and improving high quality standards that guides activities such as kaizen events. Through innovation and other lean tools, improvement guides workers in the philosophy of the organization to achieve high standards of quality.

Jishuken: Use of a consultant or other outside person (e.g., a customer) to improve a kaizen event.

Just-in-time (JIT): A system for producing and delivering the right items at the right time in the right amounts at the right place in the process.

Kaikaku: Radical improvement of an activity to eliminate muda, for example, by implementing single piece flow in a small space that reduces travel. Also called breakthrough kaizen, flow kaizen, and system kaizen.

Kaizen: The systematic, organized improvement of processes by front-line staff using straightforward methods of analysis and improvement. Kaizen can be an immediate approach to continuous, incremental improvement of an activity to create more value with less muda by establishing priorities and empowering employees to use continuous improvement tools to gain immediate results. Also can be defined as the philosophy of continuous improvement that requires every process to be continually evaluated and improved by everyone working on the process. In the TPS, kaizen applies to all aspects of life, not just work.

Kaizen event: A defined effort in which a multidisciplinary team plans and implements a significant process change to quickly achieve a quantum improvement in performance.

Kanban: A communication tool developed by Taiichi Ohno at Toyota in the "just-in-time" production and control system that authorizes production or movement. Kanban can be a card or signboard or any other authorizing device such as a light or electronic signal that is attached to specific parts in the production line signifying the delivery of a given quantity. The ideal quantity authorized for each kanban is one unit, but in many applications several units might be authorized. For example, a radiology department might authorize several patients simultaneously if several exam rooms are free. The number of circulating or available kanban for a specific unit is determined by the demand rate for the item and the time required to produce or acquire more. Unless demand changes or other circumstances intervene, the number of available kanban generally remains constant to maintain control of the process. However, more efficient, single-piece flow systems require few, if any, kanban, so the fewer kanban used, the more efficient the process. Kanban operates according to the following rules:

- All movements of production units (e.g. parts, materials, information, patients) occur only as required by a downstream operation. Thus all manufacturing, production, and procurement activities are ultimately driven by the requirements of the customer.
- Kanban have various formats and content as appropriate for their usage; for example, a kanban for a vendor is different from a kanban for an internal machining operation.

Kanban signal: A method of signaling suppliers or upstream production operations when it is time to replenish limited stocks of components or subassemblies in a just-in-time system. In the TPS, kanban signals were cards placed in specific locations to signal the need for more process units at the next step in the process. Contemporary systems often use electronic signals in place of cards or other physical elements.

Karoshi: Death from overwork. (A common problem for quality improvement professionals in health care.)

Key performance indicators: The few vital measurements that show how a business is performing throughout the production process.

Lead time: The total time a customer must wait to receive a product or service after placing an order. For example, the wait time in a physician's office would be considered lead time in a lean system environment. When a production system is running at or below capacity, lead time and throughput time are the same. When customer demand exceeds system capability, waiting time is added to the throughput so that lead time exceeds throughput.

Lean manufacturing or lean production: The philosophy of the Toyota Production System to continually reduce waste in all areas and in all forms.

Level scheduling: The use of scheduling the sequence of production units in a repetitive pattern to smooth variations in the rate of customer demand.

Life cycle costing: The identification, evaluation, tracking, and analysis of actual costs for each service or product from the point of initial research and development through the final product or service and after-service support.

Line balancing: Achievement of smooth production flow and 100% capacity utilization by equalization of cycle times for relatively small process units using proper allocation of human and physical resources.

Machine availability rate: The percent of time that equipment is available for use, divided by the maximum time it would be available if there were no downtime for repair or unplanned maintenance. This concept may be applied to other physical resources, such as operating room availability rate, emergency department room availability rate, and so on.

Manufacturing cells: A configuration of equipment and workstations in a sequence (often U-shaped) to support single-piece flow and flexible deployment of human effort. Manufacturing cells are often designed using tools such as the workflow diagram that positions equipment and other resources in a way that optimizes human interaction and decreases travel and wait time.

Manufacturing cycle time: The length of time from the start of production operations for a particular service or product to the completion of all production or service processes for a specific customer or customer order. This time does not include order-entry time or time spent on customization of nonstandard items.

Mixed-model production: The capability to produce a variety of services or variations of a product that may differ in use of human and physical resources in the same production environment; common situation for healthcare systems (e.g., pathology department that must process a variety of specimens for different customers using similar equipment and the same staff).

Muda (waste): Waste that is targeted for elimination in the lean process management system, including:

- **Overproduction:** excess production and early production leading to inventories
- **Waiting:** time spent in anticipation of the next process step
- **Transportation:** time spent in movement and transportation of production units
- **Processing:** poor process design

- **Inventory**: waste associated with inventory (e.g., storage, nonproducing assets)
- **Motion**: actions of people or equipment that do not add value to the product
- **Rework**: production of an item or service that must be discarded or requires rework

Mura: Variation.

Muri: Excessive burden due to waste or poor design.

Nagara: Smooth production flow, ideally single piece flow, with synchronization (balancing) of production processes and maximum utilization of available time, including overlapping of operations where practical. Utilization of level scheduling and line balancing to achieve smooth flow.

Nemawashi: The Japanese conduct business meetings differently from other cultures. Nemawashi, which translates to "prior consultation," is a method by which everyone involved in the meeting reviews material and make conclusions regarding the information. By gaining agreement as much as possible in advance, meetings can conclude with a decision and maintain harmony among attendees. The prior preparation allows people with differing opinions to negotiate their differences before the meeting and reduce wasted time in the meeting.

Non–value added work: Essential process steps or activities that must be performed in the present system but that do not add value to the product or service. These steps or activities are the target of lean process improvement activities.

Perfection: Complete elimination of muda and non–value added work.

Plan-do-study-act (PDSA) cycle: Shewhart's improvement cycle in which a process or system is studied and improvements planned, the improvements are initiated (do), the results of the intervention are reviewed (study), and the intervention is then either incorporated into the process or subject to the improvement cycle for another round.

Poka yoke: Mistake-proofing device or procedure to prevent a defect during the entire production sequence. Poka yoke stops a defective component from moving to the next work station by using "fail-safe" techniques to eliminate errors or quality-related production defects as far upstream in the process as possible. For example, surgical teams take a time out to review a patient's information before proceeding with a surgical procedure. The major objectives are to eliminate errors and rework.

Predictive maintenance: Practices that seek to prevent unscheduled equipment downtime by collecting and analyzing information on equipment conditions. This analysis is used to predict time-to-failure, conduct planned maintenance, and maintain equipment in good operating condition. In the manufacturing sector predictive maintenance systems typically measure parameters on machine operations, such as vibration, heat, pressure, noise, and lubricant condition, whereas in health care bioengineers monitor machine usage time and test for accuracy in parameters like fluid delivery in intravenous pumps.

Process: A series of individual operations required to create a design, completed order, product, or service.

Processing time: The time a patient is actually engaged in receiving a service or a product is being produced on a production line. Typically, processing time is a small fraction of throughput time and lead time.

Pull: A system of cascading production and delivery instructions from downstream to upstream activities in which nothing is produced by the upstream supplier until the downstream customer signals a need. For example, flexible staffing of an emergency department that allows for staff to be sent to the emergency department when volume is higher.

Pull system: A system for controlling workflow priorities in which processes requiring resources receive the resources as needed, using techniques such as kanban and just-in-time production. Contrasted with "push" systems in which material is processed and then pushed to the next stage whether or not it is really needed in the downstream environment.

Quality function deployment: A customer-focused approach to quality improvement in which customer needs (desired product or service characteristics) are analyzed at the design stage and translated into specific product, service, and design requirements for the supplier organization. Targeted customer needs may include product features, cost, durability, appearance, or other product characteristics. Quality function deployment involves carefully listening to the customer's needs and translating them into product or service design elements to create the desired customer output. The quality functions defined by the customer are then deployed throughout the organization by tying incentives and compliance activities directly to the fulfillment of these customer requirements.

Quick changeover methods: A variety of techniques that reduce equipment setup time and permit faster cycle time (e.g., as in operating room turnaround time).

Seiban: A Japanese management practice taken from the Japanese words "sei," which means manufacturing, and "ban," which means number. A Seiban number is assigned to all parts, materials, and purchase orders associated with a particular customer job, or with a project, that enables a process owner to track everything related with a particular product, service, or customer. Seiban also facilitates setting aside inventory for specific projects or priorities to accommodate nonstandard production or service requests.

Self-directed natural work teams: Autonomous teams of empowered employees that share a common work space and/or responsibility for a particular process or process segment. Self-directed natural work teams have authority for day-to-day production activities and many supervisory responsibilities, such as job assignments, production scheduling, maintenance, materials purchasing, training, quality assurance, performance appraisals, and customer service.

Sensei: A teacher or instructor.

Setup time: Work required to change over resources from one item or operation to the next item or operation, often seen as two types:

1. **Internal:** setup work that can be done only when the resource is not actively engaged in performing a service or in a production activity
2. **External:** setup work that can be done concurrently with the resource being used in a service process or in a production activity

Seven quality tools:

1. Flowcharts
2. Cause-and-effect diagrams
3. Check sheets
4. Histograms
5. Scatter diagrams
6. Pareto charts
7. Control charts

Single-piece flow: A process design in which service units or products proceed, one complete item at a time, through various operations in design, order taking, and production, without interruptions, back flows, or scrap.

Spaghetti chart: A map of the path taken by a specific product or a customer receiving a service as the item or customer travels down the value stream in a lean production organization; so called because the route typically looks like a plate of spaghetti.

Standard work: A precise description of each work activity specifying cycle time, takt time, the work sequence of specific tasks, and the minimum resources needed to conduct the activity. Standard work details the motion of the worker and the process sequence in producing an item or service. Standard work defines the most muda-free production method through the best arrangement of resources, the least amount of work in process, with indications of where measurements should be performed for quality and safety. It provides a routine for consistency of an operation and a basis for improvement. A clinical practice guideline is an example of standard work.

Statistical process control: The analysis of measure trends using graphical and statistical methods for measuring, analyzing, and controlling the variation of a process for the purpose of ensuring process performance and continuously improving the process.

Takt time: The available production time divided by the rate of customer demand. Takt time sets the pace of production to match the rate of customer demand. Used to determine targets for improvement of system output.

Throughput time: Processing and waiting time for performing a service or producing a product.

Total cost of poor quality: The aggregate cost of service or product failures (e.g., scrap, rework, and warranty costs) as well as expenses incurred to prevent or resolve quality problems (including the cost of inspection).

Total productive maintenance: A comprehensive program to maximize equipment availability in which equipment operators are trained to regularly perform routine maintenance tasks, whereas technicians and engineers handle more specialized maintenance tasks. The scope of total productive maintenance programs includes maintenance prevention (through design or selection of easy-to-service equipment), equipment improvements, preventive maintenance, and predictive maintenance (determining when to replace components before they fail).

Total quality management: A multifaceted, company-wide approach to improving all aspects of quality and customer satisfaction, including fast response and service as well as product quality. Total quality management begins with top management and ensures that all employees and managers share responsibility and accountability for managing quality.

Total quality control: Organized kaizen activities involving everyone in the company—managers and workers—in a totally integrated effort toward improving performance at every level. This improved performance is directed toward satisfying such cross-functional goals as quality, cost, scheduling, manpower development, and new product development. It is assumed that these activities ultimately lead to increased customer satisfaction.

Value: The highest quality for the lowest price. Products or services that meet a customers' needs for affordability, availability, and utility.

Value stream: The specific activities required to design, order, and provide a specific product or service from concept to final product or service.

Value stream mapping: Identification of all the specific activities occurring along a value stream for a product or service.

Visual control: The placement in plain view of all tools, parts, production activities, and indicators of production system performance so everyone involved can understand the status of the system at a glance. The use of signals, charts, measurements, diagrams, lights, and signs to clearly define the normal process flow.

Visual workplace: A work area that uses visual controls to indicate the structure and function of all processes, to the point that other instruction sets are unneeded. Characteristics of a visual workplace are as follows:

- Physical impediments to effective processing are removed; processes are tightly linked and logically ordered
- Tools and fixtures have homes: no searching for lost items
- Information and process elements travel together throughout the process flow
- Standards are clear and self-explanatory

Waste: Needless activities that do not add value to a product or service.

Work-in-process inventory: The amount or value of all materials, components, and resources representing partially completed products or services; anything on the production sequence that has not been completed.

World class manufacturing: Philosophy of being the best, the fastest, and the lowest cost producer of a product or service. It implies the constant improvement of products, processes, and services to remain an industry leader and provide the best choice for customers, regardless of where they are in the process.

Yamazumi: Meaning literally "to pile in heaps," a yamazumi board is a tool to achieve line balance, with strips of paper or cards representing particular tasks. For example, a list of patients in the emergency department kept on a white board for all to see is one type of yamazumi board.

Yield improvement: Percentage reduction in scrap or rejects. For example, if yield of a process, like x-ray film wastage improves from 95% to 98%, then the number of rejects has been reduced by 60% (from 5% waste to 2% waste), which is a yield improvement of 60%.

Six Sigma: Principles and Applications in Health Care

■ Six Sigma: Tool for Process Effectiveness

The lean process management system provides quality improvement professionals with the ability to remove non–value added work and improve process efficiency. Efficiency connotes economy of effort and expense, and the lean approach is designed to eliminate costs related to waste. Effectiveness, on the other hand, is often construed to mean doing things right (i.e., avoiding errors and eliminating mistakes). One of the goals of the healthcare industry is to eradicate errors—not just avoid errors but completely eliminate them. Society has begun to demand more from healthcare providers. No longer will 98,000 deaths from medical errors be tolerated. When the Institute of Medicine published this estimate in the seminal book, *To Err is Human* in 2000,[1] physicians and consumers were appalled, angered, and skeptical. Subsequent studies have tended to support those numbers or even suggest higher levels of patient harm[2] from medical errors.

Starting in the early part of the new century, quality improvement professionals began to delve into a new approach that had been pioneered in the manufacturing sector: six sigma. In later sections we gain a greater understanding of why this approach has great promise in promoting more effective health care, with reduced error rates and potential for making the quantum gains in patient safety that payers and society demand.

■ History of Six Sigma

When Walter Shewhart demonstrated in the 1920s that a deviation of three sigma from the mean indicated that a process required correction, many other measurement standards began to develop that culminated in the term "six sigma" being defined by Bill Smith, an engineer at Motorola, and implemented at the company in the late 1980s. In the early and mid-1980s, with impetus from CEO Bob Galvin,

Motorola engineers decided that Shewhart quality levels (i.e., three sigma levels that set defects at three per thousand) were insufficient to ensure a level of quality that was sustainable in an increasingly competitive international marketplace. Working at increasingly stringent levels, Motorola created the cultural changes and methods to achieve a new process capability standard of 3.4 defects per million—a rate that conformed to six sigma limits. This new approach helped Motorola realize robust bottom-line cost savings of more than $16 billion and successfully compete for one of the first Malcolm Baldrige National Quality Awards in 1988. Several innovators began to disseminate the techniques and culture that made six sigma successful at Motorola.

One of these visionaries, Mikel Harry, worked with Bill Smith at Motorola to create a four-stage problem-solving approach, measure, analyze, improve, control, or MAIC. This framework produced the early successes in Motorola's six sigma program that propelled quality to extraordinary levels. The company quickly broadened the approach throughout all its operations, improving quality enterprise-wide. As the six sigma paradigm spread to other companies, the concept of levels of "six sigma practitioners" evolved into a martial arts format with Six Sigma Green Belt training directed at front-line project management and Six Sigma Black Belt experts acting in supervisory positions with specific expertise in project management and statistical analysis. By 1989 Mikel Harry was leading Motorola's Six Sigma Research Institute and began to develop a program to achieve short-cycle quality knowledge transfer and rapid dissemination of quality knowledge throughout the enterprise. The resulting implementation strategy put quality tools into the hands of large numbers of workers and managers, placing ownership of those tools in the hands of everyone in the organization, not just quality engineers. This effort enhanced the quality revolution by including a wider work force to effect the changes necessary to adopting a six sigma improvement culture. As six sigma spread throughout the U.S. industry in the 1990s, the results from effective deployment caught the attention of the healthcare sector, and pioneers like Chip Caldwell (see www.chipcaldwellassoc.com) found ways of applying the methods and principles of six sigma to healthcare organization. In the past several years the use of this advanced approach has become an important tool in the quality professional's armamentarium.

Six sigma has evolved over its relatively short history. Even though it started as a quality improvement strategy, it has evolved into a business paradigm that involves setting company vision, an operational philosophy, and a measurable goal as well as an improvement methodology. Companies that have adopted the six sigma strategic approach have transformed their corporate cultures to ensure complete deployment of the program throughout the organization. Without the cultural conversion, six sigma may not be successful and may be relegated to "just another improvement project."

■ Basics of Six Sigma: Statistical Background

Sigma (the lowercase Greek letter σ) is used to represent the standard deviation, the most commonly used measure of variation of a population. The notion of a "six sigma process" connotes six standard deviations between the process mean and the nearest specification limit, leaving a very small probability that any member of the population will fail to meet specifications. FIGURE 7.1 shows a graph of the normal distribution with the relative percentages for each standard deviation in each of the divisions. For example, the mean plus one standard deviation includes about 34% of the entire population, and so about 68% of the population falls within ±1 standard deviation of the mean. As the number of standard deviations from the mean increases, the incremental percentage of the population falls off quickly, with the percentage between 5 and 6 standard deviations representing 0.00000557% of the population. If these percentages are summed, then the cumulative percentage of the population between ±6 standard deviations is 99.9999997%. In other words, the percentage of the population *outside* these six standard deviation limits is very, very small (0.0000003%, or about 3 in a million). In six sigma jargon the standard deviation is called "sigma," and so six sigma limits set a very high standard for defects. One commonly used term in six sigma is **defects per million opportunities (DPMO)**, and so six sigma limits are often termed 3 DPMO. The underlying objective of reaching six sigma goals is to ensure that the output of a process remains within specification limits that reach six

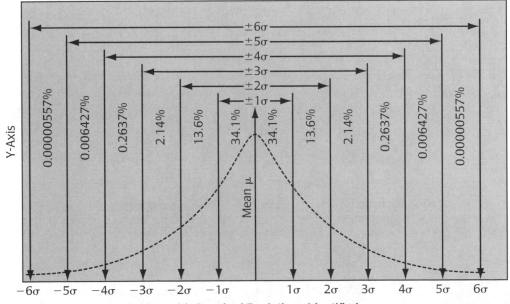

FIGURE 7.1 Normal Distribution with Standard Deviations Identified

sigma levels, that is, that nonconformities in the process output are fewer than 3 DPMO, as in FIGURE 7.2. FIGURE 7.2 represents the target of six sigma interventions, which is the centered (symmetrical) process output with upper and lower specification limits at six sigma limits.

Process capability is measured by evaluating the output of a process and comparing it to six sigma limits. In a capability study the number of standard deviations between the process mean and the nearest specification limit is calculated in terms of sigma units. If the process has a high level of variation (i.e., standard deviation is high) or if the mean value of process output varies significantly from the center of the distribution of the measurements (see FIGURE 7.3), then there are fewer standard deviations between the mean and the nearest specification limit, which decreases the sigma value and increases the likelihood of process outputs outside specification. FIGURE 7.3 demonstrates the two major problems with process output: a process mean that is not centered within specification limits and a process variation that is excessive. Either of these conditions leads to a reduced process capability as measured by the commonly used *Cpk* value.

Although there are many measures of process capability, the process capability index, *Cpk*, measures how close a process is meeting its specification limits, standardized by the process standard deviation to account for the natural variability of the process. If the *Cpk* is close to 2, then the probability is high that the process is perform-

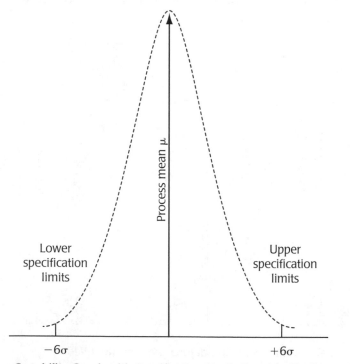

FIGURE 7.2 Process Capability Graph with Specification Limits Equal to Six Sigma Limits

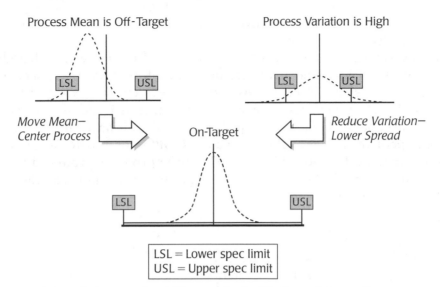

FIGURE 7.3 Variations in Process Capability and Goal of Six Sigma Interventions

ing well. The process capability is calculated to determine the index, and the calculation is performed as follows:

1. Calculate the process capability for the lower specification limit:

$$Cpl = \frac{\mu - LSL}{3\sigma}$$

   where Cpl is the process capability for the lower specification limit (LSL), μ is the process mean, and σ is the process standard deviation.
2. Calculate the process capability for the upper specification limit:

$$Cpu = \frac{USL - \mu}{3\sigma}$$

   where Cpu is the process capability for the upper specification limit (USL), μ is the process mean, and σ is the process standard deviation.
3. The Cpk is the *lower* of the two values = Min(Cpu, Cpl).

The Cpk provides a quick reference to the ability of the process to meet the specifications set by management or the customer, even if the process mean is not centered. A process that has a centered mean indicates that the mean and the median are the same and the mean lies equidistant between the upper and lower specification limits. Because the Cpk uses the smaller of the upper and lower process capabilities, it does not matter if the process mean is centered, but the further the mean performance is from the center, the less likely it is that the Cpk will be very high. Values of Cpk generally range from zero to about 2, with levels less than 1 being a red flag for needed improvements and values near or above 2 being most desirable. We see how this statistic relates to "sigma levels" shortly.

Sigma levels measure how much a process varies from perfection, based on the number of DPMO. The number of defects, or "nonconformities," that a specific sigma level represents is listed in TABLE 7.1. As should be evident the six sigma level, with DPMO of only 3.4, is most desirable, and performance at 1 or 2 sigma levels is not likely to be sustainable. In fact, some quality professionals have labeled 2σ levels as being uncompetitive, and **costs of poor quality (COPQ)** for 3 to 4σ range from 15% to 40%, or, stated differently, 15% to 40% of the products produced by 3 to 4σ processes consist of avoidable nonconformities. COPQ is the sum of all the costs that result from poor quality, including:

- Inspection
- Prevention steps in processes
- Internal failures (scrap, waste, rework)
- External failures (returns, rejects, repairs, replacement, reshipment)

When calculating these costs, all overhead charges must be included (e.g., rent, utilities, amortization for affected equipment) to ensure that the actual cost of poor quality is accurate.

Six sigma organizations use the sigma designation to compare processes throughout the enterprise. Determining sigma levels of processes (one sigma, six sigma, etc.) allows process performance to be compared throughout an entire organization using the same metric, independently of the process being measured. Additionally, sigma levels may be used to compare similar processes across different organizations or departments. The sigma level is simply a determination of opportunities for improvement regardless of the type of process that is being reviewed. Because sigma represents the standard deviation, it provides a measure of variation in the process that leads to nonconforming output. One of the easiest ways to approximate the sigma level is to use the Cpk:

$$\sigma = 3 * Cpk$$

Because Cpk can be readily calculated from process output measures, the sigma level can be quickly inferred from that value.

Table 7.1	Sigma Levels Related to DPMO and Process Efficiency	
Sigma Level	DPMO	Efficiency
1	690,000	31%
2	308,000	69.2%
3	66,800	93.32%
4	6,210	99.379%
5	230	99.977%
6	3.4	99.9997%

Specification limits are often designated as **critical to quality (CTQ)**, defined either by the customer or perhaps a regulatory or accreditation agency in health care. CTQs are the key measurable characteristics of a product or process with performance standards or specification limits that must be met to satisfy the customer. They align improvement or design efforts with customer requirements. A CTQ often must be interpreted from a qualitative customer statement to an actionable, quantitative, business specification.

Calculating sigma levels is straightforward with just a modicum of data, and the ability to calibrate processes throughout the organization using sigma levels can help managers set priorities by choosing the lowest performing (smallest σ) processes and setting targets in terms of improvements in the sigma value.

Six sigma relies on a few important assumptions:

1. The two most important causes of increased cost and lowered quality in a process, the process mean and standard deviation, are measurable and capable of being changed.

Example 7.1 Calculating Cpk and Sigma Level

Phil Medicament is the chief pharmacist at St. Perfection Hospital, and since the administration adopted the new six sigma program Phil has been given the assignment to get prescription fill errors within six sigma limits, making the CTQ value of prescription fill errors equal to 3.4 DPMO. Senior management has asked Phil to calculate the current sigma level of his prescription fill process using the statistics for the pharmacy for a typical month as follows:

- Number of prescriptions filled on the inpatient service = 50,000
- Average number of errors on fills = 65
- Upper range of errors = 125 (most errors in a month over past 24 months)
- Lower range of errors = 45 (fewest errors in a month over the past 24 months)
- Standard deviation = 22

Step 1: Calculate DPMO of the average, high, and low:

$$\text{DPMO average} = (65/50{,}000) \times 1{,}000{,}000 = 1{,}300 \text{ DPMO}$$
$$\text{DPMO high} = (125/50{,}000) \times 1{,}000{,}000 = 2{,}500 \text{ DPMO}$$
$$\text{DPMO low} = (45/50{,}000) \times 1{,}000{,}000 = 900 \text{ DPMO}$$

Step 2: Calculate upper specification limits based on total number of fills

$$3.4 \text{ DPMO} \times 50{,}000 = 0.17 \text{ errors for } 50{,}000 \text{ fills}$$

Step 3: Calculate current Cpk (use only the Cpu, because the lower specification limit lower than six sigma variation is not of concern)

$$Cpk = Cpu = |(0.17 - 65)/(3 \times 22)| = 0.98 \cong 1$$

Step 4: Calculate the current sigma level:

$$\sigma = 3 \times Cpk = 3$$

Thus the pharmacy is operating at about a 3σ level and has a lot of work to do to achieve 6σ levels of performance.

2. Senior management supports the efforts of the six sigma team(s) through appropriate deployment of resources.
3. Defects in a process are randomly distributed and approximate a normal distribution; although six sigma can be applied to other distributions, most six sigma efforts are directed at processes that have normally distributed data.
4. Process means drift over time, leading to a shift in the standard deviation, called the 1.5 sigma shift.

Over the long term processes usually do not perform as reliably as in the short term. As a result the process mean migrates toward the nearest specification limit, decreasing the *Cpk* and reducing process sigma. This change can result from a number of process features (e.g., deterioration in a measurement tool or fatigue of a critical process element). To account for this real-life increase in process variation over time, an empirically based 1.5 sigma shift was introduced into the six sigma calculation. Thus a process that presently has a *Cpk* of 2 (6σ) will likely drift toward 4.5σ, either because the process mean will move over time or because the long-term standard deviation of the process will be greater than that observed in the short term, or even more likely, both. Motorola has determined, through years of process and data collection, that processes vary and drift over time—what they call the long-term dynamic mean variation. This variation typically falls between 1.4 and 1.6. After a process has been improved using the six sigma approach, short-term process and standard deviation are used to calculate the process sigma value. Because these values are calculated over a short period of time, they are considered to include common cause variation only. However, because processes operate over a longer term and most likely will demonstrate special cause variation at various points in the future, the process capability will reduce and lead to the 1.5σ shift. In some cases long-term data collection may indicate that the shift may not be exactly 1.5σ; in that case statistical calculations can be made to compensate in the appropriate direction. However, for most cases the 1.5σ shift suffices, and the 6σ adjustment of defects to 3.4 DPMO provides the appropriate adjustment. Mikel Harry and Richard Schroeder[3] wrote the following:

> *By offsetting normal distribution by a 1.5 standard deviation on either side, the adjustment takes into account what happens to every process over many cycles of manufacturing.... Simply put, accommodating shift and drift is our "fudge factor," or a way to allow for unexpected errors or movement over time. Using 1.5 sigma as a standard deviation gives us a strong advantage in improving quality not only in industrial process and designs, but in commercial processes as well. It allows us to design products and services that are relatively impervious, or "robust," to natural, unavoidable sources of variation in processes, components, and materials.*

Measurement of process capability requires data collection, and in many cases measurement of the entire population can be incorporated into the project design.

However, in some cases the population is so big that samples must be selected because the resources needed to measure the entire population may be too costly. Sample selection is an important part of six sigma project design, because samples that are too large may waste resources, whereas samples that are too small may not yield results that are statistically significant. The following steps help determine the appropriate sample size for estimating the population mean, μ, from sample means, $\bar{x}$:

1. The difference between the sample and population means can be thought of as an error. The error, E, is the maximum difference between the observed sample mean and the true value of the population mean:

$$E = z_{\alpha/2} \bullet \frac{\sigma}{\sqrt{n}}$$

   where $z_{\alpha/2}$ is known as the critical value, the positive z value that is at the vertical boundary for the area of $\alpha/2$ in the right tail of the standard normal distribution (see FIGURE 7.4), where α is the probability of committing a type I error (i.e., rejecting a null hypothesis that is true or a false positive), σ is the population standard deviation, and n is the sample size.
2. Solving the formula for n, the equation becomes:

$$n = \left[\frac{z_{\alpha/2}\sigma}{E} \right]^2$$

Thus the sample size n can be calculated at a specific confidence level of $1-\alpha$ and margin of error. However, the formula requires that the population standard deviation also be known, which is not always the case. However, if the sample size n is over 30, then the sample standard deviation, s, can be used as an estimate for the population standard deviation, σ.

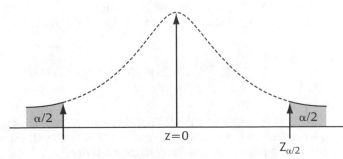

FIGURE 7.4 Error Level Determinations Using α

3. If the sample size is less than 30, then the equation is changed to use the Student's *t*-test, as follows:

$$n = \left[\frac{t_{\alpha/2} S^2}{E} \right]$$

where *n* is the estimated sample size; *t* is the positive *t*-value from the Student's *t*-table corresponding to the selected α level; $t_{\alpha/2}$ is the critical value, the *t*-value for α/2 the area under the right tail of the *t*-distribution; *s* is the sample standard deviation, and *E* is the margin of error between $\bar{x}$ and μ.

Using these approaches the two primary process parameters, the mean and standard deviation, can be collected to test the validity of the sample size and validate the sampling approach. All these methods rely on randomization of sample selection as well as a random distribution of the error in the estimate of the parameter, *E*.

Sampling may need to be modified by some practical considerations, such as how to logically divide a large population into manageable partitions that expedite analysis

---

Example 7.2 Calculating Sample Size

Problem:

Tom Sampler is evaluating the time for processing laboratory specimens and needs to estimate the average time for lab specimen handling using a 1-month time period to determine what level of performance his lab currently exhibits, as well as a sample for retesting after interventions. Because the lab performs over 50,000 tests each month, the timing measurement cannot be performed on all specimens, and so Tom needs to determine the number of tests to monitor. His goal is to have a sample large enough to be 95% sure that the sample mean is within 1 minute of the population mean μ. His prior testing has shown σ = 6.95 minutes.

Solution:

A 95% degree confidence corresponds to α = 0.05. Each of the tails in the normal distribution has an area of α/2 = 0.025. The region between the centerline (*z* = 0) and $z_{\alpha/2}$ is equal to 0.5 − 0.025, or 0.475. In the table of the standard normal (*z*) distribution, an area of 0.475 corresponds to a *z* value of 1.96. The critical value is therefore $z_{\alpha/2}$ = 1.96. Using the margin of error *E* = 1 and the standard deviation σ = 6.95, the formula for *n* then becomes

$$n = \left[\frac{z_{\alpha/2}\, \sigma}{E} \right]^2 = \left[\frac{1.96 \bullet 6.95}{1} \right]^2 = \left[13.62 \right]^2 = 185.55 = 186$$

Thus Tom will need to sample at least 186 (rounded up) randomly selected tests throughout the month to estimate the population mean at a 95% confidence level that the sample mean will be within 1 minute of the true population mean for lab test handling.

---

and improve interpretation. For example, the Medicare population of a state may be segmented by age, clinical condition, gender, or some other characteristic of interest. Creation of rational subgroups helps achieve the goal of an effective analysis. A rational subgroup can be thought of as a sample in which all sample elements are produced under conditions in which variation can be attributable only to random effects. Rational subgroups have three important characteristics:

1. Subgroup observations are independent (i.e., two observations do not influence or in any other way relate to the other). Observations that depend on each other indicate that the process has *autocorrelation*. Examples of processes that are autocorrelated include the following:
    ○ Blood samples that are taken at the same time and location (e.g., when blood cultures are drawn). Thus to avoid autocorrelation and ensure that a pathogen may be detected in a bacteremic patient, blood samples are taken from different sites and times.
    ○ Sampling waiting time in a clinic on the same day and within the same time frame. Such factors as clinic volume, staffing, and case mix may cause autocorrelation of time samples taken on the same day, whereas sampling groups on different days and times reduce the likelihood of related observations.
2. Rational subgrouping helps avoid autocorrelation by choosing samples that reduce interdependence between observations.
3. Samples are taken from a single, stable process.
4. Subgroups are collected at regular time intervals.

Rational subgroups form the basis of many types of control charts and can be important for an effective six sigma analysis. The best approach to sampling, particularly when grouping sample observations, is to ensure independence by randomizing the sampling process.

■ Six Sigma Metrics

Just as lean process management focuses on metrics like throughput and takt time, six sigma metrics reflect the drive for improved precision in process performance. Two common measurements have already been mentioned, but the list also includes the following:

- *DPMO:* The DPMO is the total number of defects divided by the total number of opportunities for a defect, multiplied by 1,000,000. Defects are critical characteristics of a sampled entity that fail to meet customer expectations. Opportunities are critical characteristics of a sample that could be defective or nondefective (i.e., meet expectations). In many health service processes there are usually multiple opportunities for not meeting customer expectations, such as staff attitude, service, safety, comfort, pain, and so on. An important differentiating factor in a six sigma environment is the need to define defects and opportunities from the customer's perspective (i.e., a defect is a failure to meet customer expectations). Defects must also be independent of each other and in general are likely to increase in number as a process becomes increasingly complex.

- *Sigma level:* Sigma is a statistical term that quantifies how much a process varies from a high performance target, based on the number of DPMO. Sigma levels are used to compare various, heterogeneous processes with each other to determine levels of performance. Organizations that apply this approach can use sigma levels of processes to prioritize opportunities for improvement, with lower sigma levels connoting worse performance and greater opportunities for improvement.
- *Defects per unit:* Average number of nonconformities per unit of output; for example, defects per unit for a radiology department may be the number of retakes required per image. For example, if 100 images are requested in a 24-hour period but 105 takes are required to complete the 100 images, then the defects per unit rate is 0.05, or five defects per 100 requests.
- *First-pass yield:* The proportion of units that, on average, go through a process the first time without defects. The first-pass yield is calculated as follows:

$$FPY = e^{-DPU}$$

The first-pass yield indicates the ability of the process to produce conforming output that satisfied customer requirements, while at the same time providing insight into the level of rework inherent in the process.

- *Rolled throughput yield:* The probability that a unit can pass through a process without defects. It is the product of the first-pass yields at each step:

$$RTY = \prod_1^n FPY$$

Thus the rolled throughput yield provides the overall probability of a product making it through an entire production process without any defects.

■ Six Sigma Improvement Model (SSIM)

When six sigma was first developed, the improvement model was MAIC, fashioned after the plan-do-study-act cycle of Shewhart and Deming. After a few years another step was added—define—to create the **DMAIC** approach that is the foundation of six sigma today. This approach consists of the following stages:

- *Define* = creation of high-level project goals and mapping the current process
- *Measure* = determine key aspects of the current process and collect relevant data

Example 7.3 Defect and Yield Calculations

Mary Cashflow is the CFO of a thriving medical center, but recently she has noticed that financial margins have been shrinking. Fee rate schedules have not changed, but she noticed that the number of unpaid claims was rising. The process of creating a claim involves:

1. Coder abstracts information from the clinical chart
2. Coder enters the associated codes into the computerized billing system
3. Clerical staff ensures that the patient's payer information is correct
4. Clerical staff selects an option to either print the claim or submit it electronically

The medical center generates an average of 1,000 electronic claims per week, of which half are printed and half are submitted electronically. Mary collected data for a month and had the following results:

Total invoices:	4,000	Total defects:	250	Total paper rejects:	65
Total scrap (paper):	85	Total electronic rejects:	100		

Further study of the process discovered that the first-pass yield (FPY) for each step was as follows:

$FPY_1 = 0.928$	$FPY_2 = 0.904$	$FPY_3 = 0.912$	$FPY_4 = 0.931$

Thus of the 250 total defects (i.e., claims scrapped for being unreadable or rejected for any number of reasons), 150 were in the paper batches and 100 were in the electronic batch. Yield calculations are as follows:

$DPU = 250$ defects per $4,000$ units $= 0.0625$ DPU

$FPY = e^{-0.0625} - 0.939$

$RTY = FPY_1 \times FPY_2 \times FPY_3 \times FPY_4 = 0.928 \times 0.904 \times 0.912 \times 0.931 = 0.717$

The rolled throughput yield (RTY) indicates only a 0.717 probability of producing a "clean claim."

- *Analyze* = evaluate the data to identify cause-and-effect relationships or specific correlations to determine existing relationship and to ensure that all pertinent factors have been considered
- *Improve* = optimize the process based on data analysis using a number of approaches like design of experiments (DOE) and pilot testing
- *Control* = institutionalize improvements to sustain gains made from the intervention and put controls into place to ensure that improvements are permanently incorporated into the process

DMAIC is the approach used for existing processes, but six sigma can be used proactively to ensure that a process is created for high performance. Design for six sigma (DFSS) uses a slightly different mnemonic, **DMADV** (define, measure, analyze, design, verify), to guide process developers. The steps in DMADV involve the following:

- *Define* = identify goals that are consistent with customer demands and organizational strategy

- *Measure* = determine characteristics that are CTQ, service or product capabilities, process capability, and risks
- *Analyze* = using the information developed in the "measure" phase, designers create a prospective design and use tools like failure mode and effects criticality analysis (see Chapter 3) to evaluate design capability and refine the new process
- *Design* = optimize the plan and develop methods of verifying and evaluating the design using techniques such as simulations and computer-assisted design
- *Verify* = validate the design through pilot testing and implement the process

The SSIM introduced an innovative approach to human resources dedicated to improvement. Rather than splintering the improvement staff into a variety of departments (e.g., statisticians in one department and project managers in another), the SSIM combined skills required for improvement into a staffing structure that promoted teamwork and appropriate skill sets to take a performance improvement initiative through the entire DMAIC or DMADV cycle. Using a martial arts framework, the SSIM defines several key roles that not only create a hierarchy of skills but also a career path for improvement professionals:

- *Six sigma champions:* executives in the top levels of management who understand the value and potential of the SSIM, who set the vision for the company's performance at six sigma levels, and who ensure that resources are available for six sigma initiatives. Champions often act as mentors to the other six sigma improvement professionals.
- *Master black belts:* experienced six sigma professionals with black belt experience and often appointed by champions to act as in-house coaches for six sigma teams. In the ideal organizational setting these experts devote all their time to six sigma activities, assisting champions, black belts, and green belts with more sophisticated statistical analyses and serving as consultants to six sigma teams across the enterprise.
- *Six sigma black belts:* operate independently or report to master black belts to manage multiple six sigma projects. Six sigma black belts devote 100% of their time to six sigma initiatives, focusing on project execution and optimizing team performance. Additionally, six sigma black belts are trained in advanced statistical techniques that are the key to six sigma analytics.
- *Six sigma green belts:* these specially trained six sigma professionals often are the backbone of a six sigma improvement program, serving the role of project management for these initiatives. Working with six sigma black belts, these staff members bring project organizational and functional skills to the team and help other team members understand and apply the advanced methods that are inherent in the SSIM. Six sigma green belts may not have the statistical depth of black belts, but they often have a broad understanding of the analytic underpinnings of the model.

- *Six sigma yellow belts:* although not an official six sigma designation, many companies provide basic training in performance improvement with emphasis on six sigma approaches and designate these trainees as "yellow belts." Six sigma yellow belts serve as team members and assist six sigma green belts in accomplishing the team's goals.

Teamwork is a key feature of any six sigma project, and all team members are steeped in the team approach described in Chapter 2.

■ Voices of Six Sigma

One of the essential tenets of six sigma is satisfying customer expectations. As part of the SSIM, customer preferences are collected and quantified to the greatest extent possible. This effort and measurement set are termed the **voice of the customer (VOC).** VOC permeates the DMAIC process, starting with define, where customer requirements determine the most important process metrics, which become CTQ features. Not only do the CTQ features drive the creation of process metrics, but failure to achieve those metrics can support the determination of the COPQ, another important six sigma concept that in most cases is one of the major sources of return in a six sigma project, as shown in FIGURE 7.5.

Other voices of six sigma are as follows:

- *Voice of the business (VOB):* the stated and unstated needs or requirements of the business/shareholders. The VOB draws from financial information and data to identify market weakness, sources and uses investment capital, research and development efficacy, and process effectiveness. Tempered with organizational strategy

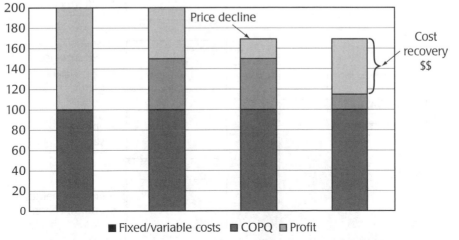

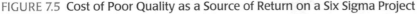

FIGURE 7.5 Cost of Poor Quality as a Source of Return on a Six Sigma Project

and direction, the VOB can be used to prioritize potential projects to aid in moving the organization closer to its goals and objectives. By identifying value levers (strategic, process, customer and financial) and prioritizing them, quality professionals can translate the VOB into opportunities for improvement, project resource needs for improvements, and apply valuation criteria that lead to project prioritization. Thus the VOB provides clarity in terms of identifying revenue growth areas, economic value added, and market value.

- *Voice of the employee:* stated and unstated needs or requirements of the employees of a business. Employees are key stakeholders in a company, and they are an important source of information on future, current, and past improvement efforts. The most effective method of hearing the voice of the employee is through employee surveys.

- *Voice of the process:* data from the process that is used to shape improvements and modifications. Voice of the process includes the average, lowest, and optimum output; capability; and status of in-control or out-of-control. Voice of the process is most often measured on a control chart (see Chapter 4), which calculates normal variation ranges mean performance, and uncovers common cause and special cause performance.

These four voices must be balanced during the design phase, as well as throughout the DMAIC cycle, when determining the parameters of a particular project, and the project management framework in Chapter 2 develops this thesis to address these issues. FIGURE 7.6 demonstrates that all four voices are important in achieving six sigma performance levels.

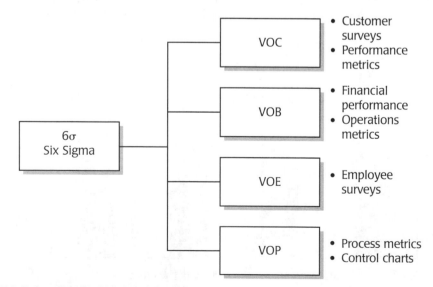

FIGURE 7.6 Balancing the Voices of Six Sigma

■ Gauge Repeatability and Reproducibility

An important aspect of six sigma is the recognition of the effects of measurement error on performance metrics. With a target of 3.4 DPMO, small measurement errors can be significant in the final assessment of performance. The approach developed by six sigma quality professionals is to include the evaluation of measurement error in the statistical analysis. Applying analysis of variance (ANOVA, see Chapter 5), the evaluation of measurement variation is termed **gauge repeatability and reproducibility (gauge R&R)**, and the approach assesses the amount of variability measurements due to the measurement system and compares this variation to the total observed variability to determine the extend to error included in the measurements. Several components affect a measurement system's variability:

- *Measuring instruments:* the gauge or instrument used to make and record measurements, including all associated mounting blocks, supports, fixtures, or any other attachment that may influence the performance of the instrument. Some sources of variation in measuring instruments include ease of use, frequency of calibration, measurement drift, and need for other measurement elements, like reagents.
- *Operators (people):* the ability and/or discipline of the measurement system operator to follow instructions on proper use of the measurement tool.
- *Test methods:* device setup, part repair and replacement, data recording techniques, or use of complementary tools.
- *Specification:* comparison of the measurement with a specification or reference value, and the range of the specification can be an important factor affecting the variation in measures using the measurement system.
- *Measurement parameter:* some items are easier to measure than others, and the measurement system will introduce errors as different samples are measured.

The two central attributes of a gauge R&R include:

- *Repeatability:* the variation in measurements taken by a single person or instrument on the same item and under the same conditions
- *Reproducibility:* the variability induced by different operators (i.e., the variation induced when different operators measure the same item)

Two important concepts in gauge R&R are accuracy and precision, illustrated in FIGURE 7.7a and b. Accuracy implies proximity to the true value, whereas precision entails the repeatability or reproducibility of the measurement. Thus a process result may be highly accurate, such as the measure in FIGURE 7.7a, but precision is lacking because measurements are scattered. On the other hand, a process result may be very precise, as in FIGURE 7.7b, but the measure may significantly miss the correct value. The gauge R&R helps measure each of these parameters and helps in the interpretation of data.

The gauge R&R is performed by measuring items using the proposed measurement system with a goal of identifying as many sources of measurement variation as

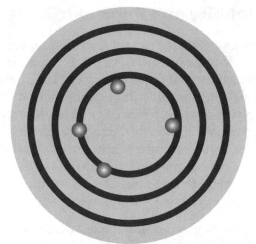

FIGURE 7.7a High Accuracy, Low Precision

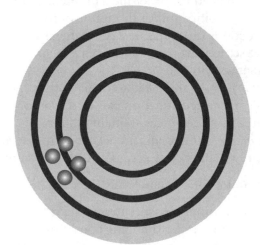

FIGURE 7.7b High Precision, Low Accuracy

possible, because a small variation detected in a gauge R&R may be a sign that an important source of error was missed during the intervention. Precision is measured by interrater reliability studies, and the American Society for Testing and Materials[4] established standards that call for at least 10 operators (or laboratories), but many situations have a practical limitation of only two or three operators performing the same measurements. To capture repeatability errors, the same item is usually measured several times per operator. In some cases one item may be more difficult to measure than another (e.g., interviews with customers regarding some issue with performance), and so 5 or 10 samples may be needed to capture interactions between operators and measured items. Although universal criteria for these reliability measurements have not been established, often a $10 \times 3 \times 3$ (10 items, 3 operators, 3 repetitions) matrix is acceptable. Frequently, cost and time attributes are important in determining these parameters, but sampling methods are important in making a final determination. However, a practical approach to gauge R&R measurement is to take one-third of the sample from the upper specification limit, midpoint (mean or median), and lower specification limit, respectively, and then having three operators make three measurements on each sample.

Although gauge R&R is very helpful to determine the accuracy and precision of a measurement process, if any of the parameters (sample size, operator, or measurement tool) changes significantly, then the gauge R&R must be repeated. Additionally, any measurement system may deteriorate over time, and so if measurement drift is suspected as a reason for process variation, then the gauge R&R procedure must be repeated. A number of software packages, such as Prolink (www.prolinksoftware.com), QI Macros (www.qimacros.com), and Symphony Freeware (www.symphonytech.com), are available to help with the calculations necessary for calculating gauge R&R.

■ DMAIC: The Six Sigma Improvement Model

Define Phase

Achieving quantum level improvements requires discipline, and DMAIC enforces the rigor required to optimize achievement within the six sigma paradigm. The DMAIC cycle ensures that data-driven meticulousness permeates every step in the SSIM. The six sigma equation resembles a multivariate equation:

$$Y = aX_1 + bX_2 + cX_3 + \dots nX_n$$

where Y is the key customer characteristic for improvement, X_n are the process elements that can be modified through improvement initiatives, and $a, b, c, \dots n$ are the multipliers for the X_n, which determines the magnitude of the effect on the customer characteristic of interest; also known as the beta, or slope coefficient in a multiple regression equation (see Chapter 5).

The statistical nature of six sigma is emphasized through DMAIC by concentrating efforts at each step on the key elements of the six sigma equation. For example, during the define phase, the key customer characteristic (Y) becomes the focus of the improvement initiative throughout the remainder of the cycle, and during the measure and analyze phases critical x measures are identified that become the targets of the improve and control phases. FIGURE 7.8 illustrates this point by detailing how the Y and critical x values are involved at each point in the DMAIC process.

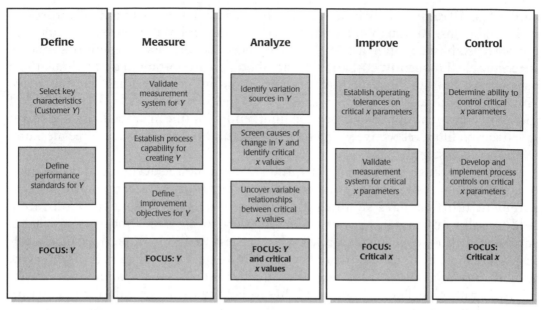

FIGURE 7.8 DMAIC and Critical X

Determination of crucial *x*'s in six sigma requires more than just brainstorming, which is one differentiating factor between six sigma and other improvement paradigms. A number of methods are used to identify critical *x* factors:

- Customer surveys
- Customer focus groups
- Individual customer interviews
- Customer complaints
- Employee feedback
- Blogs and consumer websites

Effective determination of the customer value proposition and the starting list of critical *x*'s for the six sigma project will consider all these sources and others as they become available. Customer surveys are often performed by professional companies like Press Ganey (www.pressganey.com), the Gallup Organization (www.gallup.com), NRC Picker (www.nrcpicker.com), and others or may be conducted by individual organizations using instruments like one of the CAHPS surveys discussed in Chapter 4. This information provides general insight into customer dissatisfiers, but specifics often must be discerned using other methods. For example, customers may express dissatisfaction for outpatient registration services, but the specifics of the process deficiencies often require further investigation, which may be found in comments made on the surveys or through a root-cause analysis. Customer focus groups may also surface problems with specific types of services and may be used as one of the tools to clarify findings on more formal customer surveys. Individual customers may also be willing to participate in interviews to express or amplify opinions of a company's services. In some cases these interviews may be conducted informally by employees in the course of providing services, and so effective organizations develop techniques to collect customer and employee comments that can be categorized and acted upon in a systematic manner. Staff members often hear customer comments that offer a wealth of information on customer "hot buttons" or major dissatisfiers.

An evolving method of gathering critical x's is the plethora of websites and blogs that collect comments from people who are willing to enter them on a website. These sites do not usually categorize the comments but simply offer them in list format like Angie's List (www.angieslist.com), but some are more organized and provide some classification that is directed at consumers, like HealthGrades (www.healthgrades. com). As greater rigor is introduced into online systems for collecting consumer data, these sites may become substantially more valuable for organizations as a customer information resource; however, the websites can still serve as good places to find anecdotal comments that may augment a customer information collection program.

Finally, another major resource of customer information is complaints. In fact, the criteria for the Malcolm Baldrige National Quality Award (see Chapter 8) include the existence of systems to collect and evaluate customer complaints and then to incorporate the information into improvement efforts. These systems often involve databases that either receive the information by direct customer input or provide an interface for employees to enter comments and opinions into the data set. Effective systems include the ability to classify the complaints in a number of ways (e.g., by work unit, time of day, staff member(s) involved, etc.). Many healthcare organizations have leveraged these systems for targeting improvement efforts, which not only provides a more focused effort but often reduces the cost of improvements, as well.

Once the VOC factors are ascertained, the next step prioritizes the VOC x's by collecting data that quantifies the level of significance of each factor. Each of the customer requirements has characteristics that can be quantified and probably are being collected through the venues described above, and these data elements are refined by creating operational definitions to allow specificity in data collection and effective analysis of the parameters to determine the most statistically significant factors to address in the improvement phase of DMAIC. The factors identified by this analysis create the data for a Pareto analysis and prioritization of critical x's that will be the subject for improvement efforts.

Another important objective of the define phase is to understand the target process. Frequently, black belts and green belts perform a great deal of work before chartering a new project so that everyone involved is already aware of the business needs addressed by the project and the need for a six sigma approach. However, this important project review may also be incorporated into the define phase. Criteria for using DMAIC to deal with a problem are as follows:

- Data should be easily obtainable to allow appropriate analysis.
- Senior leaders support the approach and are willing to devote resources.

- The problem's solution is either complex or difficult to ascertain.
- Project scope is well defined or can be narrowed to a workable scale.
- The project is related to a key business process or strategic goal.

The key deliverable for the define phase is the project charter, presented in more detail in Chapter 2. Six sigma projects generally adhere to aggressive timelines for each phase that are clearly outlined in the charter, as are statistics relevant to the project.

A core element of the define phase project charter is a high level description of the process, and a more thorough process mapping is part of the measure and analyze phases. The project team needs to have a clear understanding of the purpose of the process and the five elements, termed **SIPOC** (for suppliers, input, process, output, and customer), in six sigma. Although everyone involved in developing the project may believe they already comprehend these elements, explicit description of SIPOC as part of the project charter ensures that all stakeholders share a common understanding.

Measure Phase

As shown in FIGURE 7.8, the measure phase continues to focus on the Y in the customer value equation, but the critical x's also become important at this stage. Three major activities occur during this phase:

1. Validation of the measurement system(s) required to produce Y
2. Evaluation of current process capability to produce Y
3. Using the current level of performance and process capability and definition of improvement objectives for Y

Any measurement system used in a six sigma project must be able to distinguish differences that adequately differentiate high performance characteristics. In other words, the measurement system must be reliable, accurate, and precise. The approaches described in the discussion of gauge R&R are important at this stage to ensure that the inherent error levels in the measurement system are accounted for as measurements are made and analyzed. Gauge R&R was originally devised for industrial applications, but similar approaches can be applied to instruments used to collect data in health care.

The measure phase is directed at getting as much information as possible about the current process to fully understand how it currently works, how it is supposed to work, and the gap in performance. Three key tasks are necessary:

1. Creation of a detailed process map
2. Collecting baseline data
3. Summarizing and analyzing the baseline data

A detailed process map is the first step so that the team can develop or refine appropriate measures to determine the process capability and sigma level. In some cases, however, measures have already been in use and only need refinement, but as a value stream map (see Chapter 6) is created, new areas for measurement are usually found requiring the creation of new metrics. The value stream map may be created using the methods described for lean process management, through direct input from the process owners and users, by inspectors or other process observers like managers, or by suppliers and vendors who work within the process. The map should reflect the current process, not the ideal path, that will be part of the improve phase.

One of the more common measures in six sigma is cycle time, especially when process performance problems are related to delays and process completion times. Process time for key steps is usually available or can be obtained within a short period of data collection. The "process walk-through" approach of lean process management helps team members capture variation in the process implementation, because work-arounds and shortcuts become apparent when team members watch the process in action. Process variation is one of the key targets of the six sigma team, whereas lean process teams usually try to find non–value added steps that may or may not be part of process variation.

Several types of flowcharts can be used at this phase, including the workflow chart and deployment chart described in Chapter 3, but PERT charts are particularly effective here, because they include information about process times and slack times. A combination of these visual tools often helps improve understanding of the process and opportunities for improvement. The project team then reviews the diagrams to garner information about process bottlenecks and inefficiencies. At this stage process variation and non–value added work can be identified and put on a list of potential process improvement targets.

Many projects sink because of the lack of a data collection plan. Although some team members may believe data collection is intuitive, without a plan errors will occur that impair the analysis and reduce the effectiveness of later interventions. As with the other steps in DMAIC, systematic planning and execution ensure a greater likelihood for success. The focus of data collection should be to find those critical data elements that help define the quality issues and uncover factors that lead to defects. The data collection plan determines what data to collect, provides operational definitions to clarify how the data are collected, and defines steps in validating the data prior to analysis. The gauge R&R analysis helps support the data validation process. One important set of data to include in the plan relates to the CTQs identified during the define phase. Thus the data collection plan must have appropriate data elements to ensure that CTQs can be addressed.

Some key characteristics of data elements that are collected during this phase are as follows:

- Group or process worker performing the task leading to the measurement
- Time period in which the data are collected (e.g., time of day, shift, day of week)
- Type of output produced (e.g., chest x-ray, abdominal x-ray, bone x-ray)

Data are typically collected over a period of time to allow trend analysis and use of control charts in the data review. Additional benefits from time series data collection include the ability to determine if any time-related factors (e.g., time of day or weekdays/weekends or in some cases seasonality) are operational in creating variation or defects. Data analysis during the measure phase involves creating comparison graphs, like histograms and bar charts, and time series diagrams, like run charts and control charts, depending on the data and the type of analysis needed. A more complete review of these methods can be found in Chapter 5. Control charts are the hallmark tools of six sigma, because they provide both visual representation of the data and statistical analysis of variation to pinpoint opportunities for improvement initiatives. For categorical data such as complaints or types of product defect, the Pareto chart can be used to visually display the distribution of data across categories and to quickly identify priorities through Pareto analysis.

The measure phase also serves as the step in which process sigma is calculated, as described earlier in this chapter. Process sigma is one measure that can be used to determine the effect of interventions, particularly to ascertain if one targeted intervention has been offset by another change in another part of the process to prevent changes in the sigma value. The percentage of process output that meets the customer specification is calculated and used to determine the process sigma. Measure phase deliverables include:

- Process map(s)
- Detailed baseline data
- Baseline process sigma
- Clear understanding of how the process is currently performed and gaps leading to defects

Analyze Phase

During the analyze phase the team directs attention to identifying potential root causes for under-performance in the process and then to collecting data to validate the underlying issues. The project charter from the measure phase contains a problem statement that articulates the issue and circumstances hypothesized to trigger the problem as well as data to verify baseline process performance and CTQs based on customer input. The analyze phase then seeks to answer the "why" of the problem (i.e., the process fallibilities that lead to the suboptimal performance). Process improvement efforts rely on this analysis, and without this phase the team will generally find it difficult to accurately portray the root causes of problems and appropriately focus on intervention strategies.

The work completed during the define and measure phases usually offers clues to causative factors that affect performance. Team members and front-line workers frequently have a perspective that helps during the analysis, but biases often enter into these views, making an objective view equally valuable. Suspicions and conjectures must be confirmed with data: Not only must the team confirm that these perspectives are correct, but the team must also demonstrate that changes in suspected factors substantively impact outcome metrics. Several techniques that have been discussed in Chapter 3 are used by six sigma project teams to identify potential root causes:

- *Brainstorming:* with team members, enlisting the help of process workers
- *The 5 why's:* repeatedly asking "why?" until it no longer makes sense to do so (The point is to get past the surface-level answers that are likely to be put forth initially and to uncover the real underlying issues.)
- *Pareto analysis:* a method of prioritization that identifies the top 20% of causes that generally cause 80% of the problems
- *Fault tree analysis:* use of Boolean logic to track a problem to its root cause
- *Ishikawa (cause and effect) diagram:* the fishbone diagram that links a series of underlying factors to a suboptimal outcome and categorizes them to improve focus on causes
- *Barrier analysis:* used to determine barriers to effective work; may consist of physical, human, and administrative factors
- *Change analysis:* comparison of an error-free instance of a process with one in which errors occurred to determine the change in the process that led to the defect(s)
- *Causal factor tree analysis:* use of a decision tree to track an error to its root cause, often used with the 5 why's

The Ishikawa diagram (see FIGURE 3.12) is one of the most commonly used methods of organizing a list of root causes, because it allows a comprehensive, categorized view of causative factors in one diagram. The causal factor tree (see FIGURE 3.16) is another frequently used depiction, because it provides a logic tree diagram leading from cause to effect, with intermediate effects, to define the root causes of a process problem. Whichever diagram is created by the team, these diagrams help the team better organize deliberations and prioritize potential causes for investigation.

Adequate data are sometimes available from the measure phase to conduct a cause and effect analysis during the analyze phase, but it is not uncommon for the team to need to collect new data as the analysis proceeds. As in the measure phase, data analysis methods depend on the type of data collected and vice versa. Thus a data collection plan may be needed for this phase as well to ensure that the information needed for decision support is gained from the data gathered and assessed. Data display techniques such as scatter plots and frequency histograms are combined with statistical techniques discussed in Chapter 5, like ANOVA, correlation analysis, and significance testing using the *t*-test or chi-square test. In six sigma, ANOVA may be used when the output measure is continuous, like time and money, and the input measures or suspected causes are categorical, or discrete, variables, whereas correlation analysis is used when both measures are continuous and chi-square when both are discrete.

The analyze phase should culminate in at least one confirmed hypothesis regarding a root cause of the poor performance that can serve as a focus of initiatives for improvement, which are developed during the improve phase.

Improve Phase

After the thorough analyses of the DMA phases, the improve phase finally focuses on efforts to improve the process through targeted interventions based on the data and analyses performed in the first three steps of DMAIC. This phase usually starts with a complete review of the process flow and analytics, followed by brainstorming potential solutions, and then selection of solutions to test. The penultimate step in this phase is to determine which solution(s) best resolves the problem(s) and drives the process to six sigma levels of performance. The final step almost invariably involves a pilot project to ensure that the solution(s) does not have unintended consequences when put into action.

Identifying Potential Solutions

Stakeholders in the process are included in identifying potential solutions, because they often bring experience from prior improvement attempts that can save time and money as new ideas are generated. These workers and customers should be involved in this phase throughout its life cycle. Participants in brainstorming sessions must be cautioned, however, to feel free to challenge rules and assumptions, because new solutions rarely emanate from old ways of working. Brainstorming and its variants are discussed in detail in Chapter 2, but one important practice at this phase is to ensure that the idea generation sessions are open and nonthreatening for all participants. Ideas must not be judged or eliminated at this stage, because even an outlandish idea may lead to a related suggestion that evolves into a viable solution. Similar to other aspects of a six sigma project, assumptions about what can or cannot be implemented should not be accepted without data.

Selecting Solutions to Implement

The stakeholder group next establishes objective criteria, such as implementation timeline, cost factors, and barriers to improvement efforts, for evaluating the proposed initiatives. These factors are important in establishing the effectiveness of the implementation effort and reporting progress to senior management. Because the criteria may vary in importance, they may be weighted according to their relative significance to the project and to the stakeholder group. These evaluation criteria may use some of the matrix tools that were outlined in Chapter 3, such as the performance-importance matrix or the decision matrix, to clarify the issues and their relative importance to the project. The goal of this step is to objectively determine the appropriate solutions rather than using assumptions or group preferences to vet the improvement program.

Implementing Improvements

Planning the implementation is largely a matter of using the basic project management principles discussed in Chapter 2, which involves determining the budget and timeline of the implementation, assignment of roles and responsibilities, and setting up task and tracking duties. Use of software tools like Microsoft Project allow the team to produce Gantt charts, calendars, and flowcharts of tasks to guide the project as it rolls out. Additionally, the deployment flowchart provides another method of ensuring that all team members have a good understanding of individual assignments in the project. The implementation team should include a green belt with oversight by a black belt to ensure that the initiative stays on course. As in the measure phase, a data collection plan should be created to direct data collection through operational definitions, checklists, and standardization of data sources. The data sources should have been determined during the define and measure phases, and this data collection plan should provide the mechanics of managing the data during implementation of the improvement.

Failure modes and effects criticality analysis (see Chapter 3) is a useful tool to deploy before developing improvement strategies to identify and address potential problems that may arise with the improved process. The weighted list of risks and issues helps identify the most crucial issues and prioritize interventions as well as alert the team to potential problems that may arise from the interventions. The awareness created by the criticality analysis can help the team anticipate problems and design tactics to ameliorate the issues before they arise. Additionally, failure mode and effects criticality analysis can help teams foresee the impact of change on the people involved in and affected by the process. These issues can sometimes create barriers to change, and addressing staff effects before initiating the project can forestall some of these problems. Good project management principles, however, should have helped avoid the situation by involving staff at all levels during the planning stages.

Every project plan must include a system for monitoring the project's progress. Establishment of milestones as part of the project timeline lets the team gauge progress toward the project goal incrementally during implementation. As obstacles arise the team can determine how the problem will affect the project and adjust the timetable accordingly. Having a monitoring system promotes accountability and helps the team stay focused on project completion. The monitoring system should include key project metrics so the team can readily assess not just the progress of the implementation but also the effect on process performance, providing the basis for any needed midcourse corrections. One final consideration is the continuing effectiveness of the measurement system. As noted in the discussion on gauge R&R, measurement systems may drift over time, and the monitoring system must take this factor into account and have a method of evaluating and correcting for changes in the data collection and analysis plan.

Evaluating Improvements

Most projects are best served using a pilot test of the improvements before proceeding to a full-scale implementation. The benefits of a pilot test include ensuring that changes have the expected result and allow the team to gain insights into implementation challenges before a broader roll-out. Pilot tests take one of two approaches: making the intended changes in only one work unit for a longer time period or making the changes for a limited time period over several work units. During the pilot test a revised process sigma can be calculated to compare with the baseline value from the design phase. Other tools used in the evaluation of the pilot test include Pareto charts and frequency histograms to compare data from before and after the intervention, and the ever reliable six sigma tool, the control chart, can be used to graphically demonstrate changes in the process mean and degree of variation. In fact, control charts can often provide a visual representation of the process change, as both the midline and control limits may change dramatically, as shown in FIGURE 7.9. The p-chart in FIGURE 7.9 demonstrates the effect of a patient fall prevention initiative that was implemented in time period 20 on the geriatric care unit. Note that the centerline has decreased, indicating a substantial change in the fall rate (number of falls per 1,000 patient days), and the control limits have also become much tighter, indicating a more consistent level of performance with less variation. In addition to control charts, statistical significance can be demonstrated using tools like ANOVA, regression testing, and significance tests such as the chi-square and t-tests.

Multiple Interventions: Using DOE

DOE is a more sophisticated approach applied to six sigma projects that allows evaluation of multiple interventions simultaneously while testing the statistical

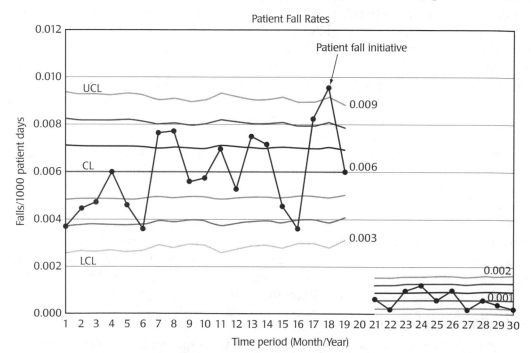

FIGURE 7.9 Control Chart Showing Pre- and Post-Intervention Values

significance of each intervention and combination of interventions. DOE was developed and first applied to experimental situations by Sir Ronald A. Fisher in the 1920s and 1930s in England. Fisher was a brilliant mathematician and geneticist who designed and supervised field trials comparing fertilizers and seed varieties, among other variables, to improve crop yields. As he performed these experiments, Fisher recognized that sources of variation external to his experimental design, such as uncontrollable variation in the soil from plot to plot and a limited number of plots available for any given trial, contributed to the variability in the results of his studies. He solved these problems by methodically arranging the two experimental elements over which he had control, the fertilizers and the seed varieties, in specific plots in the field. For example, to determine which of four varieties of wheat had the highest yield, Fisher would divide a rectangular test field into 16 plots. He then planted each of the four varieties in four separate plots, as shown in FIGURE 7.10. Each of the four varieties (A, B, C, and D) was planted just once in each row and once in each column, a design that minimized (or controlled for) the effects of soil variation in the analysis of the plot yields. As part of this concept, Fisher developed the method for analyzing designed experiments, ANOVA. In contemporary experimental designs two types of variance are recognized, termed "signals" and "noise." The signal component is measured for each controlled variation (e.g., the A, B, C, and D in FIGURE 7.10), and the noise component represents variation that is attributable to factors external to the controlled variation (e.g., soil type and pH, represented by the different matrix plots in FIGURE 7.10). The signal-to-noise ratio for a particular variation, measured by the Fisher F-test, provides the analysis of variance that helps discern which effects are from the variables of interest.

The problems Fisher encountered in conducting agricultural experiments in the 1920s prevail in a number of situations in the healthcare industry today, particularly in six sigma projects. For example, a health plan may decide to implement a variety

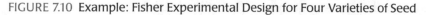

FIGURE 7.10 Example: Fisher Experimental Design for Four Varieties of Seed

of initiatives to improve member access to and use of preventive care services, such as telephone outreach calls, mailings, e-mail messages, and face-to-face home visits, but unless the plan implements the interventions sequentially one at a time in its population of members, it would be difficult to determine which has the best cost-to-benefit ratio. However, using the principles of DOE the plan can simultaneously execute the initiatives by randomizing the interventions among subgroups of the population and analyze the data to determine which individual or grouped set of interventions was most cost effective. Large experiments are usually too expensive or too time consuming, but Fisher's DOE approach can resolve these issues economically. DOE requires well-formulated data matrices, but if the experiment is well designed, then the ANOVA can deliver precise results.

Medical professionals will recognize these principles as the same used for development of medical experiments using randomized controlled trials. One major difference in the DOE approach and controlled experimental design used in randomized controlled trials is the number of variables examined and the ability to control all factors in the experimental model. Designers of medical randomized controlled trials try hard to control all outside influences by measuring these factors and including them in the model calculations, whereas the DOE approach acknowledges the existence of these outside factors and attributes their influence to the category of "noise." Because several factors vary at the same time, altering one factor usually sets off a chain reaction of modifications that may involve several factors at once, which more accurately reflects the real-world environment in which quality studies are conducted. Using statistical analyses like ANOVA and multiple regression on DOE data, the "signals" can be dissected from the "noise" to determine individual contributions of many simultaneous interventions, providing important information about the factors that are important in the improvement phase.

Because the number of combinations can become very large, most experimental designs do not exceed 8 or 16 combinations. The notation for an experimental design with two levels and three factors is 2^3, where 2 represents two levels and 3 represents three factors. Eight combinations of factors and levels is possible in this design, and the table of combinations is often created like that shown in TABLE 7.2. The three factors are represented by letters a, b, and c, and the levels for each factor are represented by +1 and −1. For example, the three factors could relate to three causes of patient satisfaction with a hospital's emergency services, like emergency department waiting time, friendliness of first provider encountered, and friendliness of physician, whereas the levels could characterize two states of the factor, for example, long waiting time versus short waiting time and friendly versus unfriendly.

TABLE 7.2 shows all potential combinations of three factors with two levels each. The design becomes much more complex as the number of factors and levels increase. Thus a 2^4 design (four factors, two levels each) requires 16 trials to evaluate all the combinations, and a 2^7 design (seven factors, two levels each) requires 128 trials to evaluate all the combinations. The number of combinations rises dramatically as the number of factors and levels increase. Not only do the trials involve the effects of the individual factors, but they also include the consequences of interactions of factors, as shown in TABLE 7.2. For instance, in the emergency department satisfaction example, if waiting times are long, then the emergency department might be very busy, leading to less friendly and more business-like providers. Thus the interaction of the factors may actually have an additive effect that must be taken into account. Experiments that run every trial combination are called **full factorial** experiments.

Statisticians have found, however, that interactions between three or more factors tend to be relatively small in their effect on an experimental outcome,[5] and so these interaction effects are often managed statistically using the **fractional factorial experimental design**. Although these techniques are beyond the scope of this text, a definitive discussion can be found in Forrest Breyfogle's book.[5] Additionally, software programs such as QI Macros (www.qimacros.com) and SAS JMP (www.sas.com) have sections that can help design fractional factorial experiments.

Measurement of the influence of each factor in a multifactorial experiment depends on the resolution of two issues: the effect of the factor alone and the effect of each factor in combination with other factors. As discussed previously, the factors may not be completely independent, and the interaction between the factors may be worth considering. The influence of each factor alone is called the **main effect** of that factor, and mathematically it is determined as follows:

- Calculate the mean for all results for which the factor is at level +1.
- Calculate the mean for all results for which the factor is at level −1.
- Subtract the mean of the results for which the results were negative from the mean of the results for which the factor was positive.

Table 7.2	Combinations for a 2^3 Experimental Design			
Trial Number	Factor a	Factor b	Factor c	Outcome Calculation
1	−1	−1	−1	$m = -a - b - c$
2	+1	−1	−1	$n = a - b - c$
3	−1	+1	−1	$o = -a + b - c$
4	+1	+1	−1	$p = a + b - c$
5	−1	−1	+1	$q = -a - b + c$
6	+1	−1	+1	$r = a - b + c$
7	−1	+1	+1	$s = -a + b + c$
8	+1	+1	+1	$t = a + b + c$

Thus the equations for calculating the main effects of each of the three factors are as follows:

$$\text{Main effect of } a = \frac{n + p + r + s}{4} - \frac{m + o + q + t}{4}$$

$$\text{Main effect of } b = \frac{o + p + s + t}{4} - \frac{m + n + q + r}{4}$$

$$\text{Main effect of } c = \frac{q + r + s + t}{4} - \frac{m + n + o + p}{4}$$

The interaction effects of the factors are similarly calculated according to the following mathematical formulae:

$$\text{Interaction effect } a \times b = \frac{m + p + s + t}{4} - \frac{n + o + q + r}{4}$$

$$\text{Interaction effect } a \times c = \frac{m + o + r + t}{4} - \frac{n + p + q + s}{4}$$

$$\text{Interaction effect } b \times c = \frac{m + n + s + t}{4} - \frac{o + p + q + r}{4}$$

$$\text{Interaction effect } (a \times b \times c) = \frac{n + o + q + t}{4} - \frac{m + p + r + s}{4}$$

Fortunately, computer programs perform these calculations, making the analysis of an experiment much easier than the work to design the experiment correctly.

Some of the bias that exists in experiments can be mitigated by randomizing distribution of the factors in the experiment. Using the example of Fisher's experiment in FIGURE 7.10, the factors were distributed throughout the matrix randomly but also so that all factors were distributed over the entire surface. Many healthcare workers will recall this issue from medical experimental designs that require randomization to reduce the possibility of experimental bias that can lead to incorrect deductions from the data. For example, an experimental design would not test one ethnic group apart from others unless the experimental hypothesis included ethnicity as an experimental variable. Randomization may not always be feasible, such as when one group of experimental subjects is only available at certain times. In those cases the study design may require more sophisticated statistical structuring to ensure validity of the results.

As demonstrated in EXAMPLE 7.4, the DOE approach can help the staff direct improvement efforts and then follow up with data collection and analysis that can be used in the improve phase to demonstrate that interventions have been effective.

Example 7.4 DOE Approach

During the analyze phase the LSS Clinic's improvement team used Pareto analysis and regression testing to identify the top three factors that appeared to have the greatest effect on likelihood of patients paying before leaving the office. These factors, use of credit card, copay over $10, and time spent in the clinic over 60 minutes, were tested in a 2^3 designed experiment using the factor assignments in TABLE 7.2. The scores and calculated effects from the experiment are shown below.

Factor 1	Factor 2	Factor 3	Score	SD of Score	Effect
Use of credit card			2.5	.8	0.30
	Copay over $10		3.2	.7	1.00
		Clinic time > 60 min	3.6	.9	0.65
Use of credit card	Copay over $10		4.1	1.0	0.45
Use of credit card		Clinic time > 60 min	3.2	.7	0.00
	Copay over $10	Clinic time > 60 min	3.8	.9	0.25
Use of credit card	Copay over $10	Clinic time > 60 min	4.2	1.1	0.05

It is clear that the three most important factors are (1) the need to remit a copay over $10, (2) time spent in the clinic over 60 minutes, and (3) the ability to use a credit card combined with a copay over $10. Thus the staff needs to design interventions that deal with patients who have larger copayments due and those who have conditions that require them to spend more time in the clinic.

By the end of the improve phase the project team will have demonstrated that the tested solutions deal with the identified root cause(s) and thus will result in substantial improvement in the CTQ metrics. The improved process is set in motion, and the team is ready to develop a plan to sustain the gains and institutionalize the improvements.

Control Phase

The control phase carries out the task of ensuring that the gains realized during the improve phase are maintained and that process changes are disseminated throughout the organization. Team members in this phase work to standardize and document procedures, set up training programs for all affected employees, and create a communication plan to spread the project's results enterprise-wide. The monitoring program must be put in place at this stage both to track metric improvements as process changes are rolled out and also to assess the new process performance going forward.

Standardizing and Documenting Improvements

Documenting and standardizing the information regarding process improvements comprise the first set of tasks in this stage. The report should include the following:

- New process map with all changes that have been validated as well as any modifications that occurred during implementation
- Deployment flowchart with clear indications of each stakeholder's role in the new process
- User's guide for the new process that details process steps and rationale, including data collection plans and communications strategies
- Training materials and guides for all affected staff members

Process Monitoring Plan

The control phase focuses on establishing a plan to monitor the new process and intervene when results are not as expected, with a goal to sustain the gains and build on the improvement initiative. This important step ensures that once the project has concluded, the system does not slip back into old habits and practices that will eliminate the effects of the intervention. The monitoring plan clarifies how process performance will be continuously monitored, who is accountable for problems, and expected responses when process performance flags.

An important focal point for the process monitoring plan is the data set to be gathered and analyzed. Metrics developed during the measure and improve phases may be used as process measures, and the CTQs acquired from customers during the define phase can serve as outcome measures. Operational definitions for the measures, as well as analysis plans and report formats, are key deliverables in the process monitoring plan. The process owner is usually assigned the task of collecting and validating the data, and larger organizations may have a business intelligence unit that can perform the necessary analyses and incorporate the metrics into reporting systems like balanced scorecards. Performance targets set by the team in collaboration with senior managers are integrated into this section of the report. As much as possible the team may try to anticipate problems with the new process and create a range of responses for any new problems, perhaps through expansion of a failure mode and effects criticality analysis performed in earlier phases.

Most process monitoring plans specify the method of reporting tracking data, and control charts are among the favorite tools to help process owners quickly identify out of control performance. Lean process management and six sigma both prefer to automate notification of an out of control process as much as possible using electronic systems or a manual kanban system. Because the process environment inevitably changes, the team should develop a method for updating the new procedures when required, including updating the process map and user guides, communicating the changes to all stakeholders, and modifying the monitoring plan to reflect the changes. Common changes that the team should plan for include evolution of employee roles, changes in customer requirements, and updates to existing technology.

Concluding the Control Phase

As the control phase concludes, deliverables are disseminated throughout the enterprise and the team's performance is evaluated against targets set by senior management as part of the project charter. Senior leaders should ensure that team members are recognized for their efforts and rewarded commensurately for their work.

■ Design For Six Sigma: Starting Right

Design for six sigma (DFSS) has become increasingly important as new processes are developed within a six sigma culture as a way to build six sigma performance into every new process or program adopted by the organization. Whereas the tools and workflow used in six sigma are designed to improve existing processes, DFSS has the objective of determining the needs of customers (VOC) and the business (VOB) and incorporating those needs into the product or service being created. The use of DFSS for innovations in a product or service category helps enhance the creative process by enforcing discipline in meeting the needs expressed in the VOC. For example, the Apple iPod replaced many other music-playing devices like portable radios and tape players because it provided specific solutions to customer requirements for portability and personal selection of a playlist. This innovation is disruptive because it caused major adjustments to the sales cycle in the music industry that have led to a paradigm shift in the way recorded music is purchased and sold. Disruptive innovation such as this is must be carefully crafted, and DFSS provides the framework within which this design process may be actuated. DMADV in the process concentrates on learning and methodical incorporation of that learning into subsequent development projects, as shown in FIGURE 7.11. DMADV also paradoxically encourages the successive generation of error, early and often, as part of the learning process to reduce the cost of later corrections.

DMADV is often used synonymously with DFSS. DMAIC is applied to existing processes, whereas DMADV aims to create a process with optimized six sigma efficiencies *before* implementation. DFSS seeks to avoid manufacturing/service process problems by using advanced VOC and systems engineering techniques to avoid process problems at the outset. When combined, these methods ascertain customer needs and derive system parameter requirements that increase product and service effectiveness in the eyes of the customer, creating greater customer satisfaction and increased market share. Just as with DMAIC, DMADV includes tools and processes to predict, model, and simulate the service or product delivery system, and the analysis of the developing system is directed at ensuring that CTQs from the VOC are satisfied in the design and final implementation of the process.

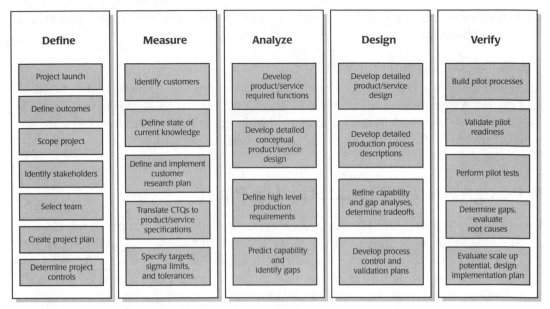

Define	Measure	Analyze	Design	Verify
Project launch	Identify customers	Develop product/service required functions	Develop detailed product/service design	Build pilot processes
Define outcomes	Define state of current knowledge	Develop detailed conceptual product/service design	Develop detailed production process descriptions	Validate pilot readiness
Scope project	Define and implement customer research plan			Perform pilot tests
Identify stakeholders	Translate CTQs to product/service specifications	Define high level production requirements	Refine capability and gap analyses, determine tradeoffs	Determine gaps, evaluate root causes
Select team				
Create project plan	Specify targets, sigma limits, and tolerances	Predict capability and identify gaps	Develop process control and validation plans	Evaluate scale up potential, design implementation plan
Determine project controls				

FIGURE 7.11 DMADV Steps and Tools

Define and Measure Phases

The define and measure phases of DMADV are very similar to those in DMAIC, with efforts to understand the VOC through surveys and other methods of gaining customer input. In the case of DMADV, however, surveys and focus groups may be directed more at what new types of services or products are desired and at finding dissatisfiers with current services or products. Focus groups may explore innovations desired by innovators and early adopters rather than pursuing the more process-centered issues that DMAIC seeks to clarify. The deliverable at this stage is still a project charter that includes a rationale for selection of this particular charter. The project charter should also contain analysis of the VOB to ensure that the business has the capability to develop and produce the new product or service.

Analyze Phase

The analyze phase of DMADV is the first stage at which this approach diverges from DMAIC. In DMADV the team starts with customer requirements but no other specifications. Thus the first task of the analyze phase is to translate the VOC and VOB into design specifications. DFSS practitioners sometimes use advanced innovation management approaches like TRIZ[6] (see EXHIBIT 7.1) to generate design specifications, but this engineering step may require technical assistance and input from legal experts to ensure that the proposed design meets all applicable standards. This phase also relies on the use of statistical software for testing hypotheses.

Exhibit 7.1 TRIZ

TRIZ is an acronym for the Russian phrase *Teoriya Resheniya Izobretatelskikh Zadatch* that is translated as the "theory of inventor problem solving" and describes an established science, method, tool set, knowledge base and model-based technology for generating innovative ideas and solutions for problem solving. Originally developed by the Russian inventor Genrich Altshuller, TRIZ is based on two primary principles:

1. All innovation can be classified, as described by Genrich Altshuller's 40 inventive principles.
2. Innovation fundamentally solves inherent or imposed conflicts. Most design is about the management of conflict, typically by trading off opposing requirements or states.

The story of TRIZ is fascinating and well documented in Altshuller's books cited in the references. TRIZ is only now being applied to issues in health care, but it has been highly useful in other industries.

DMADV's analyze phase encompasses the creation of virtual models using basic business or clinical principles in unique ways. Although sophisticated engineering approaches are used in manufacturing environments, in a healthcare setting the most commonly used tools are evidence-based models like clinical practice guidelines or new business approaches. Other methods of idea generation (e.g., quality function deployment, axiomatic design, and lateral thinking) are also useful during the creative analyze phase. For example, quality function deployment integrates market needs and business opportunities to help create or modify customer requirements, and these requirements are then used to find innovative solutions to meet customer demand.

The principles of axiomatic design advanced by Nam Suh[7] involve two axioms:

1. *The independence axiom:* The best designs occur when the functional requirements of the design are independent of one another.
2. *The information axiom:* The best designs minimize complexity.

For example, axiomatic principles can be used to reduce the cost of a clinical process without diminishing quality. The functions of cost and quality in the process are defined, and then the team works to find methods of removing cost without changing (or even improving) quality metrics. The principles that have been discussed for lean and six sigma can be applied to the specifics of each problem, and Suh and others have also provided a number of techniques to balance this optimization problem.

Another innovation generator is known as "lateral thinking," which is also called "thinking out of the box." Techniques such as those described in Chapter 2 can be applied to get teams to move into a new realm of creativity.

Design Phase

This phase requires the teamwork talents of the Black Belt in concert with the design team. Not only are creative ideas refined and concepts selected with the help of methods such as the decision matrix discussed in Chapter 3, but in the highly regulated health-care industry, issues relating to regulations and accreditation are also incorporated into the design at this stage. Many design teams thus include regulatory and legal experts on the design team either as members or as consultants to ensure all relevant constraints are included. Both lean and six sigma teams promote individual member participation to give workers a voice in the work design.

Another important function of the design phase is to identify potential risks in the new product or service. Using failure mode and effects criticality analysis (see Chapter 3), a new process or product can be evaluated for any potential failures or risks, and the team can concentrate on ensuring the design mitigates those potential problems. The design phase deliverable is a concrete product or service design that is ready for pilot testing, which has undergone basic reliability analysis to ensure it meets customer requirements, regulatory agency rules, and any legal constraints.

Verify Phase

The verify phase uses the efficiency of DOE to pilot test the new product or service and its measurement system. Because pilot testing is often expensive and involves valuable prototypes, this phase generally is associated with a fairly large part of the DMADV cost, but it is required to ensure that the design works as planned. Once pilot testing is completed and quality ensured by capability testing and reaching target sigma levels, the new product or service can be released for refinement of process and quality control programs that are critical for the implementation of the new product or service throughout the organization. This phase is the last chance to discover system integration problems—interactions that could only be evident with the innovation working within the system—and failure modes that require time for failure to occur. At the end of this phase the new product or service is ready for implementation.

DMADV's Value

In today's competitive marketplace healthcare companies, whether payer or provider, need to acquire three attributes to become innovative:

1. An environment that encourages innovative thinking
2. People with creative ideas
3. A process to ensure that good ideas become successfully implemented

DMADV provides the framework for the third requirement, and by creating a six sigma culture an organization can promote the other two requirements. A sustainable organization will have the ability to innovate continually and leverage staff and resources to encourage cutting-edge thinking. Six sigma is an approach that has created these opportunities for companies like GE and Motorola, as well as many others, and the use of six sigma in health care has tremendous potential to accomplish these same levels of performance.

■ Discussion Questions

1. Why is six sigma considered an important tool to improve process effectiveness in health care?
2. What is the meaning of the "sigma" term in six sigma? What level of performance does six sigma connote?
3. What is process capability (Cpk)? How is it related to sigma level?
4. How can sigma levels be used to compare processes throughout an organization?
5. What assumptions underlie six sigma? Why are they important?
6. Describe the 1.5 sigma shift. How does it affect the calculation of error rates?
7. Describe the process of calculating sample size required for sampling for a six sigma calculation. Why is it important to have an adequate sample size?
8. What is a rational subgroup? How is the concept used to determine sampling strategy?
9. Describe three six sigma metrics and explain their meaning.
10. Describe the six sigma improvement model. What occurs at each step in the model?
11. How is six sigma like martial arts? What do the "belts" do to accomplish the aims of a project?
12. What are the voices of six sigma? How is each important in a six sigma project?
13. How is the voice of the customer measured? What problems can arise from these methods?
14. Describe gauge reproducibility and repeatability. How does gauge R&R apply to a six sigma project?
15. What is the basic six sigma equation? Identify each of the factors in the equation and explain how they relate to the DMAIC cycle.
16. What tools are used during the measure phase of DMAIC? Explain how each contributes to this phase.
17. Describe the 5 why's. How is this tool used in six sigma?
18. Describe design of experiments. What is a factor? What is a level? How do these parameters determine experimental design?
19. What is the function of the control phase of DMAIC? What is the deliverable of the control phase and how does it guide implementation plans?
20. How does DMADV differ from DMAIC? In what circumstances is each used?

References

1. Kohn LT, Corrigan JM, Donaldson MS, eds. *To Err is Human: Building a Safer Health System*. Washington, DC: National Academy Press; 2000.
2. In hospital deaths from medical errors at 195,000 per year USA. Retrieved March 2009 from http://www.medicalnewstoday.com/articles/11856.php
3. Harry M, Schroeder R. *Six Sigma: The Breakthrough Management Strategy Revolutionizing the World's Top Corporations*. New York: Bantam Books; 2006.
4. American Society for Testing and Materials. ASTM E691-08 standard practice for conducting an interlaboratory study to determine the precision of a test method. Retrieved March 2009 from http://www.astm.org/Standards/E691.htm (fee required).
5. Breyfogle FW. *Implementing Six Sigma: Smarter Solutions Using Statistical Methods*. New York: John Wiley & Sons; 2003:578.
6. Altshuller G. *The Innovation Algorithm: TRIZ, Systematic Innovation and Technical Creativity*. Worcester, MA: Technical Innovation Center; 1999.
7. Suh NP. *Axiomatic Design: Advances and Applications*. Cambridge, UK: Oxford University Press; 2001.

Additional Resources

Anderson M, Whitcomb P. *DOE Simplified: Practical Tools for Effective Experimentation*. Danvers, MA: Productivity Press; 2007.

Caldwell C, Brexler J, Gillem T. *Lean-Six Sigma for Healthcare: A Senior Leader Guide to Improving Cost and Throughput*. Milwaukee, WI: ASQ Quality Press; 2005.

McCarty T, Bremer M, Gupta P, Daniels L. *The Six Sigma Black Belt Handbook*. New York: McGraw-Hill; 2004.

Table of the standard normal (z) distribution. Retrieved March 2009 from http://www.isixsigma.com/library/content/zdistribution.asp

Trusko B, Harrington HJ, Gupta P, Harrington J, Pexton C. *Improving Healthcare Quality and Cost with Six Sigma*. Upper Saddle River, NJ: Prentice Hall; 2007.

Zidel T. *A Lean Guide to Transforming Healthcare: How to Implement Lean Principles in Hospitals, Medical Offices, Clinics, and Other Healthcare Organizations*. Milwaukee, WI: ASQ Quality Press; 2006.

Six Sigma Glossary

Acceptance Region Alpha Risk: The region of values for which the null hypothesis is accepted.

Accuracy: (1) The degree to which an indicated value matches the actual value of a measured variable. (2) In process instrumentation, degree of conformity of an indicated value to a recognized accepted standard value, or ideal value.

Affinity Chart/Diagram: A tool for organizing large quantities of information from many people. It is often used with brainstorming and other creative-thinking activities to consolidate ideas into coherent subgroups. The ideas are usually written on sticky notes and then categorized into groupings of similar ideas.

Algorithm: (1) A prescribed set of well-defined rules or processes for the solution of a problem in a finite number of steps. (2) Detailed procedures for giving instructions to a computer.

Alpha Risk: The probability of accepting the alternate hypothesis when, in reality, the null hypothesis is true.

Alternate Hypothesis: A tentative explanation that indicates that an event does not follow a chance distribution; a contrast to the null hypothesis.

As Is Process Map: A process map that depicts a process as it is, currently. "As is" process maps are usually characterized by several input options, bottlenecks and multiple handoffs, inspections, and rework loops. This diagram is the starting point to understanding how a process is currently functioning and where opportunities for improvement might be found.

Assignable (Special) Cause: A source of variation that is nonrandom; a change in the source ("vital few" variables) produces a significant change of some magnitude in the response (dependent variable), e.g., a correlation exists; an assignable cause is often signaled by an excessive number of data points outside a control limit and/or a non-random pattern within the control limits; an unnatural source of variation; most often economical to eliminate.

Assignable Variations: Variations in data that can be attributed to specific causes.

Assumption Busting: A questioning process that helps identify and eliminate preconceptions or blind spots that hold people back from proposing or pursuing the best solution.

Attribute: A characteristic that may take on only one value, e.g., 0 or 1.

Attribute Data: Numerical information at the nominal level; subdivision is not conceptually meaningful; data that represents the frequency of occurrence within some discrete category, e.g., 42 solder shorts.

Background Variables: Variables that are of no experimental interest and are not held constant. Their effects are often assumed insignificant or negligible, or they are randomized to ensure that contamination of the primary response does not occur.

Baseline Measures: Data that reflect the performance level that exists at the beginning of an improvement project, before any solutions are initiated.

Best Practice: A completed project or other evidence that is particularly valuable for use in other situations. As evidence for a particular practice increases, it can reach the level of a best (or leading) practice when it demonstrates consistently superior outcomes and low variation.

Beta Risk: The probability of accepting the null hypothesis when, in reality, the alternate hypothesis is true.

Black Belt: The leader of the team responsible for applying the six sigma process.

Calibration: Determination of the experimental relationship between the quantity being measured and the output of the device that measures it; where the quantity measured is obtained through a recognized standard of measurement.

Cause and Effect Diagram (also Fishbone or Ishikawa): Brainstorming tool used for proposing root causes (the bones of the fish) for a specific effect (the head of the fish). Typically used in combination with the affinity diagram to determine the major categories and with the 5 why's technique to help people understand the root cause.

Center Line: The line on a statistical process control chart which represents the characteristic's central tendency.

Central Tendency: Numerical average, e.g., mean, median, and mode; center line on a statistical process control chart.

Champion: Person responsible for the logistical and business aspects of a six sigma project. Champions select and scope projects that are aligned with the corporate strategy, choose and mentor the right people for the project, and remove barriers to ensure the highest levels of success.

Charter: Team document defining the context, specifics, and plans of an improvement project; includes business case, problem and goal statements, constraints and assumptions, roles, preliminary plan, and scope. The charter is to be reviewed with the project sponsor to ensure alignment and revised or refined periodically throughout the DMAIC process based on data.

Checksheet: Forms, tables, or worksheets developed as part of the project plan for use in data collection to standardize data collection.

Common Cause (Random) Variation: Random variation inherent in a process due to process design, variability in human or machine performance, or other uncontrolled variation. This form of variation is usually harder to eliminate than special cause variation and requires changes to the process.

Complexity Matrix: A tool used to assist teams in determining the level of complexity of a project by estimating the resources required for the project.

Confidence Level: The probability that a random variable x lies within a defined interval.

Confidence Limits: The two values that define the confidence interval.

Confounding: Allowing two or more variables to vary together so that it is impossible to separate their unique effects.

Consumer Risk: Probability of accepting a lot when, in fact, the lot should have been rejected (same as beta risk).

Continuous Data: Any quantity measured on a continuous scale that can be infinitely divided; primary types include time, dollars, size, weight, temperature, and speed; also referred to as "variable data."

Continuous Random Variable: A random variable that can assume any value continuously in some specified interval. (1) Control: The state of stability, normal variation, and predictability. (2) The process of regulating and guiding operations and processes using quantitative data.

Control Chart: A graphical rendition of a characteristic's performance across time in relation to its natural limits and central tendency.

Control Specifications: Specifications called for by the product being manufactured or service being delivered.

Controlled Variable: (1) The variable that the control system attempts to keep at the set point value. The set point may be constant or variable. (2) The part of a process to be controlled (flow, level, temperature, pressure, etc.). (3) A process variable that is to be controlled at some desired value by means of manipulating another process variable.

Correlation: A measure of the degree to which two variables (such as thunder and lighting or tardiness and/or low productivity) are related (i.e., the extent to which they move together). Used to quantify the strength of the relationship between the two variables, correlation does not necessarily imply a cause-and-effect relationship. For example, daily high temperatures and ice cream sales would tend to be correlated, and so it is reasonable to conclude that hotter weather causes people to buy more ice cream. However, the conclusion cannot be made that hot weather always causes people to buy more ice cream, because other variables may affect that outcome.

Cost of Poor Quality (COPQ): Financial metrics that measure the impact of quality problems (internal and external failures) in the process; sources of costs include labor and material costs for handoffs, rework, waste or scrap, inspection, and other non–value added activities.

Cpk (**Cp, Process Capability**): The degree to which a process can meet customer requirements measured against an upper and/or lower specification limit representing the "extremes" of customer requirements or demands on the process. Values > 1 indicate a capable process; values < 1 indicate a process that is not meeting customer requirements. Values of 2 indicate the process is meeting six sigma levels of performance.

Criteria Matrix: Decision support tool used when potential choices must be weighted against key factors (e.g., cost, ease to implement, impact on customer are most relevant). Encourages use of facts, data, and clear business objectives in the decision-making process.

Critical to Quality (CTQ, Critical *Y*): The element of a process or practice that has a direct impact on its perceived quality from the customer's perspective; features that customers consider to be of the most importance in a product or service.

Customer: Any internal or external person or organization that receives the output (product or service) of a process.

Customer Requirements: The needs and expectations of the customer, translated into measurable terms and used in process improvement to ensure compliance with customers' needs. Customer requirements define CTQ (critical to quality) attributes that become the *Y* values in the six sigma equation.

Cutoff Point: The point that partitions the acceptance region from the reject region.

Cycle Time: The time it takes to complete a process from start to finish, including both value added and non–value added time.

Dashboard: A set of metrics, usually not more than five or six, that provide an "at-a-glance" summary of a six sigma project's status. Every participant in a six sigma deployment—from the CEO to a factory floor worker—should have his or her own dashboard with function- and level-appropriate data summaries.

Data: Factual information used as a basis for reasoning, discussion, or calculation; often refers to quantitative information.

Data Collection Plan: A structured approach to identifying the required data to be collected and the approach to collecting it; typically performed during the measure phase of a DMAIC project. The data collection plan includes the measure, the measure type, data type, operational definition, and the sampling plan if new data are necessary.

Defect: Source of customer dissatisfaction. Eliminating defects provides cost and quality benefits.

Defects per Million Opportunities (DPMO): Calculation used in six sigma initiatives to show how much "better" or "worse" a process is by indicating the number of defects in a process per one million opportunities to have a defect. The measure is calculated by the following equation:

$$DPMO = \frac{Number\ of\ defects}{Number\ of\ opportunities} \times 1,000,000$$

An issue for consideration is how many opportunities should be in the denominator. For example, if foreign bodies left in situ postoperatively are the measure of interest, then the number of procedures in which at least one foreign body was left in the surgical site is in the numerator and the total number of surgical procedures is in the denominator. On the other hand, the number of DPMO in a run of 1,000 medical invoices is calculated as follows: Each invoice has 20 fields that are completed, and 1,000 bills are in each batch. Thus the number of opportunities is $20 \times 1,000$ or 20,000. If 50 bills have three errors each, then the number of defects is 150 and the DPMO is calculated as follows:

$$DPMO = (150/20,000) \times 1,000,000 \text{ or}$$
$$DPMO = 7,500$$

The best guideline for counting opportunities is to use only those that directly affect the use of the final output. Thus in the billing example any of the errors would result in rejection of the claim. However, if half of those errors would not result in a rejected claim, then the calculation becomes

$$DPMO = (75/20.000) \times 1,000,000 \text{ or}$$
$$DPMO = 3,750$$

Degrees Of Freedom: The number of independent measurements available for estimating a population parameter.

Density Function: The function that yields the probability that a particular random variable takes on any one of its possible values.

Dependent Variable: A response variable; e.g., y is the dependent or "response" variable where $y = f(X)$.

Deployment Process Map: A map or graphical view of the steps in a process shows the sequence as it moves across departments, functions, or individuals. This type of process map shows "hand-offs" and the groups involved. It is also known as a functional or cross-functional flowchart or map.

Descriptive Statistics: A statistical profile of the collected data that includes measures of averages, variance, and standard deviation, that help define the level of performance and variation in the sample or population.

Design for Six Sigma (DFSS): Application of six sigma tools to product or service development with the goal of "designing in" six sigma performance capability.

Deviation: The difference between the value of a specific variable and some desired value, usually a process set point.

Discrete Random Variable: A random variable that can assume values only from a definite number of discrete values.

Distributions: Tendency of large numbers of observations to group themselves around some central value with a certain amount of variation or "scatter" on either side.

DMADV (Define, Measure, Analyze, Design, Verify): The framework for applying six sigma tools for designing new products, services, and processes. DMADV is used when

- A product or service is not yet in existence
- An existing product, service, or process has been optimized but still does not meet the level of customer specifications or a six sigma level

DMAIC (Define, Measure, Analyze, Improve, Control): Framework for continued improvement that is systematic, scientific, and fact based. This closed-loop process eliminates unproductive steps, often focuses on new measurements, and applies technology for improvement.

Effectiveness: Measures related to how well the process output(s) meets the needs of the customer (e.g., on-time delivery, adherence to specifications, service experience, accuracy, value-added features, customer satisfaction level); links primarily to customer satisfaction.

Efficiency: Measure related to the quantity of resources used in producing the output of a process (e.g., cost of the process, total cycle time, resources consumed, cost of defects, scrap, and/or waste); links primarily to company profitability.

Experiment: A test under defined conditions to determine an unknown effect; to illustrate or verify a known law; to test or establish a hypothesis.

Experimental Error: Variation in observations made under identical test conditions. Also called residual error. The amount of variation that cannot be attributed to the variables included in the experiment.

External Failure: A failure characterized by customers receiving defective units that have passed completely through the process.

Factors: Independent variables.

Five Why's: A root-cause analysis technique that consists of asking "why" five times to delve deeply into each potential cause. "Why" is asked until the root cause is revealed.

Fixed Effects Model: Experimental treatments are specifically selected by the researcher. Conclusions only apply to the factor levels considered in the analysis. Inferences are restricted to the experimental levels.

Force Field Analysis: A list of factors that support the issue juxtaposed with a list of factors that oppose the issue. Support factors are listed as "driving forces" and opposing factors are listed as "restraining forces."

Fractional Factorial Experiment: a methodically chosen subset, or fraction, of the experimental runs of a full factorial design. Each subset is chosen according to an algorithm that provides an optimum combination of factors for each run to reduce the total number of runs required for the complete experiment. A fractional factorial experiment is performed to reduce the cost of the experiment, while preserving the experimental model to ensure that the results provide the information needed to properly estimate the effects of factors and combinations of factors on the response variable.

Frequency Distribution: The pattern or shape formed by the group of measurements in a distribution.

Full Factorial Experiment: a designed experiment in which two or more factors, each with discrete "levels" (values), for which each run of the experiment tests a different combination of levels across all factors, with a design that accounts for all possible combinations being tested during the experimental runs; this type of experiment allows the experimenter to study the effect of each factor on the response variable, as well as the effects of interactions between factors on the response variable.

Goal Statement: Description of the intended target or desired results of process improvement or design/redesign activities; usually outlined during the define phase of a DMAIC project and supported with actual numbers and details once data have been obtained.

Green Belt: An individual who supports the implementation and application of six sigma tools by way of participation on project teams.

Handoff: Any time in a process when one person (or job title) or group passes the item moving through the process to another person; a handoff has the potential to add defects, time, and cost to a process.

Hawthorne Effect: An increase in worker productivity that results from the psychological stimulus of being temporarily singled out and made to feel important. A group working on a project may be receiving a lot of attention and their performance may temporarily improve; when this attention decreases, the worker motivation may decline resulting in lower productivity.

Histogram: Vertical display of a population distribution in terms of frequencies; a formal method of plotting a frequency distribution.

Homogeneity of Variance: The variances of the groups being contrasted are equal (as defined by statistical test of significant difference).

Human Factors: Human capabilities and limitations to the design and organization of the work environment; primarily attributed to errors, but also a consideration in the design of workflow and processes. The study of human factors can help identify operations susceptible to human error and improve working conditions to reduce fatigue and inattention.

Hypothesis Statement: (1) In six sigma or project management, a complete description of the suspected causes of a process problem. (2) In statistics, a testable statement of a relationship, such as a cause and effect relationship, between factors.

Impact/Effort Matrix: A matrix comparison of different projects plotted along two axes (y = impact, x = effort). The project that demonstrates the highest impact with the lowest effort is determined the best selection.

Implementation Plan: A project management tool used in the improve phase of DMAIC, compiling tools such as stakeholder analysis, FMEA, poka yoke, standard operating procedures, and pilot results (if conducted) in a consolidated format.

Independent Variable: A controlled variable; a variable whose value is independent of the value of another variable.

Interaction: The tendency of two or more variables to produce an effect in combination that neither variable would produce if acting alone.

Internal Rate of Return: The annualized effective compounded return rate that can be earned on invested capital, i.e., the yield on the investment. The internal rate of return for an investment is the discount rate that makes the net present value of the investment's income stream total to zero. This metric is used for comparing potential projects. Project planning should strive for a high internal rate of return.

Interval: Numeric categories with equal units of measure but no absolute zero point, i.e., quality scale or index.

Kano Analysis: A graph of how customer satisfaction is affected by a particular problem, change, or other variable. The graph is divided into three regions of customer reactions to the variable: "dissatisfiers," "satisfiers," and "delighters."

Line Charts: Charts used to track the performance without relationship to process capability or control limits.

Lower Control Limit: A horizontal line plotted on a control chart that represents the lower process limit capabilities.

Main Effect: In a full or fractional factorial design, a main effect represents the effect of an independent variable (factor) across multiple levels of that variable and any other independent variables.

Master Black Belt: A teacher and mentor of black belts. Provides support, reviews projects, and undertakes larger scale projects.

Measure: A numerical representation of observable data. For example, serum sodium level, number of bills sent, or rooms cleaned per shift.

Mixed Effects Model: Contains elements of both the fixed and random effects models.

Multiple Regression: Quantitative method relating multiple factors to the output of a process. The statistical study of the relationship of a combination of multiple variables ($X1$ $X2$ $X3...Xn$) to a single output Y using least-squares estimation for each coefficient of variation.

Multivoting: A method of reducing a long list of options to a shorter list by having team members cast votes on the options in multiple voting cycles one after another, dropping the options with the fewest votes at the end of each cycle, until the list is reduced to a manageable size.

Nominal: Unordered categories that indicate membership or nonmembership with no implication of quantity, i.e., number of patients with cesarean section, number of patients treated for hypertension, etc.

Nonconforming Unit: A unit that does not conform to one or more specifications, standards, and/or requirements.

Nonconformity: A condition within a unit that does not conform to some specific specification, standard, and/or requirement; often referred to as a defect; any given nonconforming unit can have the potential for more than one nonconformity.

Non–Value Added Activities: Any steps in a process that do not add value to the customer or process. Examples include rework, handoffs, inspection, and delays.

Normal Distribution: A continuous, symmetrical density function characterized by a bell-shaped curve, e.g., distribution of sampling averages.

Null Hypothesis: A tentative explanation that indicates a chance distribution is operating; a contrast to the null hypothesis.

One-Sided Alternative: The value of a parameter that has an upper bound or a lower bound, but not both.

Operational Definition: A clear, precise definition of the factor being measured or the term being used; ensures a clear understanding of terminology and the ability to collect data or operate a process consistently.

Ordinal: Ordered categories (ranking) with no information about distance between each category, i.e., rank ordering of several measurements of an output parameter.

Output/Outcome Measures: Measures related to and describing the output of the process or outcome for the customer, e.g., mortality rate, injury rate from medical errors, functional status after surgery.

Parameter: A constant defining a particular property of the density function of a variable.

Pareto Diagram: A chart that ranks, or places in order, common occurrences. A Pareto chart is a data display tool based on the Pareto principle, or 80/20 rule. It is used to help bring focus to the specific causes or issues that have the greatest impact if solved.

p-chart: Control chart used to plot percent defectives in a sample.

Poka Yoke: A Japanese term for "mistake proofing" that represents the process of empowering workers at every step in the process to seek defects and stop the defects from proceeding further in the process or allow defects to reach the customer. This concept may also involve creative thinking to develop ways to keep errors from occurring, for example, design of connecting hose ends to prevent an oxygen tube from being plugged into a vacuum outlet or labeling drugs with similar sounding names with exaggerated characters to avoid confusing the two medications.

Population: A group of similar items from which a sample is drawn. Often referred to as the universe.

Power of an Experiment: The probability of rejecting the null hypothesis when it is false and accepting the alternate hypothesis when it is true.

Precision: The degree of reproducibility among several independent measurements of the same true value.

Primary Control Variables: The major independent variables used in the experiment.

Probability: The chance of something happening; the percent or number of occurrences over a large number of trials.

Probability of an Event: The number of successful events divided by the total number of trials.

Process: A series of steps or actions that lead to a result or output. A set of common tasks that creates a product or service.

Process Average: The central tendency of a given process characteristic across a given amount of time or at a specific point in time.

Process Capability: Statistical measures that summarize how much variation there is in a process relative to customer specifications.

Process Management: The cycle of continuous review, reexamination, and renewal of fundamental work processes that contribute to an organization's performance and productivity.

Process Map: Illustrated description of the steps in a process that concisely diagrams the process flow; enables participants to visualize an entire process and identify areas of strength and weaknesses.

Process Redesign: Method of restructuring a process that addresses common cause variation using techniques to eliminate non–value added or detrimental steps that reduce process performance but do not cause the process to operate outside control limits.

Process Spread: The range of values that a given process characteristic displays; this particular term most often applies to the range but may also encompass the variance. The spread may be based on a set of data collected at a specific point in time or may reflect the variability across a given amount of time.

Producer's Risk: Probability of rejecting a lot when, in fact, the lot should have been accepted (same as alpha risk).

Project: The focus of performance improvement efforts. A defined work effort characterized by a starting point and an ending point.

r-charts: Range control chart; a plot of the difference between the highest and lowest in a sample.

RACI Matrix: A project management tool that identifies all required tasks or activities and what parties are involved in those tasks as well as their level or type of involvement. A RACI matrix is used to ensure clarity on roles and responsibilities in a team environment.

- R = Responsible—the person responsible for performing the task
- A = Accountable—the person who is accountable for the results of the process
- C = Consulted—a stakeholder involved before task completion to ensure that the task meets customer needs
- I = Informed—a stakeholder who is told the results of the process

Random: A sampling technique designed so that each item in the population has an equal chance of being selected; lack of predictability; without pattern.

Random Cause: A source of variation that is random; for example, a change in the source ("trivial many" variables) will not produce a highly predictable change in the response (dependent variable) because a correlation does not exist; random causes cannot be economically eliminated from a process, because the source of variation is inherent in the process; common cause.

Random Sample: One or more samples randomly selected from the universe (population).

Random Variable: A variable that can assume any value from a set of possible values.

Random Variation: Variation in data that results from causes that cannot be pinpointed or controlled.

Range: The difference between the highest and lowest values in a set of values or "subgroup."

Ranks: Values assigned to items in a sample to determine their relative occurrence in a population.

Reject Region: The region of values for which the alternate hypothesis is accepted.

Return on Investment: A measure of the financial returns from an investment opportunity, expressed as a percentage. All else being equal, projects with a larger return on investment are more attractive investment opportunities.

Rework Loop: Any instance in a process when the item or data moving through the process must be corrected by returning it to a previous step in the process adding time, cost, and potential for errors and more defects.

Robust: Impervious to perturbing influence.

Rolled Throughput Yield: The cumulative calculation of defects through multiple steps in a process; calculated as the product of the individual yield at each step (expressed as a percentage). For example, in an eight-step process with each step at 99%, the rolled throughput yield is $.99 \times .99 \times .99 \times .99 \times .99 \times .99 \times .99 \times .99 = 95\%$.

Root-Cause Analysis: A study of underlying reason(s) for nonconformance within a process; correction of the root cause eliminates the nonconformity.

Representative Sample: A sample that accurately reflects a specific condition or set of conditions within the universe.

Run Chart: A plot of a variable over time with a centerline (usually the median of the data set) that demonstrates the trend and provides information about trends, patterns, and special cause variation.

Sample: One or more observations drawn from a larger collection of observations or universe (population).

Sampling Bias: Collecting an unrepresentative "slice" of data that will lead to inaccurate conclusions. For instance, measuring the first five patients seen in the clinic to determine waiting times rather than taking a random sample of patients over a period of time.

Scatter Diagrams: Charts that plot two variables on a Cartesian graph that allows visual study of the relationship between two variables.

Scope: Defines the boundaries of the process; clarifies specifically where the start and end points for improvement reside; defines where and what to measure and analyze; sets the sphere of control of the team working on the project; in general, the broader the scope, the more complex and time-consuming the improvement efforts will be.

"Should Be" Process Map: A depiction of a new and improved version of a process, used in DMAIC projects, where all non–value added steps have been removed and based on:

- Everything being done right the first time
- Customer requirements built into the process
- Flexibility to meet multiple customer types or requirements
- Design with "process" versus "functional" mindset
- Limited handoffs and inspections
- Ease to document, manage, train, and control
- Several possible inputs
- Bottleneck eliminated
- Handoffs, inspection, and rework loops no longer needed

Sigma Value: Metric that indicates how well that process is performing. The higher the sigma value, the better. Sigma measures the capability of the process to perform defect-free work. A defect is anything that results in customer dissatisfaction. Sigma is a statistical unit of measure that reflects process capability. The sigma scale of measure is perfectly correlated to such characteristics as defects per unit, parts per million defective, and the probability of a failure/error.

Signal: An event or phenomenon that conveys data from one point to another.

Simple Linear Regression: The statistical study of the relationship between a single variable x to a single output, fitting a line though a set of data to reduce the variation between actual and predicted performance.

SIPOC: A high-level process map that includes suppliers, inputs, process, outputs, and customers that defines the start and end points of a process. It is used to ensure that the team members are all viewing the process in the same way and inform leadership on the process being improved.

Six Sigma: A sigma level indicating a performance level of 3.4 defects per million opportunities (DPMO).

Special Cause: Same as assignable cause.

Stable Process: A process that is free of assignable causes, e.g., in statistical control.

Stakeholder Analysis: Identifies all stakeholders impacted by a project and their anticipated and required levels of support for the project. Typical stakeholders include managers, people who work in the process under study, other departments, customers, suppliers, and finance. Used to identify potential barriers to process improvement efforts.

Standard Deviation: A statistical index of variability that describes the spread or variation in a data set.

Standard Operating Procedure: A document that compiles all procedures, job tasks, scripts of interactions with customers or others, data collection instructions and forms, and an updated list of resources to be consulted for clarification of procedures. Standard operating procedures allow the organization to maintain reproducibility of all aspects of a process improvement across shifts, time periods, and leadership changes.

Statistical Control: Process condition that is free of assignable/special causes of variation, e.g., variation in the central tendency and variance, most readily indicated on a control chart.

Statistical Process Control: The application of statistical methods and procedures to monitor a process and to determine if a process is in control; used to monitor processes over time.

Storyboard: A visual display outlining the highlights of a project and its components as well as results, storyboards are often used to track project progress or for use in presentations to managers and other stakeholders.

Stratification: Dividing data sets into groups based on key characteristics to detect patterns that relate to the characteristic. For example, a data set may be stratified into age groups by year or age group to determine the characteristics of each of the groups relative to a variable under study.

Subgroup: A logical grouping of objects or events which is used in some statistical process control charts to sample from a larger population of measurements; samples are randomly selected to decrease bias from assignable or special causes.

Subprocess: A section or subset of steps of a larger process. For example, a phlebotomy procedure may be a subprocess of a workup for a child with a fever.

Systematic Sampling: Sampling method in which elements are selected from the population at a uniform level (e.g., every half-hour, every 20th item). For example, sampling a process at fixed time intervals represents systematic sampling and ensures each sample is representative of the process because each time period is represented.

Test of Significance: A procedure to determine whether a quantity subjected to random variation differs from a postulated value by an amount greater than that due to random variation alone.

Tollgate (or Gate): A review session that determines whether activities up to that point in a project have been satisfactorily completed. Tollgates are commonly conducted to review critical decisions during a project.

Tree Diagram: A "branching" diagram that is used to break any broad goal into increasingly detailed levels of actions. Often used along with brainstorming or during project management/planning.

Type I Error: Same as alpha risk.

Type II Error: Same as beta risk.

Upper Control Limit: A horizontal line on a control chart that represents the upper limits of process capability.

Value Added Activities: Steps or tasks in a process that meet all three criteria defining value as perceived by the external customer:

- Transforms the item/service toward completion
- Customer willing to pay for it
- Done right the first time

Variable: A characteristic that may take on different values.

Variables Data: Numerical measurements made at the interval or ratio level; continuous number data. (1) Variance: A change in a process or business practice that may alter its expected outcome. (2) A statistical term that is the square of the standard deviation.

Variation: Any quantifiable difference between individual measurements; such differences can be classified as being due to common causes (random) or special causes (assignable).

Voice of the Business (VOB): The stated mission, goals, and business objectives of an organization; specific, documented statements of intent that are the guidelines by which linkages are established between six sigma projects and targeted levels of improvement. The VOB should describe what the business does and how the business intends to accomplish its mission. Combined with the voice of the customer, the VOB plays an important role in defining potential six sigma projects.

Voice of the Customer (VOC): A systematic approach for eliciting and analyzing customers' requirements, expectations, levels of satisfaction and areas of concern. The VOC is a key data source in the project selection process.

X and R Chart: A control chart that uses the values of individual x-values and the range to establish the centerline, upper control limit, and lower control limit.

Yellow Belt: Any employee who has received introductory training in the fundamentals of six sigma. The yellow belt gathers data, participates in problem-solving exercises, and adds his or her personal experiences to the exploration process.

Yield: Total number of units handled correctly through the process step(s), typically expressed as a percentage. Yield indicates how many items were delivered at the end of the process with no defect

Z-Score: Sometimes called "standard scores;" a special application of the transformation rules in which a value within a distribution is divided by the standard deviation of the distribution to provide the proportion of the standard deviation represented by the value. The Z-score for a data point indicates how far, and in what direction, that item deviates from its distribution's mean, expressed in units of its distribution's standard deviation.

Alignment and Integration of Performance Improvement Systems: The Malcolm Baldrige National Quality Award

■ History and Background

The business world in the 1980s was troublesome. Traditionally strong industries like automaking, steel, and aviation had rapidly been thrust into a highly competitive international market environment that caught managers and political leaders by surprise. The changes in the world economic environment had occurred gradually enough that the tipping point, which had previously been on the horizon, now confronted U.S. industry. President Reagan's Secretary of Commerce, Malcolm Baldrige, raised consciousness in the American business community in a number of ways, noted by Secretary of Commerce Donald Evans in his 2003 address at the National Quality Award Ceremony:[1]

- A "handshake capitalist," whose word was his bond and who knew "good enough was not good enough;"
- A visionary who saw quality management as the key to America's long-term strength and prosperity; and
- A giant who could convince vigorous competitors to work for the common goal.
- Integrity, excellence, principled leadership, sound judgment and business responsibility—Mac Baldrige stood for all these things. Our award celebrates his values, his "can-do" spirit and his abiding belief that America could rise to meet any challenge we faced.

The principle of quality management became the underpinning of the Malcolm Baldrige National Quality Award (MBNQA), created in 1987 to move U.S. industry toward a more competitive position in the international community by identifying high functioning organizations and using their examples to motivate and educate other organizations. Congress created the Foundation for the MBNQA to achieve these goals with the passage of the Malcolm Baldrige National Quality Improvement Act of 1987 (Public Law 100-107), which provided funding and oversight via the National Institute of Standards and Technology (NIST). The Foundation strives to build a permanent endowment to sustain the program into the future. Trustees are selected from major U.S. organizations to promote the mission of the Foundation and to ensure the funding base has the largest possible breadth.

NIST provides management and oversight of the program and is in a unique position because of its interface between government and industry. The agency works with U.S. industry to establish standards for measurement and to develop measurement tools, data, and services that help establish the nation's technology infrastructure (see http://www.nist.gov). Additionally, NIST partners with the private sector to facilitate development of relatively high risk technologies that may have substantial commercial returns. Businesses of all sizes benefit from the NIST Technology Extension Centers that serve all 50 states and Puerto Rico.

The American Society for Quality (ASQ, www.asq.org) works under contract with NIST to provide logistical support for MBNQA. As a leading purveyor of quality improvement educational and accreditation services, ASQ has established a strong relationship with NIST to promote the MBNQA in its publications, and the organization manages the details of such Baldrige activities as training sessions and site visits.

■ Baldrige Organizational Structure

FIGURE 8.1 illustrates the organizational structure of the Baldrige program. As mentioned previously, the program is administered for the Department of Commerce by NIST, with logistic support through a contract with ASQ. A Board of Overseers appointed by the Secretary of Commerce advises the Department of Commerce on all elements of the program, particularly its relevance to industry issues and the national interest. The Board recommends improvements to the MBNQA program that are designed to continue to make the award pertinent to current industrial trends for quality, competitiveness, and profitability. Working through the Secretary of Commerce and the Director of NIST, these recommendations impact all aspects of the program each year, leading to enhancements in the program that ensure the framework within which staff, judges, and examiners work is current.

The Board of Examiners consists of the volunteers from throughout the American business community who actually evaluate applications and prepare feedback reports. The Panel of Judges is composed of 10 examiners selected by the Secretary of Commerce, and they use the information generated by the Board of Examiners to determine an applicant's progress through the Award process. Each year, approximately 400 to 500 business, education, and healthcare experts are selected to participate in the Board of Examiners. Approximately 20% are designated as senior examiners due to their experience and tenure with the Baldrige program.

The Foundation for the MBNQA was created to provide a venue for the private sector in the United States to fund and manage an endowment that augments operational revenues from MBNQA program activities and to provide continuity for program

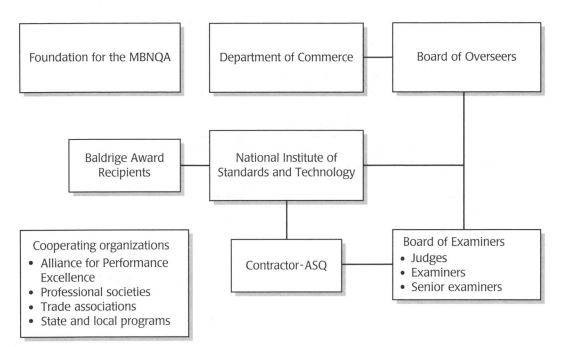

FIGURE 8.1 Baldrige Program Organizational Structure

performance review. Working with NIST, the Foundation helps pursue outside funding from the U.S. business community to ensure success of the award program. Prominent U.S. industrial leaders serve as Foundation Trustees, enhancing the profile of the MBNQA program throughout the world as well as in the United States. The Foundation has no oversight of the Baldrige program and has no involvement in the award process.

■ Baldrige Award Process

FIGURE 8.2 presents a flowchart of the Baldrige award process. The process begins in the summer of each year with the selection of a team of examiners to prepare the training case for the upcoming year. Judges, senior examiners, and examiners all take part in the annual preparation course that is held in May of each year. Each year's cycle begins in July of the previous year with a team of experienced examiners creating a "training case," which is used during the training sessions held during May of the next year. Each training case concentrates in a specific industry (e.g., health care, manufacturing, small business, education, and service). Each year a different industry is featured, and over their usual 6-year tenure, examiners will be exposed to the nuances of evaluating many different types of applications.

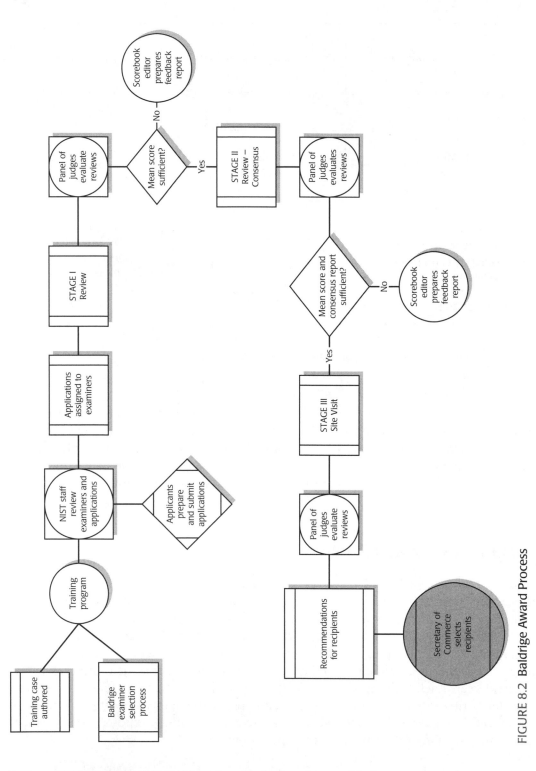

FIGURE 8.2 Baldrige Award Process

Creation of the training case requires particularly intense efforts on the part of a select group of examiners. The experienced writing team works over a 6- to 8-week period to outline, research, and craft the training case using a process similar to that used by an applicant. Senior and alumni examiners serving as team leaders then edit the case to ensure consistency in writing style and information linkages. The writers incorporate specific teaching issues into the case, so that areas of emphasis for the year's training can be incorporated into the work.

In November of each year the NIST team puts out a call for examiners, soliciting experts from throughout U.S. industries, and potential examiners complete application forms to be considered for the program. NIST staff members carefully screen the applications and fill positions to ensure an adequate number of examiners to match the expected number of applications in each sector. From these candidates, senior examiners are named to assume leadership positions in the program. Seniors are those who have demonstrated leadership potential in their first year or two of the program, and they are appointed to lead consensus review and site visit teams. Alumni examiners are highly experienced and have served at least 6 years as an examiner, and these seasoned people help with training and fill gaps where additional leaders are needed for Stage II (consensus) and Stage III (site visit).

Once the Board of Examiners has been constituted during the month of March, the training cycle begins in April of that year. Each examiner receives a packet of educational materials and access to a training website that has "just in time" video clips for each phase of the process. After reviewing the educational materials, examiners begin to dissect the training case that was so laboriously created over the preceding 9 months. The examiner completes forms for the training case that are identical to those used in Stage I (independent review), and the resulting document then is submitted to NIST at the time of training and is used by the examiner for the onsite training classes in May. Evaluation of the training case usually consumes from 20 to 50 hours of work, depending on the complexity of the case and the individual examiner's experience.

Armed with the training case analysis, examiners attend a 3-day onsite training session in May, with a 4th day added for first year examiners and for senior examiners. The additional training is directed at supplementing the written and online materials for new examiners and for leadership training for senior examiners. In addition to the training program, each new examiner is assigned a mentor to help with the independent review of the training case. The training sessions are intense, but senior examiners facilitate the sessions and try to keep them entertaining, as examiners share stories of prior experiences that produced memorable, and often humorous, anecdotes. During the training sessions examiners are taught about the three stages of the Baldrige process, the elements of a scorebook, writing style recommendations, the role of the judges, the ethics of the Baldrige program, and the mechanics of the review and selection process. Examiners get to know each other and the NIST staff, with whom they will be working closely over the next 6 months. Long-term collegial relationships are the hallmark of the Board of Examiners, all of whom share a passion for performance improvement. At the end of the training sessions NIST staff begins to assemble teams of 6 to 10 examiners who will be assigned an actual application to review.

Baldrige applicants must have their applications submitted by May, and the NIST staff carefully evaluates applications and distributes them to examiner teams during the first 2 weeks of June. Each team consists of a mix of experienced senior, alumni, and newer examiners. Although the teams have been selected and perform some early organizational work, each examiner is responsible for reviewing an entire application during the first stage of the process, independent review. Each examiner works alone to completely review the application, outline observations that will be used to write scorebook comments, and provide a tentative score based on the applicant's response to the Baldrige criteria. Once all examiners have completed Stage I, the reviews are uploaded to a secure site called the Examiner Depot, where the scorebooks can be shared with all team members. The website is heavily secured by login and password combinations, and the site is locked down for each team until all examiners have completed and uploaded their Stage I reviews.

During Stage II, consensus review, each team member is assigned one Baldrige category and one associated results item to perform an in-depth review and integration of all other team members' comments for the assigned category or item. Examiners download every other team member's worksheets from the Examiner Depot and then use the observations in the worksheets to begin creating "feedback-ready" comments. The team meets via teleconference to discuss each examiner's work at least once during Stage II, and then the team reviews and exchanges ideas on the evolving scorebook via the Examiner Depot until the comments are ready for final review and editing by the team leader and scorebook editor. Examiners evaluate the applicant's responses to the criteria with each comment, and the examiner team rates each comment using the following scale:

- Double strength (++): the applicant's response to the criterion is highly reliable, systematic, and appears to be a world-class solution that can serve as a model for other organizations
- Strength (+): the applicant's response to the criterion meets all the basic requirements and appears to be well deployed
- Opportunity for improvement (−): known as an OFI among the Baldrige cognoscenti, the applicant's response to the criterion does not meet the basic requirements or it does not seem to be effectively deployed
- Double opportunity for improvement (−−): known as a double OFI, this response does not meet criteria requirements on several points and appears to be minimally deployed

The team leader and scorebook editor thoroughly review the comments in the assembled scorebook before submission for judges' reviews, but they do not change any of the content of the comments and only ensure that grammatical errors are corrected and that the comments sound like they have been written in a "single voice." The final version of the scorebook is uploaded to the Examiner Depot for review by the Baldrige judges to determine which applicants proceed to Stage III, the site visit. The organizations that do not proceed receive the final version of the scorebook with comments to assist improvement efforts and help with preparation of another application in the future. All these activities are completed over the summer months, and the team submits the final scorebook for review toward the end of August or first week of September. Each application undergoes both Stage I and Stage II review, ensuring not only that at least 8 to 10 pairs of trained eyes see the application but also that the application is thoroughly discussed by a team of experienced examiners who come to consensus on the score for the application.

After all scorebooks have been submitted by all examiner teams, the Baldrige judges' panel begins the arduous task of reviewing all scorebooks to determine which applicants proceed to Stage III. Each judge may be responsible for several scorebooks, and they must become familiar with the application and scorebook comments so they may lead a discussion during the judges' panel meeting in September. Just as in the legal system, Baldrige judges are dispassionate and do not advocate for an applicant but strive to represent the application and scorebook to other judges on the panel to support the best decisions on which applicants will have a site visit during Stage III of the Baldrige process.

Stages I and II of the Baldrige process occur between June and September of each year, and examiners and judges work hard during those months. Each scorebook undergoes three or four edits before finalization, and during Stage II examiners work collaboratively to review each other's work and make the comments achieve a high level of quality before being submitted to the judges' panel. The teams collaborate during Stage II through teleconferences, which last from 4 to 8 hours, and some teams with more complex applications or more ambiguous responses to the criteria in the application require two consensus calls. Examiners are taught to not be wedded to their original views of the applicant, because the collective insight from the examiner team is usually better than that of a single reviewer. Consensus call discussions usually center on trying to interpret the applicant's responses, and examiners are told during training to give the applicant the benefit of the doubt ("Don't block a winner") during this stage, because interpretation of the written document can sometimes be difficult and subject to multiple interpretations. During the consensus call the team agrees on a score for each category that serves to inform the Baldrige judges of the examiner team's evaluation of the application's responses to the criteria.

The judges' panel meeting in early September is devoted to reviewing each consensus scorebook in depth, discussing the merits of the applicant based on the examiner team's assessment, and then prioritizing applicants for site visits during Stage III. Those applicants scoring well and validated by the judges can then proceed to Stage III, or the site visit. Approximately two or three applicants in each classification reach this stage. Thus from all healthcare applications submitted, only three are ultimately selected for a Stage III site visit. Much like an Academy Award nomination, selection for a site visit confers a level of recognition that is rarely recognized outside of the Baldrige staff, the examiner team involved with that applicant, and the judges' panel, because the entire Baldrige process is highly confidential until a recipient is named in November.

Usually, the same team members that participated in Stage II are involved in the site visit. Sometimes all original team members may not be able to take a week during October for the site visit, and so substitute examiners join the team. The substitute examiner usually has a demanding task of reviewing all the work done to that point, but a thorough understanding of the applicant and the team's deliberations is critical for the substitute to succeed in working with the team. Preparation for the site visit requires as much work as each of the prior stages. Comment strength and OFI ratings are reviewed, and each strength must be "verified" and each OFI "clarified" during the team's visit to the applicant's organization to ensure that the applicant's favorable responses to the criteria (strengths) can be confirmed and that any ambiguities (OFIs) regarding the applicant's satisfaction of the criteria are clearly determined to either meet or not meet the criteria conditions. By the end of the site visit there can be no ambiguities regarding the applicant's adherence to the Baldrige criteria, and so examiners must plan carefully to ensure that the short time spent with the applicant's staff and facilities is spent optimally.

Before the site visit, examiners have two or three planning teleconferences, during which they review the application and begin to formulate approaches to evaluating the organization. A plan for evaluating each comment is detailed on a "site visit issue (SVI) worksheet," which includes the following:

- Comment
- Whether the comment is a strength or OFI
- Level of the comment ("double strength," "single strength," "single OFI," or "double OFI")
- Criteria issues involved in the comment
- People who should be interviewed regarding the comment
- Questions to ask regarding the comment
- Documents to review regarding the comment
- "Walk around questions" (i.e., questions to ask regarding the comment to staff members at the organization during random walks)
- Observations to make
- Findings on site
- Conclusions

The SVI worksheet becomes one of the examiner team's primary work products for the panel of judges, and so these documents contain exhaustive detail on how specific details of the application were addressed as well as the examiners' findings and evaluation of the organization's satisfaction of the Baldrige criteria. The judges must have confidence in the information provided by the examiner team so that the panel can make an informed decision regarding the applicant's suitability for the Baldrige Award.

Examiners may spend from 10 to 20 hours preparing for the site visit, gaining deeper insight into the organization and determining which questions will help verify strengths that were identified in earlier stages, as well as clarify OFIs. This process of verifying and clarifying strengths and OFIs provides the main focus of site visit activity. The site visit team arrives at the organization's city a day or two early to finalize plans for the visit, generally during an all-day meeting on the Sunday before the site visit starts. Examiners spend a great deal of time on Sunday finalizing SVI worksheets and performing final logistical planning before arriving at the organization's facility early Monday morning. The site visit begins with a brief introductory session during which the Baldrige site visit team leader briefly describes the purpose of the site visit and introduces the team members. The applicant's staff often makes a presentation that provides the team with more in-depth background on the organization and introduces the relevant leaders who will be interacting with the Baldrige team.

During the site visit, examiners spend their days interviewing individuals at all levels of the organization, asking the "walk-around" questions of employees they encounter, reviewing pertinent documents, and discussing their findings during frequent caucuses during the day. Each evening the team meets to summarize findings and complete SVI worksheets, with a goal of "closing" or completing as many SVI worksheets as possible each day. The team leader is a critical driver of this part of the process, watching progress of the team as the SVI worksheets are completed. As SVI worksheets are completed, they are taped to the wall so that all team members can review them, a practice called "walking the wall," writing comments on sticky notes and sticking them on the sheets for the examiner's use to improve the quality of the worksheet, and sometimes identifying new issues that did not surface during the Stage I and II reviews. SVI worksheets go through many revisions during the process, and the final product becomes an important part of the judges' information during final review of the applicants who received site visits. Each SVI worksheet deals with one comment from the scorebook, and final revision of that comment is the result of the resolved SVI. The revised comment then is rewritten to reflect the applicant's strengths or OFIs, and the new comment is incorporated into the evolving final scorebook that will be used by the judges' panel to make final decisions on which applicant will receive the MBNQA.

The document is finalized on the last day of the site visit, and all examiners on the site visit sign the final document to indicate their agreement with the report. The entire site visit takes about 1 week, and, of that time, examiners usually spend 4 days—about 40 to 48 hours—at the applicant's site. Workdays during the site visit are long, often 16 to 18 hours each day, and after the team spends an 8- to 10-hour day at the applicant's facility, team members return to the hotel and spend several hours each day reviewing data, updating SVI worksheets, and "walking the wall." The team usually meets for an hour or 2 each evening to review progress and update work plans. At the end of the week team members are usually pretty exhausted, but invariably everyone on the team believes that the experience has been rewarding and highly educational.

Every effort is made to secure the information collected and reported by examiners. The meeting room in the hotel is locked and secured so that no one from outside the team can access the information, and all information recorded on examiners' computers is deleted at the end of the site visit. Any applicant information used by the team in the meeting room is returned to the organization before the team departs, ensuring that all applicant information remains secure, and any notes or other papers produced by the team are packaged and returned to NIST for shredding and secure disposal. Site visits are confidential; in fact, examiners are instructed to not even tell their spouses or significant others where they are going for a week! ASQ sets up telephone numbers for emergency contact, so examiners are not completely isolated from family during the visit. The intense work effort and need for teamwork establishes close relationships among examiners, who form strong friendships with their team members.

After the site visit cycle is completed in October, the judges' panel meets during the second week in November, reviews the final scorebooks and SVI worksheets, and comes to a final determination of the Baldrige recipients for that year. The judges' panel sometimes requires more information from the team leader to better understand any issues with the submitted materials, and team leaders may spend an hour or more on the telephone with the judges to ensure that the applicant receives the best possible review. Once the judges have deliberated, the Baldrige recipients in each category are recommended to the Secretary of Commerce, who confirms the choices and makes the announcement. The awards are presented to the recipients by the President or Vice President at the annual Quest for Excellence held in the spring of the year after the award process.

■ Baldrige Core Values

Baldrige core values provide the conceptual framework for the criteria and, as such, are embedded in the criteria requirements. These values are characteristic of high performing organizations and generate a results-oriented culture that fosters communication and feedback leading to effective action to sustain and grow the organization. The Baldrige core values are as follows:

- Visionary leadership
- Patient-focused excellence
- Organizational and personal learning

- Valuing work force members and partners
- Agility
- Focus on the future
- Managing for innovation
- Management by fact
- Societal responsibility and community health
- Focus on results and creating value
- Systems perspective

Visionary Leadership

A primary goal of senior leaders must include the establishment of a leadership system that includes all stakeholders, including healthcare providers, administrative staff, governance members, and operational leaders to align the business and healthcare functions of the organization. These key leadership groups must be deeply involved in setting organizational goals and objectives that balance stakeholder needs. Leaders must have a shared vision for the organization that translates to development of strategies, systems, and processes for achieving performance excellence and to build a knowledge-based organization to ensure long-term sustainability. Senior leaders should be dedicated to stimulating innovation among the entire work force and creating a culture that cultivates change.

Governance assumes an important role in the Baldrige value of visionary leadership. The governance body represents all stakeholders in matters of ethics and all organizational activities, and members of the board must be engaged in setting the vision. Board members and senior leaders "live the vision" and act as role models through ethical behavior and participation in activities that sustain the organization. Executives are expected to lead planning and effectively communicate the vision and to inculcate the vision in future leaders through development of a succession planning program that ensures that the vision persists. This modeling behavior reinforces expectations of the rest of the work force to demonstrate the ethics and commitment to performance excellence represented by the vision.

Patient-Focused Excellence

Healthcare organizations have become more patient (customer) focused in the past few years, partly because of increased competition but also as a result of a growing consumer movement. Multiple methods of measuring provider performance and quality have arisen, including many that assess consumers' perceptions of care, such as the CAHPS surveys discussed in Chapter 4. All aspects of patient care now are subject to some type of review, including support services like billing, transportation, and food service. The patient-focused organization addresses every aspect of patient care delivery, not just healthcare services, because every aspect of care that touches the patient is involved with creating customer value. Organizations that exhibit patient-focused excellence use data from past and current customers to anticipate the needs of future patients to improve current services and initiate new offerings to ensure competitiveness.

Patient safety has become a major consideration in the healthcare experience in recent years, and patient-focused excellence connotes attention to this critical aspect of care. The analysis of potential errors and directed preventive interventions for optimizing customer safety is one of the indications of this patient focus that show the organization's dedication to the customer experience. Additionally, methods of determining health and functional status outcomes become a natural part of the organization's approach to providing services, because optimization of the customer's results assumes increased importance in a patient-focused healthcare company. One measure of this initiative is increasing involvement of each individual and family in making decisions about their health care, which requires an effective approach to patient and family education to support informed decisions. Segmenting measurements in a variety of ways (e.g., by provider, by demographic characteristics of patients, and by clinical condition) helps the organization target areas for improvement and makes the best use of improvement resources. Measures such as access to care, breadth of healthcare services, and patient/family conveniences like easy parking, "room service" style food service, and accommodations for families often indicate a higher level of performance in this core value.

Accreditation by the appropriate oversight body is a baseline expectation for any healthcare organization, but the patient-focused enterprise seeks to achieve higher levels of performance by trying to eliminate errors and complaints. Stakeholders view certification and accreditation as a requirement to open the doors for business, but those organizations that publish their measures are more credible. In addition, the patient-focused approach includes methods of dealing with errors and service lapses that address the needs of the customer and moves to ameliorate the issue and fully inform the consumer of the problem. These approaches comprise a subset of customer-centered processes that deal not just with basic needs but also with the more advanced requirements that differentiate a healthcare organization from competitors. For example, convenience clinics have become competitive with primary care providers because of more convenient hours of operation and locations that attract families constrained by work schedules and other access issues. These factors all contribute to patients' and stakeholders' views of the organization and help define the concept of patient-focused excellence.

Patient-focused excellence creates a paradigm shift for many healthcare organizations that have traditionally concentrated on facilities, equipment, and other provider issues. Hospitals and other providers have found that obtaining and retaining patient loyalty, as well as gaining referrals of new patients, helps build market share in competitive markets and ensure sustainability. Effective application of this approach requires consistent understanding of changing patient, stakeholder, and market requirements (i.e., the voice of the customer) that enhance customer engagement. These philosophical tenets must translate into cultural changes that emphasize the needs of the customer and stakeholders over other considerations.

Organizational and Personal Learning

Businesses are recognizing that the business intelligence in the work force represents a key component of competitiveness and sustainability. Increasing emphasis on the collection, storage, and retrieval of this organizational knowledge has become a major initiative for many companies, including those in health care. Information about specific services, processes, procedures, and necessary policies must be captured and stored so it is not lost if a valued employee leaves the company. Systematic sharing of knowledge across multiple departments and divisions can be a critical element for success in complex organizations with many horizontal and vertical partitions. Not only is information sharing important, but growth in personal and organizational knowledge bases has also become crucial for organizational development and sustainability. Organizational learning involves both continuous improvement of existing approaches and quantum change or innovation, leading to new processes and objectives that take the organization to higher levels of performance. High functioning organizations have learning systems entrenched in their operations that capture both the machinations of process management and the innovative flashes that can sometimes lead to a "leap forward." Every worker in an organization should be encouraged to continually learn about the company's work processes and consider opportunities for improvement that are then entered into a system to identify the "good catches." As data are accumulated, a systematic method of collating and sharing the information among individuals, departments, and the rest of the enterprise can ensure that the knowledge is leveraged optimally to improve operations, quality, and profitability. Innovation can then be rewarded as others in the organization see the possibilities for applying the information in other areas.

A learning organization can benefit customers in a number of ways:

- New and improved healthcare services that can benefit individuals and the community
- New healthcare business opportunities that expand the organization's marketability
- Increased use of evidence-based approaches to medicine and management
- Improved business functioning through better cycle time and reduced waste
- Enhanced productivity and effectiveness in human and physical resource usage

Individual success in the workplace relies increasingly on leveraging opportunities for personal learning and for applying new acquired skills. This requirement spans the entire work force, including leaders and employees, and, importantly, other workers in the organization like volunteers. Because volunteers are innate to the healthcare industry, ensuring that these important resources are optimally trained and involved in sharing organizational learning has become even more acute in the complex medical industry today. The investments made in personal learning through education, training, and other opportunities for continuing growth and development can include tactics like job rotation and incentives such as bonuses and pay raises for the attainment of new skills that benefit patient services. Practitioners may be rewarded for continuing educational activities that build on their existing skill sets and for specialized training for new skills germane to the changing healthcare environment. Progressive learning organizations often deploy multiple methods of developing the work force, such as computer-based training and tracking systems to ensure professional educational requirements are met.

Work force development through personal learning often enhances the relationship between individual workers and the company in several ways:

- Increased staff satisfaction and engagement
- Enhanced worker versatility through job sharing and other skill-development activities
- Better retention and recruitment opportunities
- Cross-functional training that decreases overtime and work force size
- Growth in knowledge assets
- Creation of a culture of innovation

Satisfaction of this core value has the potential for not only improving the quality of services and work force productivity but also for increasing worker satisfaction, retention, and recruitment. These advantages translate directly into greater performance, profitability, and sustainability.

Valuing Work Force Members and Partners

Engaging the work force of the 21st century is a significant challenge for most organizations. Workers today seek meaningful work, clear direction from leaders, and performance accountability that includes aligned incentives. Unlike the work force just a few decades ago, today's workers are culturally diverse and have an array of skills that must be used creatively to stimulate productivity and ensure satisfaction. The core value of valuing work force members and partners involves dedicating the necessary resources to ensure that workers can engage successfully in the work effort while ensuring satisfaction and a sense of security. Related to the personal learning core value, workers also expect an organizational commitment to development of their careers through flexibility in the work system to accommodate training needs and work–life balance. Several factors must be considered in effectively addressing work force requirements:

- Leadership commitment to work force success
- Programs for recognition with incentive above the regular compensation system
- Developing opportunities for professional development and progression
- Knowledge sharing to improve communications and performance
- Creating a culture that encourages appropriate risk taking and innovation
- Supporting cultural and individual diversity

Highly effective organizations lean to partnerships with both internal and external supply chain constituents to create efficiencies that achieve goals at lower costs. In a healthcare setting internal partners include administrators, staff members, physicians and independent practitioners, and, in some cases, labor unions. External partners may involve suppliers, equipment vendors, drug companies, educational institutions, payers, community organizations, and business service providers like environmental services vendors. Integrating these various stakeholders requires prodigious skill and supreme diplomacy, but world class organizations can create the environment in which all these important organizational elements integrate synergistically to optimize customer value. Collaboration on opportunities to economize operations, develop new service lines, cross-train with various links in the supply chain, or formulate cross-functional teams leverage these associations for improving organizational effectiveness and ensuring that all stakeholders feel valued as partners.

One major challenge in healthcare organizations hinges on gaining physician engagement in organizational quality activities, but given the appropriate incentives physicians can become leaders of initiatives to promote patient safety and customer satisfaction. Increasingly, healthcare organizations are entering into strategic partnerships with other companies that may have once been considered competitors. As reimbursements shrink, the ability for every hospital to invest in high cost equipment like magnetic resonance imaging (MRI) scanners has been greatly diminished, and optimal utilization would seem to indicate that not every institution needs its own MRI scanner. Thus strategic partnerships may be formed to create imaging centers that can be used by several organizations to reduce the initial investment cost and ensure adequate volume to justify the cost of the machine.

Partnerships with other organizations also serve the need for addressing issues like public health needs, such as equity and access to care and collection of comparative performance data. Valuing partners means that all collaborators understand the importance of the relationship to each organization. As such, the partners not only address key requirements at the onset of the relationship but also revisit these requirements throughout the affiliation. Communication strategies should be designed to ensure this continual emphasis on satisfying the needs of all partners in the association.

Agility

To claim that the healthcare industry changes rapidly today is an understatement. Agility relates to the capacity for rapid change and flexibility that can keep health care viable in the present tumultuous environment. Approaches like lean and six sigma have become necessary for organizations just to compete successfully, and, applied effectively, these advanced management techniques can provide an advantage by reducing cycle time and improving responsiveness to customer requirements. Planning and introduction cycles for new services have been shortened much as in other industries, and providers, payers, and other stakeholders must be ready for any contingency by fostering a constant state of readiness and the ability to change to meet new challenges quickly. The regulatory environment can change dramatically in a very short time, forcing changes in health companies that must be swift to ensure compliance in an ever more complicated legal milieu. New approaches like lean, six sigma, and rapid cycle improvement strategies must be deployed to meet these dilemmas, and organizations adopting these approaches must develop new work systems, reducing complexity and non–value added work to streamline the organization and improve responsiveness. By using lean techniques like rapid changeover and optimized takt time, providers can become sufficiently reactive to remain competitive.

Service delivery systems must be adapted quickly to changes in clinical evidence that may alter the environment. For example, the advent of the Centers for Medicare and Medicaid Services' decision not to pay for "never events" (clinical conditions caused by lack of effective care or medical errors, like pressure ulcers, surgical infections, central line infections) required healthcare providers to take drastic action to reduce the incidence of these events or risk incurring huge, non-reimbursable costs. Systems designs must include appropriate feedback methods to ensure organizational learning to decrease cycle and response times. Measurement systems need to be sensitive enough to detect early signs of change that trigger organizational response. An agile healthcare organization thus includes cycle time as a key metric in its operations. The focus on time often drives aggressive attention to process improvement as a way of reducing cost and waste, which must always be balanced with quality and customer satisfaction.

Focus on the Future

Just as agility centers attention on the present and near term, the Baldrige core value focus on the future takes the longer term view that integrates the current environment with trends in local, regional, and national environments that influence the organization's future course of action. Sustainability requires rapid response, but that responsiveness must be placed in the context of the organization's history and future. As discussed in previous chapters, an effective leader is capable of systems thinking—being able to understand how all of the parts in a system combine to create the system's output. A focus on the future implies that leaders cannot only understand how the system's output is created in the present but also project that performance into the future and determine what system factors must be altered to ensure future performance. Long-term sustainability and growth require leaders to understand and predict the changing role of the organization in the future and simultaneously create the vision needed to ensure that all stakeholder needs are met as the external environment evolves. Strategic planning is an essential tool for this core value, and assessment of the environment becomes a key step in the strategic planning process. Understanding anticipated changes in reimbursement systems, healthcare technology, patterns of disease and clinical conditions in the population, customer expectations, and strengths and vulnerabilities of competitors and partners all become crucial elements in an appraisal of the organization's future needs. As the planning process culminates in development of strategic objectives and tactics, all these environmental elements must be considered and addressed to ensure no "blind spots" that can later make the organization unsustainable. Effective organizations demonstrate this value by developing metrics that help predict the direction of the important variables (critical x's) in the organization's environment and then preparing leaders, workers, and strategic partners for future contingencies by encouraging innovative approaches to external challenges.

Managing for Innovation

Most people would recognize the term "innovation" as meaning a new way of doing something, but most would also acknowledge that innovation connotes not just incremental change but also a revolutionary notion that contributes to a dramatic change in a process, product, or service. For example, products like the Apple iPod and Apple iPhone revolutionized the music and communications industries and are considered innovations. Healthcare researchers work toward finding innovative ways of treating diseases, and over the history of medical research, innovations have been plentiful, like the discovery of antibiotics, telemetry for monitoring complex patients, and many successful surgical techniques. These innovations often led to changes in services, processes, and even the healthcare delivery model. World class healthcare organizations not only apply innovative solutions to their operations, but they also rely on their business and work systems to develop innovations that can help the organization adapt to change quickly and effectively. Innovation can no longer be the domain of medical research but indeed must suffuse the entire industry, from business practices to delivery of health services. Thus innovative methods of creating clinical guidelines and incorporating them into clinicians' workflow using automation might represent one innovation in health service delivery. Adding a robust mechanism to align incentives with effective application of best practices completes the cycle of innovation by integrating business and clinical processes to enhance organizational performance.

Innovation may cross many domains in a healthcare company, such as clinical practice, facility design, work organization, and information system infrastructure. Baldrige examiners look for evidence that leaders create the milieu and staff members work to optimize innovative approaches to sustaining and growing the organization by staffing and work systems, knowledge management, process management, and aligned incentives. Effective deployment of this core value through incorporation of approaches to creativity as part of the work environment provides that evidence.

Management by Fact

Just as physicians are increasingly being expected to conduct patient care using evidence-based guidelines, healthcare managers are becoming equally responsible for using evidence to administer organizations. Measuring and analyzing performance has become not just a method of creating and sustaining an effective healthcare system, but it also provides the basis for accountability through reports of key measures to regulatory agencies and the general public. Measures span the gamut from clinical quality measures, like use of beta-blockers in myocardial infarction, to business metrics, like wait times in various departments or patient satisfaction levels with care. Public reporting has become more ubiquitous because of projects in states like Massachusetts, Florida, and many others that publish health provider statistics online for public viewing. Hospitals, physicians, and other institutions now have their performance reported on many key variables, providing the public with much more information than has been available in the past on effective healthcare service delivery and administrative efficiency. Thus the public has increasingly placed trust in the use of data to evaluate healthcare providers, making the need for management by fact more acute. Performance measurement involves not just process metrics but also information on healthcare outcomes. To effectively gauge organizational performance, administrators must monitor the enterprise contributions to community health using epidemiological data; organizational performance using lean metrics like throughput and wait times; clinical effectiveness though implementation rates of critical pathways, care maps, and practice guidelines; and financial performance with billing and collections measures and metrics on management of the organization's cash reserves.

Highly effective organizations not only perform these measurements and use them for decision making, but they also segment the data to ensure all stakeholder needs are being met. For example, financial data may be segmented by payer to determine which payers are providing reimbursement in a timely manner and at sustainable rates. Clinical data may be segmented by provider to determine which providers are adhering to clinical guidelines or by clinical condition to assess the organization's performance in caring for a specific disease entity. The widely accepted concept of transforming data from raw input into organizational knowledge is tackled by high performers through analysis and evaluation that includes advanced statistical approaches tempered with the human oversight that creates wisdom. The analysis performed by many organizations may be used to support a foregone conclusion, but high functioning organizations use the data analysis to find new meaning that better supports innovation and effective decision making.

In the competitive healthcare sector, benchmarks and comparisons may be difficult to find, but effective companies look to other industries for benchmarks as well. For example, many of the "hotel services" at hospitals now are compared with benchmarks from the hospitality industry, often setting higher levels of performance than available healthcare benchmarks. An important consideration for selection of measures and comparators, however, is that metrics should relate to key requirements for business effectiveness and efficiency so they can directly influence long-term sustainability. Thus, management by fact in the Baldrige framework should lead to selection of clinical and administrative measures related to those factors.

Not only should indicators address key factors and processes, but they also need to be tailored to fit the decision-making process. For example, some measures may require constant monitoring (e.g., mortality rates in the intensive care unit), whereas others may need less frequent observation, like days' receivables, which may be reviewed only monthly. The fast pace of change in health care has made timely measurement a prime consideration in the Baldrige core value of management by fact. Completion of the measurement loop must include periodic reevaluation of metrics to ensure that the measures continue to be valid, are needed to monitor organizational progress, and that measurement systems remain adequate to provide precise, accurate data.

Societal Responsibility and Community Health

Medical organizations irrefutably have a significant responsibility to society as well as to the populations each one serves. Care for individual consumers must be safe and high quality, and the contribution to community health is manifold—from improving immunization rates and use of primary screening procedures to ensuring that medical waste does not seep into a community's environment. This responsibility is manifest in a number of ways within a medical provider organization. For example, as part of ongoing communications to the enterprise, leaders should help coworkers understand public responsibilities. Additionally, leaders are involved in community activities and demonstrate ethical behavior in their relationships with other community entities. Strategic planning processes include consideration of community needs and well-being as part of the prioritization process as well as the effects of organizational activities on community health. Operational metrics at responsible organizations include those that measure environmental impact and community health measures to monitor the organization's social footprint. Good business operations (i.e., exercising economical management approaches) also demonstrate conservation of resources to optimize community or stakeholder benefits. The waste reduction that was the topic of Chapter 6 demonstrates good management as well as stewardship of resources.

Organizations that demonstrate effective planning and measurement ensure that information systems and work systems reinforce the aims for ensuring social responsibility. Information systems must be designed to monitor community impact and detect detrimental changes before they become widespread. Early detection implies having operational responses in place to mitigate any untoward effects as well as having work systems that encourage workers to respond effectively. Baseline expectations require healthcare providers to meet local, state, and federal laws and to be accredited by the appropriate oversight agency (e.g., The Joint Commission for hospitals), but world class organizations view these requirements as springboards for higher levels of performance by exceeding the requirements as frequently as possible.

Social responsibility also implies a high level of ethical behavior. Indications of a concentration on ethics include clear expectations of behavior among leaders and staff, with methods of detecting and reporting ethical lapses that are anonymous and effective. Workers should never feel threatened when reporting apparent ethical issues, and so anonymity is usually a prerequisite to an effective reporting system. Not only is the reporting system ubiquitous and robust, but the methods by which workers interact with all stakeholders are steeped in ethical principles and monitored for adherence to the corporate behavioral expectations. Ultimately, the governance body is accountable for organizational ethics, and so a clear line should be evident between front-line behavior and board understanding of adherence to guidelines. In a healthcare organization ethical conduct subsumes both business and clinical circumstances, and the organization's reporting system should ensure that all applicable Health Insurance Portability and Accountability Act (HIPAA) regulations regarding protected health information are observed.

These elements of corporate citizenship should suffuse the entire industry: not just providers but payers and suppliers like drug companies and other vendors as well. Ensuring societal well-being must be a goal of all health-related organizations, because peoples' lives literally depend on this attribute. Thus providers, vendors, and payers might collaborate to ensure meeting the health needs of those with impeded access to care through such venues as free clinics or subsidized health insurance or medication programs. World class organizations not only understand their local market needs for these types of programs but also have a systems view to promote such efforts on a larger scale through participation in professional organizations that can expand these community action programs to a larger scale. In the vein of "you can't manage what you don't measure," these high performing organizations ensure that metrics are developed to ensure organizational compliance with these efforts.

Focus on Results and Creating Value

Making "focus on results" one of the core values of the MBNQA indicates the importance of actually demonstrating that an organization is performing the tasks that it purports to do. Just as the healthcare industry has turned from a process orientation to outcomes, so does the MBNQA emphasize results as a key feature of a high performing organization. In fact, of the 1,000 potential points tallied by examiners on an applicant's submission, 450 points relate to category 7. Thus a Baldrige applicant's metrics must focus on results and outcomes. The concept of "creating value" also holds organizations to understanding and then satisfying the many stakeholder value propositions as part of its determination of success. Creating balance between all the different value propositions is one of the key leadership tasks and demonstrates the effectiveness of the organization's structure and operations. Nearly all stakeholders are most interested in operational results rather than the processes needed to achieve the results. Thus creating high performing outcomes can be used to build market share, customer loyalty, and community benefits. However, to achieve high levels of performance, organizational planning must clearly recognize key stakeholder requirements as part of the strategic plan and design strategies and tactics with metrics to meet those expectations and ensure that corporate operations are developed to meet these sometimes conflicting needs.

Systems Perspective

Just as healthcare providers are increasingly called on to understand the systems perspective of their work, leaders must share the systems perspective to understand the "anatomy and physiology" of the organization. Imbuing and sharing the systems perspective requires understanding of the business and clinical systems through metrics and process management oversight as well as a dedicated communications infrastructure to disseminate the information. The Baldrige criteria span six system-oriented categories that must be integrated to ensure proper functioning across the enterprise. Successful performance management mandates alignment and integration across operations and departments within the organization. Many organizations have used the Baldrige criteria as a basis for developing a systems perspective and achieving the integration that leads to alignment and streamlined operations. This application of the criteria (i.e., as a strategic business approach) ensures that measures, indicators, core competencies, and organizational knowledge are all integrated as guide operations yet also builds on strengths to promote continuous improvement. Linking and aligning resources to achieve organizational strategic goals can result in greater efficiencies and an enhanced value proposition.

■ Baldrige Criteria: Basis for Evaluation

The Baldrige criteria provide the framework examiners use to analyze applications and are related to the core values shown in TABLE 8.1. Each of the results items relates to one or more of the first six categories, usually termed the "approach/deployment" categories because they answer the question "How does your organization…?." Each of the results items has an equal score, except for item 7.1, which is weighted slightly more heavily because it relates to the organization's core business results.

Table 8.1	Baldrige Criteria and Core Values	
Results Item Number	Organizational Functional Area	Approach/Deployment Category
7.1	Health care outcomes	All
7.2	Customer-focused outcomes	3
7.3	Financial and market outcomes	All
7.4	Work force systems outcomes	5
7.5	Process effectiveness outcomes	6
7.6	Leadership, governance, societal responsibility results	1, 2

Criteria Are Nonprescriptive

Another important characteristic of the Baldrige criteria is that they are nonprescriptive, that is, the criteria do not have specific elements that must be present to attain a specific score. Thus the criteria do not serve as a checklist to be met but rather provide guidance for the attributes expected of a high performing organization. It is the job of applicants to match their organizational structure and processes to those attributes. The criteria do not prescribe organizational structure or governance, such as the need for specific departments or board of directors' composition. Rather the criteria specify that the structure implemented by senior leaders should satisfy the requirements of the criteria to address specific issues such as ethics monitoring and compliance. The criteria do not specify the use of a particular management style or use of a certain quality framework. As long as the management system provides the ability for organizational leaders to articulate the vision and implement the organization's mission and values to achieve high performance, the actual structure is not at issue. Thus the criteria do not specify an ideal "Baldrige company" but rather provide a framework within which an organization can attain world class performance by ensuring that the tenets of exemplary performance are met. The Baldrige framework focuses on results attained by the enterprise, not on particular procedures, tools, or a specific organizational structure. The Baldrige program is designed more to learn about innovative business practices than to outline the practices that might work.

The MBNQA program recognizes that multiple factors underlie the selection of a management style or tools and approaches to improvement. For example, the business environment that is detailed in the organizational profile section of each application can be a powerful force in determining some of the acceptable approaches to management and improvement. Organizational relationships with other companies and stakeholders in the industry can influence decisions regarding management reporting tools and ethical requirements. The Baldrige focus on common requirements, rather than on specifying procedures or structures, allows latitude that encourages diversity and creativity.

Criteria Are Adapted to Health Care

When the business criteria were first designed in 1988, the award was primarily directed toward the manufacturing sector. When the healthcare sector was added to the award program in 1998, the business criteria were adapted to reflect the unique nature of the healthcare industry. For example, organizational missions vary substantially between payers and providers or between teaching and research institutions. The relationship between providers and patients has distinctive properties that differ from typical vendor–customer relationships. Physician roles in the system vary from vendor to customer to primary stakeholder in some cases. In short, the criteria for health care have been crafted to accommodate these differences between the various entities in health care and the rest of the business community.

Criteria Promote a Systems Perspective

As discussed previously, cogent business leaders have the ability to view a business system and understand the parts and how they interact, much as a health professional understands anatomy and physiology as the basis for improving a patient's health. The criteria are designed to view an organization as a system, with multiple components that function within the major criteria categories (leadership, strategic planning, market knowledge, knowledge management, work force systems, process management, and results). Rather than simply evaluating each of the functional areas, however, the criteria are written to determine that leaders and work force have integrated the functional areas to ensure optimum performance. The Baldrige program values integration as one of the important characteristics of high performing organizations, reflected in higher scoring levels for demonstrated integration. FIGURE 8.3 is an adaptation of a Baldrige diagram that shows the importance of integration in determining the scoring "band," or range, for each category. Examiners use this diagram to conceptualize the relationship between systematization in an applicant organization and the level of scoring that the organization earns.

The criteria promote linkages between individual items and across categories to support the systems perspective that exemplifies Baldrige recipients. For example, the strategic planning process relies on senior leaders to balance short- and long-term challenges (item 2.1(b)(2)), work systems (item 2.1(a)(5)), market knowledge (item 2.1(a)(2), measurement systems (item 2.2(b)), and process management (item 2.2). Most criteria items cross all categories, emphasizing the systematic nature of the criteria and the integration expected of a world class organization. One of the primary linkages occurs in the results category (category 7, items 7.1–7.6). Integration between business units is often reflected in process and outcome measures that are related because processes link and depend on each other. With the interdependencies that accompany integration, shared or cross-unit metrics demonstrate the level of integration. The criteria anticipate cycles of improvement based on the metrics, requiring agility and innovation to align efforts to continually improve. In addition to the project improvement stages discussed in earlier chapters, the criteria also request evidence of organizational learning and feedback loops that demonstrate these learning cycles.

Criteria Have 18 Performance-Oriented Requirements

Once examiners have evaluated an application, the next step is to assign a score to each of the items within each category. Scoring guidelines assist with this task. Guidelines have been created for the approach/deployment categories (categories 1–6) and the results category (category 7). These guidelines for the 2009 Healthcare Criteria are presented in TABLE 8.2 and can be found on the Malcolm Baldrige website at http://www.baldrige.gov/HealthCare_Criteria.htm. Using the criteria and the scoring guidelines, examiners are able to assess each application and assign scores according to a standardized, objective process. Examiners evaluate each of the criteria items (e.g., item 2.1 or item 3.2) and select a scoring band from the guidelines. Each item is

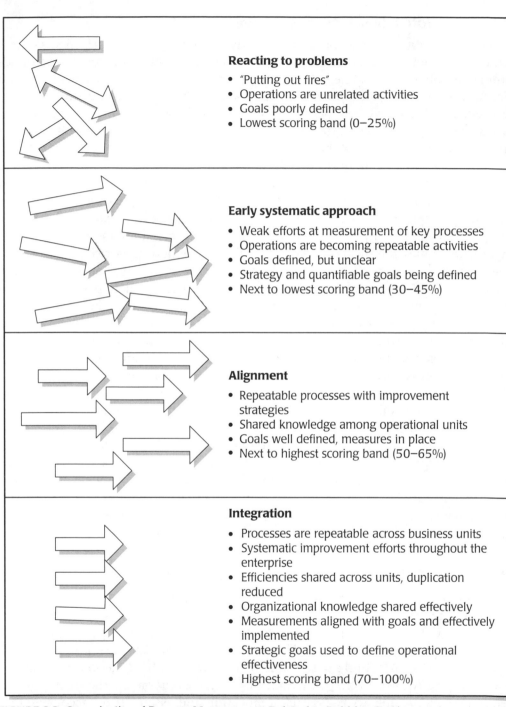

Reacting to problems

- "Putting out fires"
- Operations are unrelated activities
- Goals poorly defined
- Lowest scoring band (0–25%)

Early systematic approach

- Weak efforts at measurement of key processes
- Operations are becoming repeatable activities
- Goals defined, but unclear
- Strategy and quantifiable goals being defined
- Next to lowest scoring band (30–45%)

Alignment

- Repeatable processes with improvement strategies
- Shared knowledge among operational units
- Goals well defined, measures in place
- Next to highest scoring band (50–65%)

Integration

- Processes are repeatable across business units
- Systematic improvement efforts throughout the enterprise
- Efficiencies shared across units, duplication reduced
- Organizational knowledge shared effectively
- Measurements aligned with goals and effectively implemented
- Strategic goals used to define operational effectiveness
- Highest scoring band (70–100%)

FIGURE 8.3 Organizational Process Management Related to Baldrige Scoring

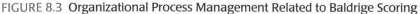

Table 8.2	Scoring Guidelines	
Score	Process (For Use With Categories 1–6)	Results (For Use With Category 7)
0% or 5%	• No SYSTEMATIC APPROACH to Item requirements is evident; information is ANECDOTAL. (A) • Little or no DEPLOYMENT of any SYSTEMATIC APPROACH is evident. (D) • An improvement orientation is not evident; improvement is achieved through reacting to problems. (L) • No organizational ALIGNMENT is evident; individual areas or work units operate independently. (I)	• There are no organizational PERFORMANCE RESULTS and/or poor RESULTS in areas reported. (Le) • TREND data either are not reported or show mainly adverse TRENDS. (T) • Comparative information is not reported. (C) • RESULTS are not reported for any areas of importance to the accomplishment of your organization's MISSION. No PERFORMANCE PROJECTIONS are reported. (I)
10%, 15%, 20%, or 25%	• The beginning of a SYSTEMATIC APPROACH to the BASIC REQUIREMENTS of the Item is evident. (A) • The APPROACH is in the early stages of DEPLOYMENT in most areas or work units, inhibiting progress in achieving the BASIC REQUIREMENTS of the Item. (D) • Early stages of a transition from reacting to problems to a general improvement orientation are evident. (L) • The APPROACH is ALIGNED with other areas or work units largely through joint problem solving. (I)	• A few organizational PERFORMANCE RESULTS are reported, and early good PERFORMANCE LEVELS are evident in a few areas. (Le) • Some TREND data are reported, with some adverse TRENDS evident. (T) • Little or no comparative information is reported. (C) • RESULTS are reported for a few areas of importance to the accomplishment of your organization's MISSION. Limited or no PERFORMANCE PROJECTIONS are reported. (I)
30%, 35%, 40%, or 45%	• An EFFECTIVE, SYSTEMATIC APPROACH, responsive to the BASIC REQUIREMENTS of the Item, is evident. (A) • The APPROACH is DEPLOYED, although some areas or work units are in early stages of DEPLOYMENT. (D) • The beginning of a SYSTEMATIC APPROACH to evaluation and improvement of KEY PROCESSES is evident. (L) • The APPROACH is in the early stages of ALIGNMENT with your basic organizational needs identified in response to the Organizational Profile and other Process Items. (I)	• Good organizational PERFORMANCE LEVELS are reported for some areas of importance to the Item requirements. (Le) • Some TREND data are reported, and a majority of the TRENDS presented are beneficial. (T) • Early stages of obtaining comparative information are evident. (C) • RESULTS are reported for many areas of importance to the accomplishment of your organization's MISSION. Limited PERFORMANCE PROJECTIONS are reported. (I)

(continues)

Table 8.2	Scoring Guidelines (continued)	
Score	Process (For Use With Categories 1–6)	Results (For Use With Category 7)
50%, 55%, 60%, or 65%	• An EFFECTIVE, SYSTEMATIC APPROACH, responsive to the OVERALL REQUIREMENTS of the Item, is evident. (A) • The APPROACH is well DEPLOYED, although DEPLOYMENT may vary in some areas or work units. (D) • A fact-based, SYSTEMATIC evaluation and improvement PROCESS and some organizational LEARNING, including INNOVATION, are in place for improving the efficiency and EFFECTIVENESS of KEY PROCESSES. (L) • The APPROACH is ALIGNED with your organizational needs identified in response to the Organizational Profile and other Process Items. (I)	• Good organizational PERFORMANCE LEVELS are reported for most areas of importance to the Item requirements. (Le) • Beneficial TRENDS are evident in areas of importance to the accomplishment of your organization's MISSION. (T) • Some current PERFORMANCE LEVELS have been evaluated against relevant comparisons and/or benchmarks and show areas of good relative PERFORMANCE. (C) • Organizational PERFORMANCE RESULTS are reported for most KEY student, STAKEHOLDER, market, and PROCESS requirements. PERFORMANCE PROJECTIONS for some high-priority RESULTS are reported. (I)
70%, 75%, 80%, or 85%	• An EFFECTIVE, SYSTEMATIC APPROACH, responsive to the MULTIPLE REQUIREMENTS of the Item, is evident. (A) • The APPROACH is well DEPLOYED, with no significant gaps. (D) • Fact-based, SYSTEMATIC evaluation and improvement and organizational LEARNING, including INNOVATION, are KEY management tools; there is clear evidence of refinement as a result of organizational-level ANALYSIS and sharing. (L) • The APPROACH is INTEGRATED with your organizational needs identified in response to the Organizational Profile and other Process Items. (I)	• Good to excellent organizational PERFORMANCE LEVELS are reported for most areas of importance to the Item requirements. (Le) • Beneficial TRENDS have been sustained over time in most areas of importance to the accomplishment of your organization's MISSION. (T) • Many to most TRENDS and current PERFORMANCE LEVELS have been evaluated against relevant comparisons and/or BENCHMARKS and show areas of leadership and very good relative PERFORMANCE. (C) • Organizational PERFORMANCE RESULTS are reported for most KEY student, STAKEHOLDER, market, PROCESS, and ACTION PLAN requirements, and they include some PROJECTIONS of your future PERFORMANCE. (I)

Table 8.2		
Score	Process (For Use With Categories 1–6)	Results (For Use With Category 7)
90%, 95%, or 100%	• An EFFECTIVE, SYSTEMATIC APPROACH, fully responsive to the MULTIPLE REQUIREMENTS of the Item, is evident. (A) • The APPROACH is fully DEPLOYED without significant weaknesses or gaps in any areas or work units. (D) • Fact-based, SYSTEMATIC evaluation and improvement and organizational LEARNING through INNOVATION are KEY organization-wide tools; refinement and INNOVATION, backed by ANALYSIS and sharing, are evident throughout the organization. (L) • The APPROACH is well INTEGRATED with your organizational needs identified in response to the Organizational Profile and other Process Items. (I)	• Excellent organizational PERFORMANCE LEVELS are reported for most areas of importance to the Item requirements. (Le) • Beneficial TRENDS have been sustained over time in all areas of importance to the accomplishment of your organization's MISSION. (T) • Evidence of education sector and BENCHMARK leadership is demonstrated in many areas. (C) • Organizational PERFORMANCE RESULTS fully address KEY student, STAKEHOLDER, market, PROCESS, and ACTION PLAN requirements, and they include PROJECTIONS of your future PERFORMANCE. (I)

associated with a point value, as shown in TABLE 8.3. The scoring bands provide a range of percentages of the total possible points for each item; thus the scoring band from 30% to 45% when applied to item 1.2 indicates that the numeric score falls between 15 and 22.5 (rounded to 23). Examiners are trained to narrow the item score into one of the bands using the ADLI (approach-deployment-linkages-integration) standards for categories 1 to 6 and the LeTCI (levels-trends-comparisons-integration) for category 7. Each of the questions or statements in the guidelines allows the examiner to determine which of the standards within each band is most appropriate and, once a band is selected, to decide if the application's responses fit in the upper, middle, or lower part of the band. The score that is entered into the examiner's scorebook is the percentage that best fits with the applicant's responses to the criteria language.

The criteria define 18 specific areas of focus, each of which requires responses to specific questions regarding the approaches and methods of deployment for the objective. For an applicant this clearly defined and integrated set of objectives provides a comprehensive management tool to determine the organization's level of performance. For the examiner the information in the application serves as the basis for the assessment of performance. The examiner's evaluation includes determination of the applicant's strengths (things that the organization does well) or OFIs that indicate a difference between the applicant's response and the criteria requirements. The resulting profile is an effective management tool to guide leaders in directing improvement efforts. Because a panel of six or more experienced examiners performs the evaluation, the

Table 8.3				Scores by Item for the Baldrige Criteria	
Item Number	Approach	Deployment	Results	Description	Points
1.1	X			How senior leaders demonstrate leadership	70
1.2	X	X		Governance and social responsibility	50
2.1	X			Strategy development	40
2.2		X		Strategy deployment	45
3.1	X	X		Stakeholder/patient engagement	40
3.2	X	X		Obtaining and using patient information	45
4.1	X	X		Measure, analyze, and improve performance	45
4.2	X	X		Knowledge management and information infrastructure	45
5.1	X	X		Work force engagement, leadership development	45
5.2	X	X		Work force capability and capacity, work environment	40
6.1	X	X		Work systems design, key work processes, emergency readiness	35
6.2	X	X		Design, manage, improve work processes	50
7.1			X	Health care services results	100
7.2			X	Patient and stakeholder satisfaction results	70
7.3			X	Financial and market results	70
7.4			X	Work force performance results	70
7.5			X	Process effectiveness results	70
7.6			X	Leadership and social responsibility results	70

resulting feedback report, based on a consensus of all examiners who reviewed the application, can serve as a high level consultants' report on the business.

■ Structure of a Baldrige Application

Understanding the Current State: Organizational Profile

Every Baldrige application starts with an organizational profile (OP) designed to provide a relatively high level overview of the applicant's enterprise. Several points are covered in the OP:

- Organization's business environment
- Key organizational relationships

- Market characteristics and competition
- Key collaborators
- Strategic context of the organization's business model
- Performance improvement system

This structured description helps examiners understand the nature of the business and the key factors that distinguish the organization and marketplace. This information is critical for the examiner team and judges to understand the business and to interpret the application in the appropriate context. In fact, the examiner's first task is to review the OP and craft a list of key factors that will be related to the responses in the application in each of the categories. As the examiner then compares the application responses to the criteria, the review is made in the context of four to six key factors that relate the applicant's important business concerns to each criteria item. This relationship is also helpful as applicant's review the final report (called the "feedback report"), because it demonstrates that the examiner team understood the applicant's responses.

For many applicants in the early stages of the Baldrige process, the OP may be the first time that managers and staff have taken the 30,000-foot view of the organization. Responding to the questions in the OP requires understanding critical elements like key internal and external influences in the business, as well as the central nature of the mission, vision, and values (often abbreviated to MVV in Baldrige-speak). Another important area of focus in the OP involves recognition of core competencies and how they relate to internal and external business factors within the context of the organization's competitive environment. The OP also requires identification of key competitors and enterprise partners, particularly those who directly influence the supply chain. The Baldrige framework has been constructed to acknowledge the importance of suppliers and other partners in a number of areas, from extension of business ethics (category 1) to process management and improvement (category 6). In short, the OP provides examiners, judges, and often organizational leaders, with a better understanding of the applicant's organization and its milieu, including the business factors needed for future growth.

P.1 Organizational Description: What Are Your Key Organizational Characteristics?

The first section of the OP addresses the organization's business fundamentals. Applicants must respond to questions regarding the MVV and identify core competencies, which when done properly can be difficult. Smaller businesses (e.g., medical practices) may not have gone through the exercise of creating a mission, vision, and statement of values; however, this part of the application may help them realize they have been operating with a de facto MVV that has simply been unstated and prompt leaders to codify these important business principles. This issue emphasizes the value of the Baldrige criteria and the application process as a substantive improvement tool, providing a framework for high performance.

Another important question to be answered in P.1 is that of core competencies. Many organizations grow through an evolutionary process, adding processes and services in response to perceived customer demand, with little regard as to the sustainability of the services or the net value to the organization and its customers. By identifying core competencies, leaders can determine if the most important business requirements are being met or if scarce resources are being wasted on less important products or services. By defining core competencies and melding them with MVV, leaders can best understand the fundamental nature of the organization and where to concentrate human and financial resources for sustainability and market differentiation. For that reason these items are the first to be requested as part of the Baldrige application.

As perhaps the most regulated U.S. sector, healthcare organizations must be accredited by organizations like The Joint Commission and pass inspections by a large panoply of federal, state, and local governmental agencies. Thus accreditations and certifications are considered by most health professionals as baseline requirements for doing business; however, high performing organizations look at these requirements not as pinnacles to be reached but as springboards for further improvement. Many regulations have varying levels of compliance, and world class organizations set the upper limits of these requirements as goals rather than a simple "passing score." In other words, satisfactory is not good enough. Examiners reviewing applications seek evidence of this philosophy as an indication that the organization is trying to reach higher performance levels. Exceptional performance in these business requirements usually translates to other areas of the organization, but it also demonstrates a commitment to quality as well as a greater likelihood of sustainability and risk mitigation.

Governance systems, including reporting relationships throughout the organization, have become particularly important in the past several years, and accountability of governing boards has become the subject of countless corporate debacles. High performing organizations have clearly defined functions and communications plans so that the MVV are clear to everyone, ethical standards are deployed effectively, and each member of management and the governance body understand their accountabilities in the system. Increasingly, board independence has become a major factor in ensuring true arms-length oversight that creates stakeholder confidence and attenuates legal liability. Because every healthcare organization deals with individual and population health, the need for every stakeholder, payer, and patient to feel confident that the organization is operating to ensure patient safety, outcomes, and satisfaction must be a key customer requirement. As noted above, suppliers and other business partners must participate in this accountability to ensure that the services delivered by the organization meet the highest quality standards.

P.2 Organizational Situation: What Is Your Organization's Strategic Situation?

In the past two decades competition in the healthcare industry has reached new heights. Few providers in leadership positions today could have foreseen the extent that competition has engulfed the industry, from the addition of marketing divisions in most good-sized healthcare organizations to the competitive advertising that now fills billboards and airwaves. This section of the OP requires an applicant to delve deeply into the business environment, whether it be within a city, a state, a region, or larger, to assess the competition and to identify partners. Health care is particularly intriguing from this standpoint: A local competitor might also be a collaborator in a public health program, such as community emergency preparedness. Thus leaders often walk a fine line between competition and cooperation, trying on one hand to create community value while on the other hand not disclosing those business "secrets" that maintain differentiation from competitors.

Additionally, an applicant must also identify key strategic assets and vulnerabilities. These important attributes are useful in understanding responses to the category items, because the organization's structure and processes reflect its approach to dealing with challenges by deploying its assets. Some of the more typical challenges are as follows:

- *Operational costs*: The cost of healthcare supplies is constantly rising.
- *Capital expenses*: Advancing technology demands investment to keep up and retain a competitive advantage.
- *Staffing*: Shortages of nurses and some medical specialties require organizational focus on work systems to effectively mitigate.
- *Market competition*: New developments like walk-in clinics or specialty hospitals create new competitive challenges that must be met.
- *Economic conditions*: The cyclical economy generates changes in demand and often the rapidity with which organizations are paid.
- *Public health and bioterrorism*: New investments are needed to ensure that a healthcare organization is ready for any eventuality, including environmental or human-produced disasters.
- *Compliance with changing regulations*: Regulations change constantly, requiring monitoring and response systems to ensure business continuity.
- *Major industry trends*: Operating patterns (e.g., a move to outpatient care for traditional inpatient services) are changing.

The criteria inquire more deeply into the specifics of these approaches and how well they are applied to meet the organization's challenges. Examiners focus on these approach/deployment descriptions and, coupled with the results attained (category 7), can decipher the effectiveness of the organization's operations. Additionally, this section of the OP allows applicants to distinguish themselves from others in the marketplace. Each company has unique characteristics, and understanding the assets and vulnerabilities helps examiners and judges better comprehend those distinctions.

Section P.2 also asks for sources of comparative and competitive data. Healthcare organizations often have difficulty finding and using comparative or competitive data, and the competitive environment in today's industry makes this effort even more challenging. However, high performing organizations often find data sources such as those discussed in Chapter 4, or even others that may provide comparisons in similar, but not the same, industries. For example, some Baldrige recipients have found customer satisfaction data in the hospitality industry to be effective in supplying comparisons for services like housekeeping and food services. Industrial production comparators may help with process-related issues in materials management, and medical service comparisons may be found with some of the organization's suppliers or customers (e.g., managed care organizations). High performing organizations find the need to compare themselves with others and reach for the highest levels of performance, and so invariably these world class companies find the most challenging comparisons possible.

Applicants must include a description of the performance improvement system in this part of the OP. Regardless of which of the concepts described in previous chapters has been deployed, the organization should have a systematic approach to improvement that ensures a continuous review and update for nearly all organizational processes. Metrics should incorporate methods of data collection and analysis that make indicators credible, and the use of the metrics is described in more detail in the criteria items. Additionally, applicants describe their approaches to improvement (e.g., using cycles of refinement and techniques for fostering innovation). A key element of the improvement approach, and a linkage between category 4 and category 6, is the use of improvement data to enhance organizational learning.

The OP provides a company overview for examiners and judges, but it also helps each applicant to concretely define its MVV, operations, and environment. Many applicants find that just creating the OP helps identify opportunities for improvement, whereas others find this effort frequently binds the team into a cohesive group to begin work on the improvement effort.

Leadership (Category 1, 120 points)

The fact that the leadership category is associated with the highest number of points of all the approach/deployment categories is no accident. The Baldrige program recognizes the importance of the leadership and governance structures in helping an organization achieve world class performance. Through a series of "how" questions, this category addresses senior leaders' involvement in providing guidance in areas such as ensuring deployment of the MVV and setting performance objectives. Communications strategies are of particular importance because they define the methods by which leaders exert influence and help determine the effectiveness of leadership efforts. Additionally, leaders are expected to work to continually improve their own performance and encourage others to continually learn and grow in the organization, including ensuring sustainability by grooming the next generation of leaders through succession planning and mentoring. Leaders are also the symbol of ethics for the organization, making the leaders in this effort especially consequential. Finally, governance structure and influence are considered key components of the leadership system and are described in this category.

Item 1.1 Senior Leadership: How Do Your Senior Leaders Lead? (70/120 Points)

The approaches that senior leaders use to exert their influence throughout the organization are the focus of this item. Responses address the issues of the leaders' roles in setting values and directions based on the MVV as well as how these key items are communicated in a manner to cause the organization to respond. Leaders must provide the vision that leads the organization into the future and ensure that a strong customer focus pervades the work force. The ability to set an environment that rewards innovation and promotes empowerment for the work force distinguishes leaders in this item, as does promotion of a continuous learning system that allows workers to expand their horizons and grow in the company. Healthcare organizations present a special challenge, however, because the leadership structure is often bifurcated into an administrative branch and a medical branch, consisting of physician leaders. The harmonization of these two groups of leaders is one of the key determinants of success, because the administrative and medical staff must be aligned to ensure that the MVV are served and objectives achieved. Unresolved conflict between these two parallel leadership cadres can prove devastating to a healthcare entity.

World class leaders commit their own efforts and organizational resources to developing future leaders through education and mentoring and to ensuring recognition for outstanding contributions by administrative and professional staff alike. As with any professional, the most effective senior leaders also participate in educational and personal development programs to enhance their own skills but also readily share those experiences with others. Their example sets the tone for organizational learning as a method of developing workers into a more effective force for organizational improvement and future leadership. This caliber of leader is not only a capable learner but is also effective as a teacher and mentor.

Item 1.2 Governance and Societal Responsibilities: How Do You Govern and Fulfill Your Societal Responsibilities? (50/120 Points)

Governance structure and function is the subject of the second item in the leadership category. Because governance bodies are ultimately accountable for the performance of the organization, issues such as legal and ethical monitoring and management are addressed, along with the processes used to ensure that the board is informed of operations and other critical programmatic issues. Governance boards should represent key stakeholders and, as such, provide guidance about how the organization can meet stakeholder needs most effectively and efficiently. Transparent communication between senior leaders and the board is a topic in this item, because that interaction provides the necessary information for effective board engagement. Although closely linked to senior leaders, the board must maintain a level of independence that ensures stakeholders that governance will protect stakeholder interests through vigilance and independent performance audits.

Governance members in healthcare organizations have increasing accountability in a number of areas:

- Ensuring high performance throughout the organization, from senior leaders to front-line workers to the most specialized providers
- Ensuring compliance with legal, regulatory, and accreditation requirements are met or exceeded
- Mitigating of risk factors, such as malpractice risk, biohazards, and public safety problems

Thus governance board members must be apprised of performance through reports of indicators but also often by personal commitment to spending time with staff members throughout the organization who can inform them of burgeoning issues. For many board members this responsibility entails learning about arcane healthcare measurement systems and issues that may not be within their scope of knowledge, and so the organization must have a method for board members to learn and understand technical issues in a way that makes sense to them. This learning experience is never a one-time event but rather a continuous effort to make certain that the board comprehends the issues facing the organization.

Commitment to the community (i.e., considering the system in which the organization operates) now includes such issues as resource conservation. "Green" technologies must be considered important by healthcare organizations because of the potential damage that can occur from disposing of hazardous wastes or contaminated fluids. Business operations must now contemplate energy conservation and "clean" energy sources, not only as a way of demonstrating social responsibility but also as a way of being economically sensible. Waste management is no longer a minor inconvenience but rather a significant issue to be managed. Compliance with regulators and accreditation activities are considered minimum requirements for operations, and high performing healthcare entities must exceed those baseline requirements to demonstrate exceptional performance.

The other major issue that this item subsumes is the community involvement expected of any contemporary, socially responsible company. These efforts obviously benefit the community, but, importantly, they should also be designed to provide some return for the company as well. For example, a hospital might sponsor a health fair that provides blood pressure screening and also distributes information about cardiovascular services. By emphasizing areas related to the organization's core competencies, there is a high likelihood that the activity may benefit both the organization and the community. Senior leaders' activities are also important in community outreach, because they often are asked to participate in a number of community organizations and events. Because their time is often scarce, a systematic approach to selecting beneficial activities can often produce substantive benefits. Aligning community outreach with the organization's MVV becomes an important function of the planning process.

Strategic Planning (Category 2, 85 Points)

Development of strategic plans has become a somewhat standard process in many larger healthcare organizations, but effective planning for and achievement of deployment are less pervasive. Creation of a strategic plan involves the following:

- Development of strategies based on data and organizational MVV
- Design of action plans that focus on resource optimization and high return on investment
- Deployment plans with realistic timelines and expectations of changes in metrics
- Assignment of resources to ensure plan success but avoid waste
- Change strategies that accommodate changing circumstances
- Measures of accomplishment
- Plans to sustain gains

Strategic plans generally include short-term and long-term goals and strategies, with timeframes that are realistic. For example, a short-term time horizon of 1 month is too short, whereas a short-term horizon of 4 years is typically too long. The short-term time horizon should be of sufficient duration to allow implementation of strategic initiatives and time to determine whether the initiatives changed associated metrics. Similarly, a long-term time horizon must be set with a timeframe that allows the organization to determine if longer term strategies (e.g., capital investments in property or equipment) have had a positive effect on associated measures. Long-term time horizons tend to allow time to focus on long-term sustainability, whereas short-term horizons are designed to concentrate on more rapid improvements due to strategic initiatives. Identification of core competencies often is used to start the strategic planning process, because that understanding is integral to determining the subjects of the planning process to ensure sustainability.

As noted above, execution of strategic plans can be foiled because of a lack of organizational agility in a rapidly changing marketplace. For example, loss of a key provider might decimate a service line strategy that has substantial revenue impact, and thus the planning process must include plans for such a contingency or the organization must be able to change quickly to accommodate such a devastating blow. Execution strategies are a hallmark of high performing organizations, providing workers with the ability to concentrate on implementing the organizational strategy with a minimum of distraction. These criteria factors are consistent with the Baldrige core values of patient-focused excellence, innovation, agility, and organizational/personal learning. Organizations that are patient focused maintain the appropriate vision of achieving the highest quality care, and innovation, agility, and learning simply provide the basis on which the patient care model can be built.

The strategic planning criteria request an explanation of how the organization deals with a number of issues:

- Strengths, weaknesses, opportunities, and threats
- Core competencies
- Ability to execute strategy
- Optimization of resources
- Availability of a skilled work force
- Management of short- and longer-term plans, like capital expenditures, technology development or acquisition, supplier development, and new healthcare partnerships or collaborations
- Communication plans to meet plan requirements and achieve alignment at the senior leader level, work system and process level, and the work unit level for individuals and departments

Importantly, the criteria do not call for a specific type of planning system or structure but simply ask for a description of the process in effect. As in many organizations the strategic plan concentrates on the key strategic requirements for organizational growth and sustainability, recognizing that many other processes and improvement efforts are necessary for day-to-day operations. Thus the Baldrige criteria do not anticipate that all organizational activities are subsumed in the strategic planning effort. A key part of the plan, however, is the presence of strategic thinking and a focus on the future as well as the present. Another key factor in the consideration of the strategic planning process is the consideration of the budget as part of the process.

2.1 Strategy Development: How Do You Develop Your Strategy? (40/85 Points)

The basic elements of the strategic planning process are the subject of this item, including the primary risks, anticipated problems, and internal and external environmental influences on the strategic planning process. Examiners evaluate responses to this item for evidence of long- and short-term management of the organization's challenges and opportunities. The approach to strategic planning is reviewed to ensure that the applicant has a systematic method for understanding and responding to stakeholder requirements, market influences, and resource allocation that addresses the strategic opportunities and challenges presented in the OP. Criteria for item 2.1 elicit the organization's orientation to the future through responses to questions about competitive and collaborative strategies, approaches to planning, and development of plans. Although no specific planning process or dedicated planning staff are requisites for this item, the key to applicant responses is an indication of an approach that the organization defines performance objectives based on the MVV and then determines essential actions and measures to ensure deployment.

Effective strategy development is characteristic of high performing organizations, and applicants must articulate a process that documents the current status of the organization through an environmental assessment while concurrently exhibiting a focus on the future that transcends the existing situation to evoke visions of long-term prospects. Healthcare industry leadership requires a vision of the future that considers all aspects of the criteria, such as markets, work force, knowledge management and access, process excellence, and leadership. Understanding strengths and weaknesses helps position an organization in the marketplace and often helps identify opportunities for collaboration as well as requirements for effective competition.

Organizations in all industries must have projections of future marketplace challenges. The use of data to perform an environmental assessment is a key element of strategic planning, but data analysis must also provide a basis for understanding the direction of competitors as well as the stability and availability of collaborative opportunities. Knowing the marketplace and having methods of listening and learning from a variety of sources, including customers, competitors, and collaborators, are key features of strategic plans that help ensure sustainability. Leveraging data for business intelligence is generally evidenced by analytic techniques that extract knowledge from data.

2.2 Strategy Deployment: How Do You Deploy Your Strategy?

Ask nearly any leader: Deploying strategy is immensely more difficult than almost any other management task. Item 2.2 explores the methods of actually making the strategic plan come alive throughout the organization. Not only must a robust structure for implementation be created, but it must include metrics to assess progress to plan goals. World class organizations make this aspect of the strategic planning process one of their key success factors, because failure to implement plans subverts the ability of the organization to grow and improve.

A common failure in this item is not involving the entire work force and other key stakeholders in the supply chain (e.g., suppliers and other vendors) in the deployment process. Item 2.2 questions are directed at how action plans are deployed not only to the organization's staff but also to key suppliers and other partners. For example, a strategic objective of reducing surgical site infections must include nursing staff and others involved in a patient's care, but it must also involve other key stakeholders, like physicians and surgical supply vendors. All key process owners and users must have metrics that help them determine success or opportunities for improvement as well as appropriate resources to ensure that the tasks can be completed.

Aligning all these staff members, partners, and suppliers is a key factor to ensure successful implementation of an initiative. This part of the strategic plan focuses on achieving consistency through standardization of work, as discussed in the chapters on lean and six sigma. Understanding and involving work systems and work processes and aligning key measures with these process elements are the keys for ensuring alignment of all these work components. Communication systems must be designed and implemented to ensure that priorities, processes, and requisite knowledge are adequately deployed to every worker involved in the process. Finally, alignment of work incentives must be part of the plan implementation to gain buy-in at all levels of the organization.

Resource allocation is a critical management task, and item 2.2 requires a description of the methods by which leaders ensure that financial and human resources are available to those responsible for implementing the action plans. Financial analyses that involve straightforward, as well as complex, economic assessments should be evident to demonstrate that resource deployment issues are addressed. Action plans must be considered as investments for growth and improvement, and use of financial tools like return on equity, or return on invested capital may be helpful in demonstrating that resources adequately deployed and used in a way that increases value.

This item also calls for projections of short- and long-term outcomes and comparisons with competitors' performance as a way to better understand the organization's execution of action plans. Performance projections could include the changes in outcomes due to new partnerships, new customer groups, use of new technologies, or innovations that provide the organization with a competitive advantage. This information is often reflected in the results catogory and typically becomes an important management barometer of performance.

Customer Focus (Category 3)

Just as with lean and six sigma paradigms, the Baldrige criteria place a great deal of emphasis on the customer. Category 3 exemplifies the six sigma concept of the "voice of the customer," seeking to elicit ways that the organization obtains feedback and prospective data from customers to build the client base and meet patient and other stakeholder needs. Many healthcare organizations have discovered that building customer loyalty is a key component to ensuring revenue flow and reducing marketing costs, and so the customer focus highlights efforts at not only attracting but also retaining key customer segments. Techniques of listening and learning become important methods of this customer cultivation process, and high performing organizations have reliable ways of two-way communications with customers that incorporate each segment's unique needs. Measurement of patient and stakeholder satisfaction *and* dissatisfaction results in an ability to better understand and respond to customer needs in a timely, effective, and efficient manner. Aggregating this information across market segments provides a much more robust view of the entire marketplace that then feeds into the strategic planning process.

Healthcare organizations have many stakeholders, although patients are generally considered to be the most important group. However, other stakeholders include employees, providers, payers, employers, and suppliers of various types. Hospitals, for example, often rely heavily on volunteers for a number of service needs, and so the hospital's volunteer corps must be considered another important stakeholder group. Successful responses to category 3 include all important stakeholder groups and how the institution balances the needs of all segments in its environment.

3.1 Customer Engagement: How Do You Engage Patients and Stakeholders to Serve Their Needs and Build Relationships?

The first item in category 3 assesses the institution's methods of identifying and segmenting stakeholder groups and then designing services and products to meet the needs of each group. Building relationships with multiple stakeholder groups is often the biggest challenge for healthcare organizations, and innovative approaches to serving the needs of the many constituencies has become a crucial competency of high performance organizations. Improving patient and other stakeholder connections enhances sustainability and enables the healthcare organization to make better decisions regarding future services and improve the effectiveness of existing services.

Building customer engagement achieves the strategic goal of customer loyalty that places stakeholders in the role of advocates who aid marketing efforts through word-of-mouth support of the organization. The work force culture must be directed at serving customer needs to an extent that delights customers rather than just satisfying their needs. If this philosophy pervades the strategic plan, then the likelihood of succeeding in fostering customer loyalty grows significantly. Building these types of relationships may not be possible with all stakeholders, and in nearly every case stakeholder groups require tailored approaches to ensure creation of a lasting relationship. Thus high functioning organizations often have a relationship building approach that accounts for the unique needs of each stakeholder segment as well as each stage of the relationship.

3.2 Voice of the Customer: How Do You Obtain and Use Information From Your Patients and Stakeholders?

Item 3.2 focuses on the voice of the customer, that is, how the organization communicates and learns from customers. Unlike many customer listening programs, this item does not just seek methods of assessing satisfaction, but the criteria also try to determine approaches to determining causes of dissatisfaction and ways of dealing with dissatisfiers. Use of this information can help both retention of current customers and recruitment of new customers, making these approaches important to sustainability. This item helps evaluate the organization's methods of listening to customers, aggregation of data, and then use of the data to create value for all stakeholders. In all cases voice of the customer strategies must align with organizational key factors (i.e., they should correlate with key customer requirements in the OP). Selection of voice of the customer strategies depends on your key organizational factors. For example, if a key constituency is contacted via outreach programs to skilled nursing facilities, then the organization should have effective methods of managing that communication channel. Importantly, the organization should tailor its listening and learning methods to its customer segments and allocate resources to ensure effective interactions. Several typical communication methods include:

- Focus groups
- Interviews with lost and potential patients and stakeholders
- Use of the complaint process to understand customer issues and opportunities for improvement
- Win/loss analysis relative to competitors and other similar organizations
- Survey or other feedback data

Information from these processes should be actionable, such that the data collected in the feedback process should lead to responses and interventions that improve the stakeholder relationship. Such information can be used to direct initiatives that improve the cost and quality of the organization's services and processes. Listening and learning approaches need to be aligned with the organization's strategic planning process to ensure that the data lead to stakeholder focused planning and implementation of improvements, with direct impact on customer value.

Gaining knowledge of stakeholder groups and market segments provides the organization with opportunities to more specifically craft interventions to focus the work force, information systems, and the planning process on enhancing systems to meet customer requirements. Managing this, at times, flood of information through aggregation methods that incorporate complaints, suggestions, and other feedback can lead to elimination of the root causes of customer dissatisfaction and help set priorities for improvement efforts. Information systems are a key component of this effort, effectively linking this category to category 4. Thus methods of deploying satisfaction of information throughout the enterprise should be an important part of the effort to manage customer interactions. Additionally, comparisons with competitors provide the work force and leaders alike with an idea of the effectiveness of customer relationship management approaches. Because these data are often difficult to find, some healthcare organizations perform broad market surveys to gain insight into competitors' performance. Competitor information is particularly valuable in determining which services may be most in need of intervention.

Measurement, Analysis, and Knowledge Management (Category 4)

Modern businesses rely on data to support decisions, and the healthcare industry is no exception. Category 4 subsumes measurement, analysis, and knowledge management, which serve as the foundation for the other categories. Although measurement and analysis are key elements of this category, in recent years greater emphasis has been placed on knowledge management and integration of information into the organization's management structure to improve decision making, increase worker knowledge, facilitate processes, and track performance. Information quality and availability are key characteristics of any decision support system, and user interfaces must expedite, rather than obstruct, access to information. Knowledge management systems leverage the experience and insight of the work force and share this information in a way that enhances competitive advantage and productivity growth; this category also includes consideration of such strategic issues.

4.1 Measurement, Analysis, and Improvement of Organizational Performance: How Do You Measure, Analyze, and Then Improve Organizational Performance?

Item 4.1 seeks to identify methods used to apply data resources to performance improvement and strategic planning. The selection of data sources is an important first step in creating an infrastructure for decision support. Ensuring that these sources are accurate is critical to information reliability, increasing the confidence of end users that decisions based on the information are indeed valid. Analytic methods applied to the data to produce reports must also be credible, and this item seeks to elicit details of these analyses. Selection of statistically valid indicators, analyzed appropriately, and reported in a coherent manner are important to supporting high quality care and outcomes. Such factors as linking the data to specific providers to help focus improvement efforts can enhance the utility of a decision support system and lead to use of data in management of the business as well as clinical care. Integration of financial and clinical data has become particularly important for assessing the value proposition for a variety of stakeholders, including patients, payers, and providers. The goal of these systems, however, is to create the infrastructure for both evidence-based management and evidence-based medicine.

Alignment and integration of the data with user needs must be considered crucial in determining the success of an information infrastructure. Thus the involvement of users in system configuration presents an opportunity for organizations to incorporate features that will lead to greater confidence and use by staff members from senior leaders to front-line staff. Consistency and reliability of information dictates a large component of user acceptance, and clinical care decisions must be based on accurate information. From a management perspective, senior leaders and other managers require this level of data integrity to ensure proper alignment of organizational performance with strategic goals as well as precise allocation of scarce resources.

Comparative data sources must also be vetted for accuracy and reliability. Because comparative and competitive data come from disparate sources, the reliability of those sources must be verified. Accurate assessment of the organization's competitive position and understanding best practices for directing improvements provide compelling reasons for affirming the validity of external comparators. Thus, as the organization considers which comparisons to use, issues such as ensuring compatible operational definitions and data sources become important considerations in discerning the quality of the comparative information. These comparisons may determine important strategic directions, such as outsourcing certain services, intervening in clinical care patterns, and contracting with outside vendors and payers, and so comparative data must be matched to the organization's metrics as well as an accurate method of assessing performance. Selection and use of comparative data require a number of considerations:

- Needs and priorities of the organization, i.e., comparative data are selected for higher priority items that are likely to be targeted for improvement.
- Creation of criteria for seeking specific sources for comparisons, i.e., what data resources are available for the comparisons. For example, some measures like satisfaction with food quality may not have comparison data within the healthcare industry but may have comparable information from other sectors, like the hospitality industry.
- Data sources that help set stretch goals to stimulate innovative approaches for breakthrough improvements. For example, the "star" performer in the industry is chosen to set goals that require nonincremental improvement.

Chapter 4 discusses a number of sources of comparative data, which might include other organizations in the marketplace, large national data sets, medical and management literature, and federal and state agencies. Item 4.1 also calls for the organization's approach to analyzing trends and making predictions of future performance. Additionally, the projections must be tied to action plans that are directed at achieving the projected goals.

This item also requires a description of analyses conducted to better recognize trends and opportunities for improvement. Some examples of these analyses might include the following:

- Correlation of health service performance with stakeholder requirements, e.g., customer satisfaction with a business unit correlated with clinical performance
- Effect of stakeholder problem resolution on net margin
- Staff satisfaction across the enterprise correlated with customer loyalty
- Operational performance trends in key business areas, like wait time in the emergency department, length of stay on specific clinical units or by provider, average daily census by clinical unit or provider
- Staff satisfaction related to specific personal learning opportunities, such as online computer-based training systems
- Cost-to-benefit relationships associated with improved knowledge management and sharing of important organizational performance data throughout the work force
- Factors in the benefit structure that relate most strongly to retention, motivation, and productivity
- Relationship of worker productivity and speed of complaint or grievance resolution
- Cost trends relative to competitors' trends, such as cost/diagnosis-related group code for key diagnosis-related groups

- Rates of compliance with Health Effectiveness Data Information Set (HEDIS) measures (see Chapter 4) related to other providers with a particular health plan
- Analysis of expected cost-to-benefit outcomes of different improvement projects used to prioritize resource allocation
- Cost of quality and cost of poor quality to determine the actual return on improvement projects
- Ranking of quality interventions by the effects on factors like patient satisfaction and loyalty
- Relationship of market share with profits and other financial returns, including the cost of increasing market share incrementally
- Trends in economic, market, and stakeholder measures of value

These are just examples of many types of analyses that could be performed using transactional data, and the increasing prevalence of electronic medical record systems provides numerous opportunities to include clinical information as part of these reviews. Improving understanding of relationships between financial and administrative data and clinical outcomes aids healthcare organizations in making better appraisals of resource needs and allocation, and so these analyses will increasingly become important for enhancing stakeholder value. Although cause and effect relationships may not be defined by these analyses, the associations provided by statistical analysis may in fact define high performance in the near future.

4.2 Management of Information, Knowledge, and Information Technology: How Do You Manage Your Information, Organizational Knowledge, and Information Technology?

Part of any information system is the hardware and software backbone. Item 4.2 examines the organization's approach to ensuring that hardware and software are reliable, user friendly, and protected from internal and external disasters. Not only do examiners determine these features for the applicant's own work force, but the systems must also be robust in supporting suppliers and partners. Thus patient and provider portals, supplier extranets, and other methods of sharing information are included as part of this review.

Information management now consumes increasing resources, and the function has become a critical component of nearly all organizations. Data storage and resources have grown dramatically in the past several years, to the point that access to information can be considered a key business requirement, and the systems used to ensure that access must be reliable and secure. E-mail communications have become standard in most healthcare organizations, and ensuring the free exchange of this communication modality constitutes an important information technology function. Additionally, systems must be easily learned and readily accessible for staff members who often require the information for their daily work. Thus assurance of hardware and software access and reliability must be a core competence of high performing organizations.

Item 4.2 also includes a review of information security and privacy relating to HIPAA regulations. Increasingly, supply chain management relationships require the ability of vendors and other partners to access parts of the information system to expedite movement of supplies and equipment into and out of the organization. All these system interactions require vigilance to comply with legal and regulatory rules encompassing security and privacy.

Disaster planning has become a factor for the entire U.S. business community, but the need is particularly acute as healthcare organizations become increasingly automated. With patient records stored on disk drives rather than in chart racks, continuing access to the records in spite of climatic or other emergencies is a factor that must be guaranteed. Disaster planning has become an important strategic planning component, but it is especially important for the organization's electronic records. Plans must deal with all stakeholder needs, including the work force, patients, suppliers, and partners, and the plan must be coordinated with the overall plan for operational continuity in the event of a disaster

Work Force Focus (Category 5)

Scarcities of healthcare professionals like nurses and some subspecialists have emphasized the need to focus management attention on work force systems. The work force system involves the physical work environment, but it also includes important work elements like engagement and empowerment. Enabling of the work force has long been a challenge for high performing enterprises, but these organizations have designed systems to deal with these issues. These organizations integrate the work system by incorporating work force engagement, development, and oversight into the strategic plan and then developing action plans to ensure these objectives are achieved. Effective strategic planning involves evaluation of the work effort and staff needed to accomplish the organization's work each year, with appropriate adjustments in training and hiring to attain strategic goals. Thus work force management should be closely related to strategy development and implementation (Category 2).

5.1 Work Force Engagement: How Do You Engage Your Work Force to Achieve Organizational and Personal Success?

A key challenge in contemporary work force management is engaging employees in the organization's operations at a level that creates a win–win for the worker and the organization. Work force engagement is accepted as a key factor in organizational performance, and item 5.1 examines an applicant's work systems for approaches to engagement of the work force and for methods used to enable and empower employees to optimize performance. Approaches in this item are evaluated for their ability to encourage high performance in the organization's core competencies and to provide incentives to achieve the goals in action plans. Healthcare organizations have a unique challenge due to the heterogeneity of the work force: The staff varies from physicians and other health professionals with particular requirements to front-line staff like environmental services workers, who have significantly different work requirements and expectations. Additionally, staff members may be employees or independent members of the medical staff who have no employment relationship with administrators but who have tremendous influence on the organization's business. Work systems must be designed to encompass all these worker needs to be successful, and these accommodations must be detailed in the responses to this item.

High performing organizations have a number of characteristics in work force design, including flexibility in work design, incentives for innovation, systems for knowledge and skill sharing, processes for communication and information flow, work processes that align with strategic objectives, patient and other stakeholder focus, and agility in responding to healthcare industry and business needs.

Engagement is generally defined by the following characteristics:

- Performing meaningful work
- Clear organizational direction
- Accountability for work products and outcomes
- Efficiency
- Safe, trusting, and cooperative work environment

Importantly, this item includes volunteers, who often find meaning in the services they provide, and independent practitioners on the medical staff, who can present special issues for administrators and managers. Barriers to engagement should be evaluated and addressed as part of work force system design (e.g., by employee satisfaction surveys, focus groups, or exit interviews).

Compensation and recognition have become especially problematic in contemporary health care because of restrictions on financial relationships with physicians, worker shortages in some categories (like nursing), and shrinking revenues due to payer changes in reimbursement. Work systems design must consider these issues not only to ensure equity but also to ensure adequate staffing for the organization's work requirements. Methods of rewarding high performing employees are also part of work system design and should be tied to organizational objectives and goals. Incentives may also include profit sharing, benefit design, cash or time off rewards for teams or work unit staff exhibiting high performance, or perhaps linkage to customer satisfaction measures.

Ensuring staff competence is of utmost importance in work system design. Healthcare professionals have continuing education requirements, and all staff members must understand the hazards inherent in patient care work units. Exposures to infectious diseases should be controlled through application of timely educational programs for all staff with patient care responsibilities, and all staff members now require annual updates on patient health information due to HIPAA regulations. Professional and institutional licensure depend on satisfying clinical education requirements, but high performing organizations exceed these baseline requirements by establishing systems (see item 4.1) for knowledge sharing and collaboration. As new technologies are adopted, in-service education programs are needed to optimize incorporation of the equipment or procedure into workflow. In some instances educational programs may be developed to enhance basic skills for those workers who need remedial support. These programs may be developed by the organization or through collaboration with local educational institutions (e.g., colleges or trade schools). To help workers achieve their full potential, an organization might collaborate to create individual development plans to address the worker's career and learning objectives.

Training programs must also include volunteers, because their work often brings them in contact with patients, with the attendant risks of contracting infectious diseases or other care-related injuries. Volunteer orientation programs often include:

- The organization's healthcare services
- Patient confidentiality and privacy
- Listening skills to learn from patients and other stakeholders
- Managing and reporting problems or service failures
- Organizational approaches to meeting patient and stakeholder expectations

As noted in category 4, the knowledge management system in high performing organizations has become an important vehicle for sharing information throughout the enterprise. Work system deployment should include systematic plans for ensuring that each worker has access to the information of greatest importance to effectively complete his or her work. As workers gain experience at a job, they should have the ability to share the experience through the knowledge management system to help others learn from that experience.

As with other Baldrige categories, measures should be part of the work system plan to allow assessment of the effectiveness and efficiency of all elements of the system. These metrics might gauge the impact of educational programs on productivity and innovation or worker satisfaction with the work environment. Metrics are often integrated into the organizational measurement system so that senior managers can continually evaluate the work system and its relation to other key measures. Other measures that are considered important to healthcare systems include turnover rates, particularly among professional staff; grievances; and absenteeism.

5.2 Work Force Environment: How Do You Build an Effective and Supportive Work Force Environment?

One of the key steps in strategic planning involves understanding work force capability and capacity and then identifying gaps that require intervention. Item 5.2 addresses this issue as well as the enterprise work environment, including safety and security. High performing organizations seek to create an environment in which workers can feel secure and achieve self-actualization. Almost every organization, regardless of size, has opportunities to support the work force, such as personal and career counseling to help in career development, recreational and cultural activities, formal and informal recognition for exemplary performance, educational opportunities, day care, family leave time, and flexible work hours or benefits. Although every organization must meet some regulatory standards for worker safety and accommodation of physical challenges, world class organizations exceed these minimum standards and act proactively to secure the workplace.

Process Management (Category 6)

Implementation of strategic plans requires reliable and repeatable processes, and category 6 focuses on the ways in which an organization manages processes to support reliability, flexibility, and sustainability. The information provided in this category deals with the approaches that the organization has put into place to actualize core competencies and all the related work required to deliver services. Core competencies are addressed specifically, as are the organization's ability to respond to emergency situations and disasters. The goal of reliable processes is high quality customer service and long-term sustainability, but continuity of operations must also be a key competence of healthcare organizations today. Sustainable work systems require effective design, which includes considerations of a number of factors:

- Value creation for all stakeholders
- Operational performance factors
- Focus on organizational mission (e.g., providing preventive services or responding to emergencies)
- Measurement systems to determine efficiency and effectiveness, like cycle time, takt time, nonconformity rates, error rates, and sigma levels
- Improvement strategies based on data
- Innovation strategies
- Information capture systems to foster organizational learning

Agility is another key feature of effective process management, because change in the healthcare industry continues to challenge leaders. The ability to quickly adapt key processes to new technology or changes in payments is one of the hallmarks of highly effective organizations. For example, an organization may need to quickly decide whether to outsource certain services when a third-party payer changes the payment amounts for a service that has traditionally been provided in-house. Lagging performance may require rapid cycle improvements using lean or six sigma tools, and the agile organization has procedures in place to identify performance lapses.

6.1 Work Systems: How Do You Design Your Work Systems?

The first item in Category 6 examines work systems, core competencies, and work process decisions and how these systems are designed and implemented to create value for stakeholders. The goals of successful work systems in health care ensure that stakeholder needs are met and the organization is sustainable and ensure adequate preparation for contingencies such as emergencies or other unexpected changes in the environment. The subject of item 6.1 is the overall design of work systems and methods of systematizing delivery of healthcare services. Key processes form the basis of core competencies and as such play a critical role in the organization's success. Thus all the elements of success, like competitiveness and sustainability, depend on how a company manages its processes.

Item 6.1 begins with a request for a description of key work processes and their specific requirements. Most of these processes will certainly be health care related, but in most medical/surgical organizations these approaches are associated with a number of support processes as well. For example, a seemingly simple respiratory therapy treatment requires a number of supporting processes, such as equipment cleaning and maintenance, supply ordering, staff scheduling, and so on. Key business processes may not only be health care related, however. Some healthcare organizations consider processes that encourage innovation or research and development to be key business processes, because they help the organization maintain or advance its competitive position. Some examples of key processes that may not be related to the direct provision of healthcare services include those designed to address:

- Innovation
- Research and development
- Technology acquisition
- Information and knowledge management
- Supply chain management
- Supplier partnering
- Outsourcing
- Mergers and acquisitions
- Project management
- Sales and marketing
- Fundraising
- Media relations
- Public policy advocacy

Thus healthcare organizations may have a number of processes that can be considered key to the business but are not directly related to the delivery of healthcare services. Because of the variety of activities and business units involved, the requirements and performance attributes for these processes may vary and will require description in an application.

Business activities that support ongoing operations are usually considered to be key work processes as well, but these activities may not be dependent on health service characteristics. For example, a physician's office billing function supports the business through collection of revenue, but it is not directly related to the provision of healthcare services. Design and operation of these services may require consideration of different requirements and performance expectations but typically use the same process management procedures, such as those described in previous chapters, that are applied to design and improvement of healthcare processes. Some other examples of support processes include:

- Housekeeping and environmental services
- Medical records
- Finance and accounting
- Facilities management
- Legal services
- Human resources
- Public relations
- Community relations
- Administrative services, such as secretarial or clerical support

Increasingly, supply chain management approaches are being applied to improve operations and decrease costs. Vendors and other business partners have become important collaborators in strategic and operational planning to ensure continuity and reliability of core competencies. For example, a vaccine supplier's logistical operations for vaccine delivery can be important for a health department facility that provides immunizations to the public. Disruptions in the vaccine supplier's operations can have a significant effect on the health facility's ability to provide services to its stakeholders. Because even minor changes in the supplier's performance can impair the facility's services, including the supplier in planning may help mitigate the risk of shortages. Managing the supply chain includes selection of a limited number of preferred suppliers based on characteristics like reliability, cost, and compatible business ethics and practices. Limiting the number of suppliers may seem counterintuitive and noncompetitive, but supply chain management approaches have been validated in a number of industries and can lower overall costs and increase revenue by ensuring operational continuity.

A supply chain management strategy must establish work system and process design requirements for vendors and other partners. Process design must include all stakeholders throughout the value stream, and so the design process may become complex and require substantial management coordination. In many cases this coordination may span multiple facilities and involve shared equipment and staff services. The synchronization of all these "moving parts" may require a management structure that ensures control and efficient operations.

Another important aspect of item 6.1 is an emphasis on continuity of operations, particularly in a community emergency. Emergency planning starts by determining which processes are crucial for maintaining operations in the event of a catastrophe and then creating the infrastructure to ensure that these processes are sustained. Healthcare organizations are key to any community during an emergency, and so this planning effort is important not just to the institution but also to the community as a whole. Although all of an organization's services may not be sustained in these situations, the key operations that are important to the community and the organization's mission should be the focus of planning and resource allocation. In many cases this planning effort is done collaboratively with other similar organizations, some of whom may be competitors, which differentiates the healthcare industry from many others without a similar societal mission.

6.2 Work Processes: How Do You Design, Manage, and Improve Your Key Organizational Work Processes?

The second item in category 6 is directed at ascertaining the methods by which processes are designed, managed, and improved. As discussed in Chapter 7, with systematic approaches to process design incorporating frameworks like design for six sigma and tools like failure mode and effects analysis, organizations can ensure that new processes meet customer requirements for effectiveness, safety, and efficiency. Improvement approaches, such as lean, six sigma, or other systems, must be adaptable to a variety of process types, environments, and economic constraints. Modifications of services involve important issues that must be considered in process improvement:

- Target health outcomes for a clinical condition
- Safety of the current and improved processes
- Mitigation of risk
- Throughput and access
- Care model (e.g., to provide continuity of care)
- Shared decision making with patients and families
- Range of customer expectations
- Environmental impact of process changes
- Measurement systems
- Human resource availability
- Efficiency measures (e.g., cycle time, takt time, etc.)

All the process management and improvement approaches that have been subjects of prior chapters are germane to this category, and tools like value stream mapping can be used to evaluate existing processes and create new processes. Importantly, item 6.2 requires a systematic approach to improvement that is applied consistently to improvement and design.

In-process measurements are those that determine effectiveness at various points along the process. For example, treatment of a patient with chest pain in the emergency department may include administration of an adult aspirin tablet, and the in-process metric would be the percent of patients with chest pain who received aspirin within 1 hour of presenting in the department. By identifying critical points in the process and creating operational definitions for metrics at each of these points, an organization can monitor key processes in real time and make corrections as necessary. As discussed in Chapter 6, these modifications can be performed by human input or, when available, by technologic solutions. In-process measures must be tailored to the time factors in the process; for longer processes, more in-process metrics might be necessary to ensure that the process is following expected performance tracks. Metrics must assess the most important parts of the process (e.g., cycle time, gaps in specifications during the process, and customer satisfaction).

Results (Category 7)

Results and outcomes are the keys to a successful healthcare organization, and so the results category had the highest point value in the criteria. Society has placed greater emphasis on outcomes in recent years after years of focusing on structure and process, and so the results category in the criteria has assumed greater importance as well. However, category 7 goes beyond health outcomes to include all aspects of a healthcare institution's structure and operations. As shown in TABLE 8.1, every approach/deployment category has a corresponding results category to ensure linkage of what an applicant says and the actual results realized by the organization. Category 7 thus provides the reality check of the organization's management and deployment efforts. Additionally, the results category should reflect many, if not all, of the measures noted in category 2 for strategic planning and throughout the other categories if metrics are mentioned. For example, if retention rates are noted as important in category 5, then examiners expect to see that metric reported in item 7.4.

Scoring in category 7 relies on the mnemonic "LeTCI," which connotes levels-trends-comparisons-integration. Each result that is reported in this category is evaluated by examiners to determine how it meets these conditions:

- *Level:* numerical information that places or positions an organization's results and performance on a meaningful measurement scale to permit evaluation relative to past performance, projections, goals, and appropriate comparisons.
- *Trend:* numerical information that shows the direction and rate of change for an organization's results, providing a time sequence of organizational performance. A minimum of three historical (not projected) data points generally is needed to begin to ascertain a trend.
- *Comparisons:* numerical evaluation of data to determine the organization's performance in relationship to a benchmark or best practice from the industry or from competitors and/or collaborators. Comparisons allow the organization to determine if its performance meets or exceeds the top level in its industry or peer group.

- *Integration:* harmonization of plans, processes, information, resource decisions, actions, results, and analyses to support key organizational results. Examiners look for a relationship between the approach/deployment categories and results as evidence of integration.

Just as ADLI influences the scoring range for approach/deployment categories, LeTCI serves as the basis for determining the scoring range for results items.

7.1 Healthcare Outcomes: What Are Your Healthcare Results?

Because health outcomes represent the most important customer value for any healthcare organization, the first item in category 7 focuses on these metrics. Outcomes measures should be applicable to the organization's MVV and operations. For example, a hospital that features a cardiac care unit as a core competence would be expected to have one or more measures relating to care in that unit. Additionally, the data should include comparisons to national, regional, or local organizations as relevant to demonstrate performance relative to external benchmarks as well as trends in performance. Many sources of comparative data are available, as discussed in Chapter 4. Additionally, health outcome measures may include customer health status survey data (e.g., through instruments like the SF-36) or metrics that involve patient safety, adherence to clinical guidelines or critical pathways, medication administration, timeliness of care, and coordination of care across practitioners and settings. Other potential patient outcome measures include:

- Pain score management
- Functional outcomes, like resumption of activities of daily living
- Time to return to work or school
- Elimination of "never events"
- Rate of use of physical restraints
- Effectiveness of care measures (e.g., the HEDIS measure for "control of blood pressure")
- Mortality and morbidity rates
- Long-term survival rates

Some applicants correlate healthcare service performance with stakeholder indicators to better understand drivers for stakeholder satisfaction and to differentiate performance from other providers in the marketplace. This analysis sometimes reveals emerging market segments or changing requirements in current segments.

7.2 Customer-Focused Outcomes: What Are Your Patient and Stakeholder-Focused Performance Results?

As health care has become more patient focused, the importance of customer outcome measures has grown commensurately. Customer and stakeholder opinions of performance have become key metrics for high performing healthcare entities, with associated targets that are translated into strategic plans and objectives. Patient and stakeholder loyalty has become a major factor in health care, leading to greater financial stability and sustainability. Measures of patient and stakeholder satisfaction are among the most important metrics used by healthcare organizations to focus improvements on substantive issues. Additionally, a number of parameters have become commonly used to identify stakeholder issues:

- Patient and stakeholder dissatisfaction
- Patient retention rates
- Gains and losses of patients and other stakeholders
- Complaints
- Patient and stakeholder perceptions of healthcare quality
- Patient and stakeholder assessment of access
- Patient and stakeholder likelihood to recommend the institution
- Patient and stakeholder ratings by independent organizations

The number of measures of stakeholder value has increased, and high performance organizations optimize their use of these metrics to improve customer service and stakeholder value.

7.3 Financial and Market Outcomes: What Are Your Financial and Marketplace Performance Results?

The maxim "no margin, no mission" exemplifies the importance of this item. Financial and market outcome measures provide senior leaders with the ability to assess financial performance and organizational health. Financial indicators include the typical income statement, balance sheet, and fund flow data but can also include financial ratios, like debt-to-equity ratio, days' receivables, earnings per share, return on equity, collection ratios, and many other such metrics. Financial measures are key to ensuring that value is delivered to customers as well as ensuring long-term sustainability.

Market performance is often measured as growth rates in services or numbers of patients served. These metrics indicate the effectiveness of the organization's market outreach activities as well as the methods used to build the organization's reputation. These metrics might include:

- Market share
- Donations and grants
- New services
- New market service areas
- New patient populations served
- Incremental income from new market growth

Trends and levels of these measures are important in determining the effectiveness of the organization's strategic planning and deployment of operational and improvement initiatives.

7.4 Work Force-Focused Outcomes: What Are Your Work Force-Focused Performance Results?

This item measures the effectiveness of approaches and deployment strategies described in Category 5. Not only are process metrics typically reported, but outcomes of effective work system implementation may be included as well. Thus measures for this item may involve work force engagement and satisfaction, like satisfaction with involvement in decision making, acceptance of organizational change initiatives, comfort with organizational culture, and knowledge sharing. Applicants usually include the results of reward systems (e.g., the number of incentives awarded), but other important measures often involve changes in worker retention, segmented by classification. For example, retention rates may be stratified by professional and nonmedical staff members, which leads to design of specific interventions to improve employee satisfaction and willingness to stay with the organization. Other measures that are frequently reported for this item are:

- Work unit staffing levels
- Safety
- Absenteeism
- Satisfaction
- Complaints and grievances
- Training rates
- Licensure rates
- Cross-training rates
- Volunteer hours

Comparative data are sometimes difficult to find, but local and regional comparators are sometimes available through sources.

7.5 Process Effectiveness Outcomes: What Are Your Process Effectiveness Results?

Determining the effectiveness of processes is performed to ensure that process management and efforts at improvement are successful. Many processes are unique, requiring specific metrics to demonstrate effectiveness, but some measures may be more generally applied to all processes, such as the sigma level. Key areas of healthcare service delivery and operational performance, such as error rates for pharmaceutical administration or nonrecyclable waste produced by medical processes, are typical measures in this item, but measures should be chosen because they are relevant to core competencies and related processes. Measures might also focus on productivity of specific processes reported as throughput or takt time or even trends in cost per unit of output. Many other potential measures can demonstrate process effectiveness:

- Utilization rates of specific key services
- Reduction in rework (e.g., repeat tests and imaging studies)
- Time to new service introduction

- Increased use of e-technology, such as patient or provider portals
- Supply chain indicators (e.g., inventory reductions)
- Changes in process sigma levels

Process effectiveness measures provide important information across processes to ensure that the organization's process management and improvement systems are functioning effectively. By using metrics that are applicable across processes (e.g., sigma level), the organization can use these data to prioritize intervention targets and better refine use of scarce resources to improve operations.

7.6 Leadership Outcomes: What Are Your Leadership Results?

The importance of leadership was discussed in category 1, and this item provides the venue for reporting measures of leadership effectiveness, including measures for issues like compliance and accreditation. Although organizations may have difficulty designing measures of leadership, progress measures can be created by determining progress to goals in major strategic categories. For example, many organizations assign specific operational responsibilities to each leader, and achievement of goals by that leader can be used to measure leadership effectiveness. Fiscal accountability and ethics have become a preoccupation throughout U.S. industry, including health care, and measures of ethical lapses and effectiveness of resolution of compliance problems can be used to determine effectiveness in this area. This item seeks evidence that the governance bodies and senior leaders effectively measure and use data to improve their own performance as well as that of the organization.

Organizations usually report results of their key accreditation requirements (e.g., The Joint Commission for hospitals or National Committee for Quality Assurance for health plans), but other data include patient safety results, staff licensure and credentialing results, and external audit reports. Other important results indicating effective leadership activities include noteworthy achievements, such as awards for excellence or state excellence awards. Finally, the organization's contribution to the community is also an indication of the satisfaction of the criteria in item 2.2, which calls for participation in relevant community activities. For example, the organization may have a United Way campaign each year that solicits employee support of that community service organization. Importantly, the organization should report any untoward sanctions or other adverse actions (e.g., a malpractice suit) in the past 5 years.

■ Healthcare Recipients 2002–2008

A list of healthcare recipients with year of award is presented in TABLE 8.4, and summaries of the applications of two of the early recipients are shown in TABLES 8.5 and 8.6. Organizational characteristics of the recipients vary significantly, from single hospitals to multi-hospital systems. Summaries of all of the recipients may be found

Table 8.4	Baldrige Health Care Recipients 2002–2008	
Recipient		Award Year
SSM Healthcare, St. Louis, MO		2002
St. Luke's Hospital, Kansas City, MO		2003
Baptist Hospital, Jacksonville, FL		
Robert Wood Johnson University Hospital, Hamilton, NJ		2004
Bronson Methodist Hospital, Kalamazoo, MI		2005
North Mississippi Medical Center, Tupelo, MS		2006
Mercy Health System, Janesville, WI		2007
Sharp Health System, San Diego, CA		
Poudre Valley Health System, Fort Collins, CO		2008

Table 8.5	Baldrige Healthcare Recipient Profiles: SSM Healthcare, St. Louis, MO

SSM is a Catholic healthcare system in the Midwest, with acute and chronic care facilities and other healthcare business operations. SSM's largest facilities are in St. Louis, MO, where the corporate headquarters are housed. SSM's mission is simply stated as "Through our exceptional healthcare services, we reveal the healing presence of God."

Category	Innovation
1: Leadership	• Mission, vision, and values (MVV) were determined through a system-wide effort, involving all employees across the system.
	• The system-wide Performance Management Process relies on the quality report that directs improvement efforts using data from current performance and benchmarking.
	• The Leadership Development Process is based on a 360 evaluation of leaders at all levels of the system and provides a basis for accountability and learning.
	• Public accountability is achieved in a number of ways, including the Corporate Responsibility Process, which provides structure for legal and regulatory issues, and the SSM Policy Institute, which studies and anticipates changes in public issues for corporate planning.
2: Strategic planning	• Mission Awareness Teams throughout the enterprise focus on ensuring that the planning and work efforts of each entity in the system maintains efforts toward serving the mission.
	• Leaders deploy elements of the strategic plan through "Passports" specific to each employee at all levels. Managers cascade the plans to each of their direct reports in an annual process of plan deployment.
3: Market knowledge and customer focus	• Multiple listening and learning data sources are collated to inform the Strategic, Financial, and HR Planning Process (SFPP) each year; these information sources are reviewed semiannually to determine the impact of operations on customer satisfaction.

Table 8.5	
Category	Innovation
	• Customer satisfaction survey results and information from the Complaint Management Process are combined to identify opportunities for improving customer service.
	• Managers empower employees to "fix it now" when confronted with a customer complaint, and when unable to deal with a specific issue, employees refer the problem to someone who can provide immediate relief.
4: Information and knowledge management	• The SSM Information Center (SSMIC) integrates data from multiple sources into the Performance Improvement Report, including 16 measures that are common to all entities and rolled up into a system report for senior management. Most metrics are compared with benchmarks from national data sources.
	• The SPPP includes the Information Management Planning Process, which ensures that information systems are maintained at high levels of performance for data management requirements.
	• A multidisciplinary, cross-system Information Management Council oversees the Information Management Planning Process and makes certain that the needs of all stakeholders are met as information systems are revised.
5: Staffing	• SSM has engendered a culture of continuous quality improvement as the basis for staff relations and human resource management. The result of this approach has been the development of Shared Accountability, Diversity Mentoring, and Executive Career Development programs to enhance staff opportunities and satisfaction.
	• A number of efforts have been implemented to deal with the impact of shortages in key staff positions, such as nursing. These programs have included shared accountability, training and education, access to technology, improved professional collaboration, and development of better benefits for key staff members.
6: Process management	• The PDCA cycle serves as the quality improvement model for the organization and is deployed system-wide. This approach is used as the basis for Clinical Collaboratives, which help the organization enhance medical and surgical services.
	• The Physician Partnering and Supply Chain Management Processes are key to SSM's business strategy and are paid particular attention during development and implementation of the strategic plan. Focusing on physicians and strategic suppliers has created an environment that fosters improvement and contains costs.
	• Measures for both medical and business support processes include outcome and in-process metrics to facilitate day to day management of the system.
7: Results	• Although SSM presents a small sample of results from its healthcare and business processes, the levels and trends are favorable for such important attributes as unplanned readmissions and patient satisfaction. Additionally, clinical measures like percent of orders with dangerous abbreviations also showed satisfactory levels and appropriate trends.

Table 8.6	Baldrige Healthcare Recipient Profiles: St. Luke's Hospital, Kansas City, MO

St. Luke's Hospital is the flagship institution of a healthcare system in Kansas City, with 7 other hospitals, 14 outpatient facilities, 7 employee assistance program facilities, 5 behavioral health clinics, 3 wellness/fitness locations, 5 home health/hospice services, and 4 other affiliated institutions. The organization's vision is "The best place to get care, the best place to give care."

Category	Innovation
1: Leadership	• Leaders set and deploy the MVV and elements of the strategic plan through three major venues: Very Important Principles, Performance Management Program, and the Balanced Scorecard.
	• The leadership structure includes a strong community-based Board, an Executive Council of senior leaders, a Medical Staff Executive Committee and Medical Staff Board, the Hospital Leadership Group, and the Performance Improvement Steering Committee. These groups work closely together to ensure effective execution of the strategic plan.
	• Senior leaders have a number of ways of maintaining contact with the hospital and medical staff, such as the explicit instructions in the Plan for Care and Services Manual, Administrator On Call program, an Open Door Policy, Administrative Rounding, and the Customer Satisfaction Research Program.
	• The Leadership for Performance Excellence (LPE) program is a highly developed method that integrates leadership responsibilities throughout the organization with each of the Baldrige categories to ensure leadership involvement throughout the enterprise.
2: Strategic planning	• A seven-step strategic planning process is deployed throughout each year, and each step subsumes a specific portion of the process. The entire organization becomes involved in the process, which leads to deployment through the Balanced Scorecard system.
	• The Balanced Scorecard is used to track deployment of the plan throughout the year, with changes occurring as needed. Use of the metrics on the scorecard ensures data-driven management.
3: Market knowledge and customer focus	• Listening and learning methods are segmented according to customer type, and the information is integrated with other customer information during the strategic planning process environmental scan. This information is also used to refine the approach to customer segmentation.
4: Information and knowledge management	• Integrated system of balanced scorecard measures that relate individual process measures to departmental measures, which are then aggregated into a system balanced scorecard.
	• Balanced scorecard is the key approach to aligning organizational analysis with key performance results.
	• Benchmark and comparative data from a number of sources are used to enrich the analysis for strategic planning, setting future goals and targets, and improvements for clinical and administrative processes.

Table 8.6

	• The Performance Improvement Steering Committee ensures that collection, analysis, and use of the data are all performed in a timely and accurate manner. The organization recognizes the strategic value of data in achieving excellence. The entire data evaluation is assembled into an Environmental Assessment for planning.
	• Information and analyses are disseminated in regular leadership and staff meetings throughout the year, with particular emphasis during the strategic planning process.
	• The data systems that have been built to support this effort include e-portals for physicians and other staff members to access clinical and administrative data, and these systems meet all applicable security and confidentiality regulations.
5: Staffing	• Work systems are based on a matrix architecture that aligns work according to product lines, clinical departments, administrative departments, nursing units, cross-functional work teams, and multidisciplinary committees.
	• Management of the matrix structure occurs through a Performance Management Process that identifies primary customers at all levels and then delineates expectations and competencies required to meet the core values of the organization for the target customers. The Performance Management Process supports a pay-for-performance approach to providing incentives for employees reaching high achievement in reaching goals.
	• SLH retains recruits and retains employees using traditional methods of salary and benefits but also through an active reward program that recognizes employee excellence during regular ceremonies and through spot awards, e.g., the "Angel for an Angel" Award.
	• Education and training programs span mandatory training for hospital personnel to high level continuing medical education, and program delivery is accomplished through a wide variety of approaches from individual mentoring to classroom education and Internet-based instruction. Training is evaluated through the Kirkpatrick model.
	• Employee wellness and safety are key elements of the work system and include fitness programs, prenatal programs for parents, and ongoing assessment of employee health needs.
6: Process management	• The "PI Model" consists of five phases, Plan, Design, Measure, Assess, and Improve, and is used throughout the organization as the basis for achieving performance excellence in clinical and administrative processes. All staff members are trained in the model, which is reinforced through "VIP Cards" carried by every employee.
	• All process improvements and new process design includes steps to gather evidence for the proposed approach, through literature or empirical data collection through pilot programs. Patient expectations are factored into healthcare service design, to ensure that SLH addresses its core values.

(continues)

Table 8.6	Baldrige Healthcare Recipient Profiles: St. Luke's Hospital, Kansas City, MO (continued)
Category	Innovation
6: Process management *(continued)*	• The Multidisciplinary Care Process underlies all clinical process design and ensures participation of all stakeholders in the design and implementation of new processes as well as the improvement of existing processes. This approach has led to use of clinical pathways for 60% of the organization's patients. Feedback from patients and families through listening and learning methods provides feedback into process improvements (assess and improve steps).
	• Caregivers and support staff are accountable and empowered to make regular improvements in processes using the PI Model. The organizational infrastructure for improvement ensures that senior leaders support efforts for improving services.
7: Results	• SLH's mortality and Length of Stay results place it among the highest performers, and performance on Centers for Medicare and Medicaid Services and The Joint Commission reportable measures are among the highest in the country.
	• The organization ranks first in its market area for overall quality, best doctors, best nurses, best heart care, and best orthopedic care for 3 consecutive years in a consumer survey.
	• Patient satisfaction results have consistently been high (above 85th percentile) in most departments and has ranked high in patient willingness to recommend for 5 years.
	• SLH financial performance has remained in the top 5% of a national comparison group for several years, and financial success has been coupled with increased market share and a growing market index.
	• Employee satisfaction has remained very high, as measured by "high box" (Outstanding or Exceeds Expectations) responses on employee surveys.
	• Measures of effectiveness, such as laboratory precision, radiology turnover time, admitting waiting time, and pharmacy stockout rates, have shown benchmark performance and favorable trends.
	• The organization has achieved all salient compliance and accreditation certifications and has contributed to the community through a number of activities and educational programs.

on the MBNQA web site (www.mbnqa.gov). The applications demonstrate systematic approaches with effective deployment and results that exceed those of competitors in many instances.

■ Conducting a Self-Assessment

The criteria are used to develop and then assess an application for the MBNQA, but they also serve to provide the framework for an effective management system for nearly any organization. Conducting a Baldrige self-assessment entails developing an

Table 8.7	Team Assignments for Self-Assessment	
Team	Approach Deployment Category	Results Category
1	1	7.6
2	2	7.3
3	3	7.2
4	4	7.1
5	5	7.4
6	6	7.5

OP and then creating teams for each category and results item. A senior leadership team can provide oversight for the teams, with each senior leader becoming the "champion" for one or more of the criteria. For example, the chief executive officer might champion category 1 and item 7.6, whereas the chief information officer might support category 4 and item 7.5, which relates to process outcomes.

The teams can "double up" on the approach/deployment categories and results items because the results items are tied to the approach/deployment categories. A suggested team assignment matrix is shown in TABLE 8.7, but any combination of categories and results items can be used. Each team is given responsibility for responding to each item requirement in the assigned categories, with a report to the senior leader champion for that category. From this report the senior leader oversight team can determine opportunities for improvement and begin to design strategic programs for addressing gaps in structure and performance. Many organizations that never intend to apply for the MBNQA have found the criteria to be a highly effective tool for assessment and directing improvement strategies.

■ Summary

The MBNQA has achieved a great deal in its first three decades of existence. The healthcare industry has adopted the Baldrige Award as a premier indicator of performance excellence, and the recipients of the Award have become models for the industry to emulate. Bringing a coherent structure to the delivery of health care has been one of the great contributions that the Award has made to the healthcare industry, and organizations that adopt the criteria to guide their management systems have found that the systematic approach has provided the impetus to improve that would be hard to achieve otherwise. As the MBNQA program expands to other industries, the effect on U.S. competitive leadership in the world will continue to grow and help maintain the U.S.'s preeminent role in world commerce.

Discussion Questions

1. Why is the Malcolm Baldrige National Quality Award (MBNQA) program important to the business world of the United States?
2. How has the MBNQA influenced state and international award programs?
3. What government agency oversees the MBNQA? What other agencies and contractors are involved?
4. Briefly describe the Baldrige Award cycle. Why is the cycle so long?
5. How are Baldrige application scores assigned? How are the scores used?
6. Which approach/deployment category has the highest point value? Why?
7. Which results category has the highest point value? Why?
8. What is the significance of a double strength in a Baldrige scorebook? A double OFI?
9. What is the function of the judges' panel in the Baldrige process?
10. Briefly describe the Baldrige core values and their meaning.
11. What is the organizational profile? Why is it an important part of the application? Why is it important in a self-assessment?
12. Why would an organization perform a Baldrige self-assessment?
13. Define ADLI. What significance does ADLI have in the Baldrige process?
14. Define LeTCI. What significance does LeTCI have in the Baldrige process?
15. Describe the six approach/deployment categories.
16. Describe the six results items.
17. Using the examples of the Baldrige recipients in this chapter, describe some of the unique characteristics of these organizations.

Reference

1. Evans D. Remarks by U.S. Secretary of Commerce Donald L. Evans, Malcolm Baldrige National Quality Award. Retrieved February 2009 from http://www.nist.gov/public_affairs/newsfromnist_evans052103.htm

Baldrige Award Glossary

I thank the Baldrige National Quality Program at the National Institute of Standards and Technology for use of the glossary from the criteria for performance excellence (Gaithersburg, MD, 2009).

Action Plans: Refers to specific actions that respond to short- and longer term strategic objectives. Action plans include details of resource commitments and time horizons for accomplishment. Action plan development represents the critical stage in planning when strategic objectives and goals are made specific so that effective, organization-wide understanding and deployment are possible. The criteria deployment of action plans includes creating aligned measures for all departments and work units. Deployment also might require specialized training for some staff members or recruitment of personnel. An example of a strategic objective for a health system in an area with an active business alliance focusing on cost and quality of care might be to become the low-cost provider. Action plans could entail designing efficient processes to optimize length of hospital stays, reduce the rework resulting from patient injuries and treatment errors, analyze resource and asset use, and analyze the most commonly encountered diagnosis-related groups with a focus on preventive health in those areas. Deployment requirements might include training for all department/work unit caregivers in setting priorities based on costs and benefits. Organizational-level analysis and review likely would emphasize process efficiency, cost per patient, and healthcare quality. See also the definition of "strategic objectives."

Alignment: Refers to consistency of plans, processes, information, resource decisions, actions, results, and analyses to support key organization-wide goals. Effective alignment requires a common understanding of purposes and goals. It also requires the use of complementary measures and information for planning, tracking, analysis, and improvement at three levels: the organizational level, the key process level, and the department or work unit level. See also the definition of "integration."

Analysis: Refers to an examination of facts and data to provide a basis for effective decisions. Analysis often involves the determination of cause and effect relationships. Overall, organizational analysis guides the management of work systems and work processes toward achieving key organizational performance results and toward attaining strategic objectives. Despite their importance, individual facts and data do not usually provide an effective basis for actions or setting priorities. Effective actions depend on an understanding of relationships, derived from analysis of facts and data.

Anecdotal: Refers to process information that lacks specific methods, measures, deployment mechanisms, and evaluation, improvement, and learning factors. Anecdotal information frequently uses examples and describes individual activities rather than systematic processes. An anecdotal response to how senior leaders deploy performance expectations might describe a specific occasion when a senior leader visited all of the organization's facilities. On the other hand, a systematic process might describe the communication methods used by all senior leaders to deliver performance expectations on a regular basis to all organizational locations and work force members, the measures used to assess the effectiveness of the methods, and the tools and techniques used to evaluate and improve the communication methods. See also the definition of "systematic."

Approach: Refers to the methods used by an organization to address the Baldrige criteria item requirements. Approach includes the appropriateness of the methods to the item requirements and to the organization's operating environment as well as how effectively the methods are used. Approach is one of the dimensions considered in evaluating process items.

Basic Requirements: Refers to the topic criteria users need to address when responding to the most central concept of an item. Basic requirements are the fundamental theme of that item (e.g., your approach for strategy development for item 2.1). In the criteria the basic requirements of each item are presented as the item title question.

Benchmarks: Refers to processes and results that represent best practices and performance for similar activities, inside or outside an organization's industry. Organizations engage in benchmarking to understand the current dimensions of world class performance and to achieve discontinuous (nonincremental) or "breakthrough" improvement. Benchmarks are one form of comparative data. Other comparative data organizations might use include information obtained from other organizations through sharing or contributing to external reference databases, information obtained from the open literature (e.g., outcomes of research studies and practice guidelines), data gathering and evaluation by independent organizations (e.g., Centers for Medicare and Medicaid Services, accrediting organizations, and commercial organizations) regarding industry data (frequently industry averages), data on competitors' performance, and comparisons with other organizations providing similar healthcare services.

Collaborators: Refers to those organizations or individuals who cooperate with your organization to support a particular activity or event or who cooperate on an intermittent basis when short-term goals are aligned or are the same. Typically, collaborations do not involve formal agreements or arrangements. See also the definition of "partners."

Core Competencies: Refers to your organization's areas of greatest expertise. Your organization's core competencies are those strategically important capabilities that are central to fulfilling your mission or provide an advantage in your marketplace or service environment. Core competencies frequently are challenging for competitors or suppliers and partners to imitate, and they may provide a sustainable competitive advantage. Core competencies may involve unique service offerings, technology expertise, a marketplace niche, or a particular business acumen (e.g., healthcare delivery start-ups).

Customer: In the healthcare criteria, a customer is an actual and potential user of your organization's services or programs (referred to as "healthcare services" in the healthcare criteria). Patients are the primary customers of healthcare organizations. The criteria address customers broadly, referencing current and future customers as well as the customers of your competitors and other organizations providing similar healthcare services or programs. Patient-focused excellence is a Baldrige core value embedded in the beliefs and behaviors of high performing organizations. Patient focus impacts and should integrate an organization's strategic directions, its work systems and work processes, and its organizational performance results. See the definition of "stakeholders" for the relationship between customers and others who might be affected by your healthcare services.

Customer Engagement: Refers to your patients' and/or stakeholders' investment in or commitment to your organization and healthcare service offerings. It is based on your ongoing ability to serve their needs and build relationships so they will actively seek and provide positive referrals for your healthcare services. Characteristics of customer engagement include their loyalty, their willingness to make an effort to seek healthcare services from your organization, and their willingness to actively advocate for and recommend your organization and healthcare service offerings.

Cycle Time: Refers to the time required to fulfill commitments or to complete tasks. Time measurements play a major role in the criteria because of the great importance of time performance to improving competitiveness and overall performance. "Cycle time" refers to all aspects of time performance. Cycle time improvement might include test results reporting time, time to introduce new healthcare technology, order fulfillment time, length of hospital stays, call-line response time, billing time, and other key measures of time.

Deployment: Refers to the *extent* to which an approach is applied in addressing the requirements of a Baldrige criteria item. Deployment is evaluated on the basis of the breadth and depth of application of the approach to relevant departments and work units throughout the organization. Deployment is one of the dimensions considered in evaluating process items. For further description, see Scoring System.

Diversity: Refers to valuing and benefiting from personal differences. These differences address many variables, including race, religion, color, gender, national origin, disability, sexual orientation, age and generational preferences, education, geographic origin, and skill characteristics as well as differences in ideas, thinking, academic disciplines, and perspectives. The Baldrige criteria refer to the diversity of your work force hiring and patient and stakeholder communities. Capitalizing on these communities provides enhanced opportunities for high performance; patient, stakeholder, work force, and community satisfaction; and patient, stakeholder, and work force engagement.

Effective: Refers to how well a process or a measure addresses its intended purpose. Determining effectiveness requires (1) the evaluation of how well the process is aligned with the organization's needs and how well the process is deployed or (2) the evaluation of the outcome of the measure used.

Empowerment: Refers to giving people the authority and responsibility to make decisions and take appropriate actions. Empowerment results in decisions being made closest to the patient or business front line, where patient and stakeholder needs and work-related knowledge and understanding reside. Empowerment is aimed at enabling people to satisfy patients and stakeholders on first contact, to improve processes and increase productivity, and to improve the organization's health care and other performance results. An empowered work force requires information to make appropriate decisions; thus an organizational requirement is to provide that information in a timely and useful way.

Ethical Behavior: Refers to how an organization ensures that all its decisions, actions, and stakeholder interactions conform to the organization's moral and professional principles. These principles should support all applicable laws and regulations and are the foundation for the organization's culture and values. They distinguish "right" from "wrong." Senior leaders should act as role models for these principles of behavior. The principles apply to all people involved in the organization, from temporary members of the work force to members of the board of directors, and need to be communicated and reinforced on a regular basis. Although there is no universal model for ethical behavior, senior leaders should ensure that the organization's mission and vision are aligned with its ethical principles. Ethical behavior should be practiced with all stakeholders, including the work force, patients, partners, suppliers, and the organization's local community. Although some organizations may view their ethical principles as boundary conditions restricting behavior, well-designed and clearly articulated ethical principles should empower people to make effective decisions with great confidence.

Goals: Refers to a future condition or performance level that one intends to attain. Goals can be both short and long term. Goals are ends that guide actions. Quantitative goals, frequently referred to as "targets," include a numerical point or range. Targets might be projections based on comparative or competitive data. The term "stretch goals" refers to desired major, discontinuous (nonincremental) or "breakthrough" improvements, usually in areas most critical to your organization's future success. Goals can serve many purposes, including clarifying strategic objectives and action plans to indicate how you will measure success, fostering teamwork by focusing on a common end, encouraging "out-of-the-box" thinking (innovation) to achieve a stretch goal, and providing a basis for measuring and accelerating progress.

Governance: Refers to the system of management and controls exercised in the stewardship of your organization. It includes the responsibilities of your organization's owners/shareholders, board of directors, and senior leaders (administrative/operational and health care). Corporate or organizational charters, bylaws, and policies document the rights and responsibilities of each of the parties and describe how your organization will be directed and controlled to ensure (1) accountability to stakeholders and other owners/shareholders, (2) transparency of operations, and (3) fair treatment of all stakeholders. Governance processes may include the approval of strategic direction, the monitoring and evaluation of senior leaders' performance, the establishment of executive compensation and benefits, succession planning, financial auditing, risk management, disclosure, and shareholder reporting. Ensuring effective governance is important to stakeholders' and the larger society's trust and to organizational effectiveness.

Healthcare Services: Refers to all services delivered by the organization that involve professional clinical/medical judgment, including those delivered to patients and those delivered to the community.

High Performance Work: Refers to work processes used to systematically pursue ever-higher levels of overall organizational and individual performance, including quality, productivity, innovation rate, and cycle time performance. High performance work results in improved service for patients and stakeholders. Approaches to high performance work vary in form, function, and incentive systems. High performance work focuses on work force engagement. It frequently includes cooperation between administration/management and the work force, which may involve work force bargaining units; cooperation among departments/work units, often involving teams; the empowerment of your people, including self-directed responsibility; and input to planning. It also may include individual and organizational skill building and learning; learning from other organizations; flexibility in job design and work assignments; a flattened organizational structure, where decision making is decentralized and decisions are made closest to the patient or business front line; and effective use of performance measures, including comparisons. Many high performing organizations use monetary and nonmonetary incentives based on factors such as organizational performance, team and individual contributions, and skill building. Also, high performance work usually seeks to align the organization's structure, core competencies, work, jobs, work force development, and incentives.

How: Refers to the systems and processes that an organization uses to accomplish its mission requirements. In responding to "how" questions in the process item requirements, process descriptions should include information such as approach (methods and measures), deployment, learning, and integration factors.

Indicators: See "measures and indicators."

Innovation: Refers to making meaningful change to improve healthcare services, processes, or organizational effectiveness and to create new value for stakeholders. Innovation involves the adoption of an idea, process, technology, product, or business model that is either new or new to its proposed application. The outcome of innovation is a discontinuous or breakthrough change in results, healthcare services, or processes. Successful organizational innovation is a multistep process that involves development and knowledge sharing, a decision to implement, implementation, evaluation, and learning. Although innovation is often associated with healthcare research and technological innovation, it is applicable to all key organizational processes that would benefit from change, whether through breakthrough improvement or a change in approach or outputs. It could include fundamental changes in organizational structure or the business model to more effectively accomplish the organization's work and to improve critical pathways and practice guidelines, facility design, the administration of medications, the organization of work, or alternative therapies.

Integration: Refers to the harmonization of plans, processes, information, resource decisions, actions, results, and analyses to support key organization-wide goals. Effective integration goes beyond alignment and is achieved when the individual components of a performance management system operate as a fully interconnected unit. See also the definition of "alignment." Integration is one of the dimensions considered in evaluating both process and results items. For further description, see the scoring system in TABLE 8.3.

Key: Refers to the major or most important elements or factors, those that are critical to achieving your intended outcome. The Baldrige criteria, for example, refer to key challenges, key patient and stakeholder groups, key plans, key work processes, and key measures—those that are most important to your organization's success. They are the essential elements for pursuing or monitoring a desired outcome.

Knowledge Assets: Refers to the accumulated intellectual resources of your organization. It is the knowledge possessed by your organization and its work force in the form of information, ideas, learning, understanding, memory, insights, cognitive and technical skills, and capabilities. Your work force, databases, documents, guides, policies and procedures, software, and patents are repositories of your organization's knowledge assets. Knowledge assets are held not only by an organization but reside within its patients, stakeholders, suppliers, and partners as well. Knowledge assets are the "know-how" that your organization has available to use, to invest, and to grow. Building and managing its knowledge assets are key components for your organization to create value for your stakeholders and to help sustain overall organizational performance success.

Leadership System: Refers to how leadership is exercised, formally and informally, throughout the organization; it is the basis for and the way key decisions are made, communicated, and carried out. It includes structures and mechanisms for decision making; two-way communication; selection and development of leaders and managers; and reinforcement of values, ethical behavior, and directions. Capitalizing on these communities provides enhanced opportunities for high performance; patient, stakeholder, work force, and community satisfaction; and patient, stakeholder, and work force engagement.

Learning: Refers to new knowledge or skills acquired through evaluation, study, experience, and innovation. The Baldrige criteria include two distinct kinds of learning: organizational and personal. Organizational learning is achieved through research and development; evaluation and improvement cycles; work force, patient, and other stakeholder ideas and input; best-practice sharing; and benchmarking. Personal learning is achieved through education, training, and developmental opportunities that further individual growth. To be effective, learning should be embedded in the way an organization operates. Learning contributes to organizational performance success and sustainability for the organization and its work force. For further description of organizational and personal learning, see the related core value and concept. Learning is one of the dimensions considered in evaluating process items.

Levels: Refers to numerical information that places or positions an organization's results and performance on a meaningful measurement scale. Performance levels permit evaluation relative to past performance, projections, goals, and appropriate comparisons.

Measures and Indicators: Refers to numerical information that quantifies input, output, and performance dimensions of processes, programs, projects, services, and the overall organization (outcomes). The healthcare criteria place particular focus on measures of healthcare processes and outcomes, patient safety, and patient functional status. Measures and indicators might be simple (derived from one measurement) or composite. The criteria do not make a distinction between measures and indicators. However, some users of these terms prefer "indicator" (1) when the measurement relates to performance but is not a direct measure of such performance (e.g., the number of complaints is an indicator of dissatisfaction but not a direct measure of it) and (2) when the measurement is a predictor ("leading indicator") of some more significant performance (e.g., increased patient satisfaction might be a leading indicator of a gain in health maintenance organization member retention).

Mission: Refers to the overall function of an organization. The mission answers the question, "What is this organization attempting to accomplish?" The mission might define patients, stakeholders, or markets served; distinctive or core competencies; or technologies used.

Multiple Requirements: Refers to the individual questions criteria users need to answer within each area to address. These questions constitute the details of an item's requirements. They are presented in black text under each item's area(s) to address.

Overall Requirements: Refers to the topics criteria users need to address when responding to the central theme of an item. Overall requirements address the most significant features of the item requirements. In the criteria, the overall requirements of each item are presented in one or more introductory sentences printed in bold.

Partners: Refers to those key organizations or individuals who are working in concert with your organization to achieve a common goal or to improve performance. Typically, partnerships are formal arrangements for a specific aim or purpose, such as to achieve a strategic objective or to deliver a specific healthcare service. Formal partnerships are usually for an extended period of time and involve a clear understanding of the individual and mutual roles and benefits for the partners. See also the definition of "collaborators."

Patient: Refers to the person receiving health care, including preventive, promotional, acute, chronic, rehabilitative, and all other services in the continuum of care. Other terms organizations use for "patient" include member, consumer, client, or resident.

Performance: Refers to outputs and their outcomes obtained from processes, healthcare services, and patients and stakeholders that permit evaluation and comparison relative to goals, standards, past results, and other organizations. Performance can be expressed in nonfinancial and financial terms. The Baldrige healthcare criteria address four types of performance: (1) healthcare processes and outcomes, (2) patient and stakeholder focused, (3) financial and marketplace, and (4) operational. "Health care process and outcome performance" refers to performance relative to measures and indicators of healthcare delivery important to patients and stakeholders. Examples of healthcare performance include reductions in hospital admission rates, mortality and morbidity rates, nosocomial infection rates, length of hospital stays, and patient-experienced error levels, as well as improvements in functional status. Other examples include increases in outside-the-hospital treatment of chronic conditions, culturally sensitive care, and patient compliance and adherence. Healthcare performance might be measured at the organizational level, the diagnosis-related groups–specific level, and the patient- and stakeholder-segment level. "Patient- and stakeholder-focused performance" refers to performance relative to measures and indicators of patients' and stakeholders' perceptions, reactions, and behaviors. Examples include patient loyalty, complaints, and survey results. "Financial and marketplace performance" refers to performance relative to measures of cost, revenue, and market position, including asset utilization, asset growth, and market share. Examples include returns on investments, value added per staff member, bond ratings, debt-to-equity ratio, returns on assets, operating margins, performance to budget, the amount in reserve funds, days cash on hand, other profitability and liquidity measures, and market gains. "Operational performance" refers to work force, leadership, organizational, and ethical performance relative to effectiveness, efficiency, and accountability measures and indicators. Examples include cycle time, productivity, waste reduction, work force turnover, work force cross-training rates, accreditation results, regulatory compliance, fiscal accountability, community involvement, and contributions to community health. Operational performance might be measured at the department and work unit level, key work process level, and organizational level.

Performance Excellence: Refers to an integrated approach to organizational performance management that results in (1) delivery of ever-improving value to patients and stakeholders, contributing to improved healthcare quality and organizational sustainability; (2) improvement of overall organizational effectiveness and capabilities as a healthcare provider; and (3) organizational and personal learning. The Baldrige healthcare criteria for performance excellence provide a framework and an assessment tool for understanding organizational strengths and opportunities for improvement and thus for guiding planning efforts.

Performance Projections: Refers to estimates of future performance. Projections may be inferred from past performance, may be based on competitors' performance or the performance of other organizations providing similar healthcare services that must be met or exceeded, may be predicted based on changes in a dynamic healthcare environment, or may be goals for future performance. Projections integrate estimates of your organization's rate of improvement and change, and they may be used to indicate where breakthrough improvement or innovation is needed. Although performance projections may be set to attain a goal, they also may be predicted levels of future performance that indicate the challenges your organization faces in achieving a goal. Thus performance projections serve as a key management planning tool.

Process: Refers to linked activities with the purpose of producing a healthcare service for patients and stakeholders within or outside the organization. Generally, processes involve combinations of people, machines, tools, techniques, materials, and improvements in a defined series of steps or actions. Processes rarely operate in isolation and must be considered in relation to other processes that impact them. In some situations processes might require adherence to a specific sequence of steps, with documentation (sometimes formal) of procedures and requirements, including well-defined measurement and control steps. In many service situations, such as healthcare treatment, particularly when patients and stakeholders are directly involved in the service, process is used in a more general way (i.e., to spell out what must be done, possibly including a preferred or expected sequence). If a sequence is critical, the service needs to include information to help patients and stakeholders understand and follow the sequence. Such service processes also require guidance to the providers of those services on handling contingencies related to the possible actions or behaviors of those served. In knowledge work, such as healthcare assessment and diagnosis, strategic planning, research, development, and analysis, process does not necessarily imply formal sequences of steps. Rather, process implies general understandings regarding competent performance, such as timing, options to be included, evaluation, and reporting. Sequences might arise as part of these understandings. In the Baldrige Scoring System, your process achievement level is assessed. This achievement level is based on four factors that can be evaluated for each of an organization's key processes: approach, deployment, learning, and integration.

Productivity: Refers to measures of the efficiency of resource use. Although the term often is applied to single factors, such as the work force (labor productivity), machines, materials, energy, and capital, the productivity concept applies as well to the total resources used in producing outputs. The use of an aggregate measure of overall productivity allows a determination of whether the net effect of overall changes in a process—possibly involving resource trade-offs—is beneficial.

Purpose: Refers to the fundamental reason that an organization exists. The primary role of purpose is to inspire an organization and guide its setting of values. Purpose is generally broad and enduring. Two organizations providing different healthcare services could have similar purposes, and two organizations providing similar healthcare services could have different purposes.

Results: Refers to outputs and outcomes achieved by an organization in addressing the requirements of a Baldrige criteria item. Results are evaluated on the basis of current performance; performance relative to appropriate comparisons; the rate, breadth, and importance of performance improvements; and the relationship of results measures to key organizational performance requirements.

Segment: Refers to a part of an organization's overall patient, stakeholder, market, healthcare service, or work force base. Segments typically have common characteristics that can be grouped logically. In results items the term refers to disaggregating results data in a way that allows for meaningful analysis of an organization's performance. It is up to each organization to determine the specific factors that it uses to segment its patients, stakeholders, markets, healthcare services, and work force. Understanding segments is critical to identifying the distinct needs and expectations of different patient, stakeholder, market, and work force groups and to tailoring healthcare service offerings to meet their needs and expectations. As an example, market segmentation might be based on geography, distribution channels, healthcare service volume, or technologies used. Work force segmentation might be based on geography, specialties, skills, needs, work assignments, or job classifications.

Senior Leaders: Refers to an organization's senior management group or team. In many organizations this consists of the head of the organization and his or her direct reports. In healthcare organizations with separate administrative/operational and healthcare provider leadership, "senior leaders" refers to both and the relationship between those leaders.

Stakeholders: Refers to all groups that are or might be affected by an organization's services, actions, and success. Examples of key stakeholders might include patients, patients' families, the community, insurers and other third-party payers, employers, healthcare providers, patient advocacy groups, departments of health, students, the work force, partners, collaborators, governing boards, stockholders, investors, charitable contributors, suppliers, taxpayers, regulatory bodies, policymakers, funders, and local and professional communities. See also the definition of "customer."

Strategic Advantages: Refers to those marketplace benefits that exert a decisive influence on an organization's likelihood of future success. These advantages frequently are sources of an organization's current and future competitive success relative to other providers of similar healthcare services. Strategic advantages generally arise from either or both of two sources: (1) core competencies, which focus on building and expanding on an organization's internal capabilities, and (2) strategically important external resources, which are shaped and leveraged through key external relationships and partnerships. When a healthcare organization realizes both sources of strategic advantages, it can amplify its unique internal capabilities by capitalizing on complementary capabilities in other organizations. See the definitions of "strategic challenges" and "strategic objectives" for the relationship among strategic advantages, strategic challenges, and the strategic objectives an organization articulates to address its challenges and advantages.

Strategic Challenges: Refers to those pressures that exert a decisive influence on an organization's likelihood of future success. These challenges frequently are driven by an organization's future collaborative environment and/or competitive position relative to other providers of similar healthcare services. Although not exclusively so, strategic challenges generally are externally driven. However, in responding to externally driven strategic challenges, an organization may face internal strategic challenges. External strategic challenges may relate to patient and stakeholder or healthcare market needs or expectations; healthcare service or technological changes; or financial, societal, and other risks or needs. Internal strategic challenges may relate to an organization's capabilities or its human and other resources. See the definitions of "strategic advantages" and "strategic objectives" for the relationship among strategic challenges, strategic advantages, and the strategic objectives an organization articulates to address its challenges and advantages.

Strategic Objectives: Refers to an organization's articulated aims or responses to address major change or improvement, competitiveness or social issues, and healthcare advantages. Strategic objectives generally are focused both externally and internally and relate to significant patient, stakeholder, market, healthcare service, or technological opportunities and challenges (strategic challenges). Broadly stated, they are what an organization must achieve to remain or become competitive and ensure long-term sustainability. Strategic objectives set an organization's longer term directions and guide resource allocations and redistributions. See the definition of "action plans" for the relationship between strategic objectives and action plans and for an example of each.

Sustainability: Refers to your organization's ability to address current organizational needs and to have the agility and strategic management to prepare successfully for your future organizational, market, and operating environment. Both external and internal factors need to be considered. The specific combination of factors might include healthcare—wide and organization-specific components. Sustainability considerations might include work force capability and capacity, resource availability, technology, knowledge, core competencies, work systems, facilities, and equipment. Sustainability might be affected by changes in the marketplace and patient and stakeholder preferences, changes in the financial markets, and changes in the legal and regulatory environment. In addition, sustainability also has a component related to day-to-day preparedness for real-time or short-term emergencies. In the context of the Baldrige healthcare criteria, the impact of your organization's healthcare services and operations on society and the contributions you make to the well-being of environmental, social, and economic systems are part of your organization's overall societal responsibilities. Whether and how your organization addresses such considerations also may affect its sustainability.

Systematic: Refers to approaches that are well ordered, are repeatable, and use data and information so learning is possible. In other words, approaches are systematic if they build in the opportunity for evaluation, improvement, and sharing, thereby permitting a gain in maturity.

Trends: Refers to numerical information that shows the direction and rate of change for an organization's results. Trends provide a time sequence of organizational performance. A minimum of three historical (not projected) data points generally is needed to begin to ascertain a trend. More data points are needed to define a statistically valid trend. The time period for a trend is determined by the cycle time of the process being measured. Shorter cycle times demand more frequent measurement, whereas longer cycle times might require longer time periods before meaningful trends can be determined. Examples of trends called for by the healthcare criteria include data related to healthcare outcomes and other healthcare service performance; patient, stakeholder, and work force satisfaction and dissatisfaction results; financial performance; marketplace performance; and operational performance, such as cycle time and productivity.

Value: Refers to the perceived worth of a product, process, asset, or function relative to cost and to possible alternatives. Organizations frequently use value considerations to determine the benefits of various options relative to their costs, such as the value of various healthcare service combinations to patients and stakeholders. Organizations need to understand what different stakeholder groups value and then deliver value to each group. This frequently requires balancing value for patients and other stakeholders, such as third-party payers, investors, your work force, and the community.

Values: Refers to the guiding principles and behaviors that embody how your organization and its people are expected to operate. Values reflect and reinforce the desired culture of an organization. Values support and guide the decision making of every work force member, helping the organization accomplish its mission and attain its vision in an appropriate manner. Examples of values might include demonstrating integrity and fairness in all interactions, exceeding patient and stakeholder expectations, valuing individuals and diversity, protecting the environment, and striving for performance excellence every day.

Vision: Refers to the desired future state of your organization. The vision describes where the organization is headed, what it intends to be, or how it wishes to be perceived in the future.

Voice of the Customer: Refers to your process for capturing patient- and stakeholder-related information. Voice of the customer processes are intended to be proactive and continuously innovative to capture stated, unstated, and anticipated patient and stakeholder requirements, expectations, and desires. The goal is to achieve customer engagement. Listening to the voice of the customer might include gathering and integrating various types of customer data, such as survey data, focus group findings, and complaint data, that affect patients' and stakeholders' relationship and engagement decisions.

Work Force: Refers to all people actively involved in accomplishing the work of your organization, including paid employees (e.g., permanent, part-time, temporary, and telecommuting employees, as well as contract staff supervised by the organization), independent practitioners not paid by the organization (e.g., physicians, physician assistants, nurse practitioners, acupuncturists, and nutritionists), volunteers, and healthcare students (e.g., medical, nursing, and ancillary), as appropriate. The work force includes team leaders, supervisors, and managers at all levels.

Work Force Capability: Refers to your organization's ability to accomplish its work processes through the knowledge, skills, abilities, and competencies of its people. Capability may include the ability to build and sustain relationships with your patients, stakeholders, and your community; to innovate and transition to new technologies; to develop new healthcare services and work processes; and to meet changing health care, business, market, and regulatory demands.

Work Force Capacity: Refers to your organization's ability to ensure sufficient staffing levels to accomplish its work processes and successfully deliver your healthcare services to your patients and stakeholders, including the ability to meet varying demand levels.

Work Force Engagement: Refers to the extent of work force commitment, both emotional and intellectual, to accomplishing the work, mission, and vision of the organization. Organizations with high levels of work force engagement are often characterized by high-performing work environments in which people are motivated to do their utmost for the benefit of their patients and stakeholders and for the success of the organization. Work force engagement also depends on building and sustaining relationships between your administrative/operational leadership and your independent practitioners. In general, members of the work force feel engaged when they find personal meaning and motivation in their work and when they receive positive interpersonal and workplace support. An engaged work force benefits from trusting relationships, a safe and cooperative environment, good communication and information flow, empowerment, and performance accountability. Key factors contributing to engagement include training and career development, effective recognition and reward systems, equal opportunity and fair treatment, and family friendliness.

Work Processes: Refers to your most important internal value creation processes. They might include healthcare service design and delivery, patient support, supply chain management, business, and support processes. They are the processes that involve most of your organization's work force and produce patient and stakeholder value. Your key work processes frequently relate to your core competencies, to the factors that determine your success relative to competitors and organizations offering similar healthcare services, and to the factors considered important for business growth by your senior leaders.

Work Systems: Refers to how the work of your organization is accomplished. Work systems involve your work force, your key suppliers and partners, your contractors, your collaborators, and other components of the supply chain needed to produce and deliver your healthcare services and your business and support processes. Your work systems coordinate the internal work processes and the external resources necessary for you to develop, produce, and deliver your healthcare services to your patients and stakeholders and to succeed in your marketplace. Decisions about work systems are strategic. These decisions involve protecting and capitalizing on core competencies and deciding what should be procured or produced outside your organization to be efficient and sustainable in your marketplace.

Index